QUICK WINS

Healthy Cooking for Busy Lives

QUICK WINS

Healthy Cooking for Busy Lives

75+ NO-FUSS RECIPES

8 WEEKLY MEAL PLANS

ELLA MILLS

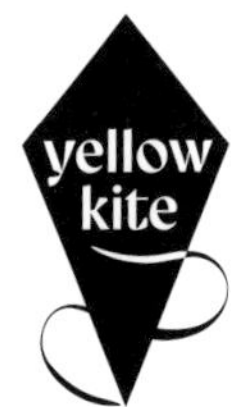

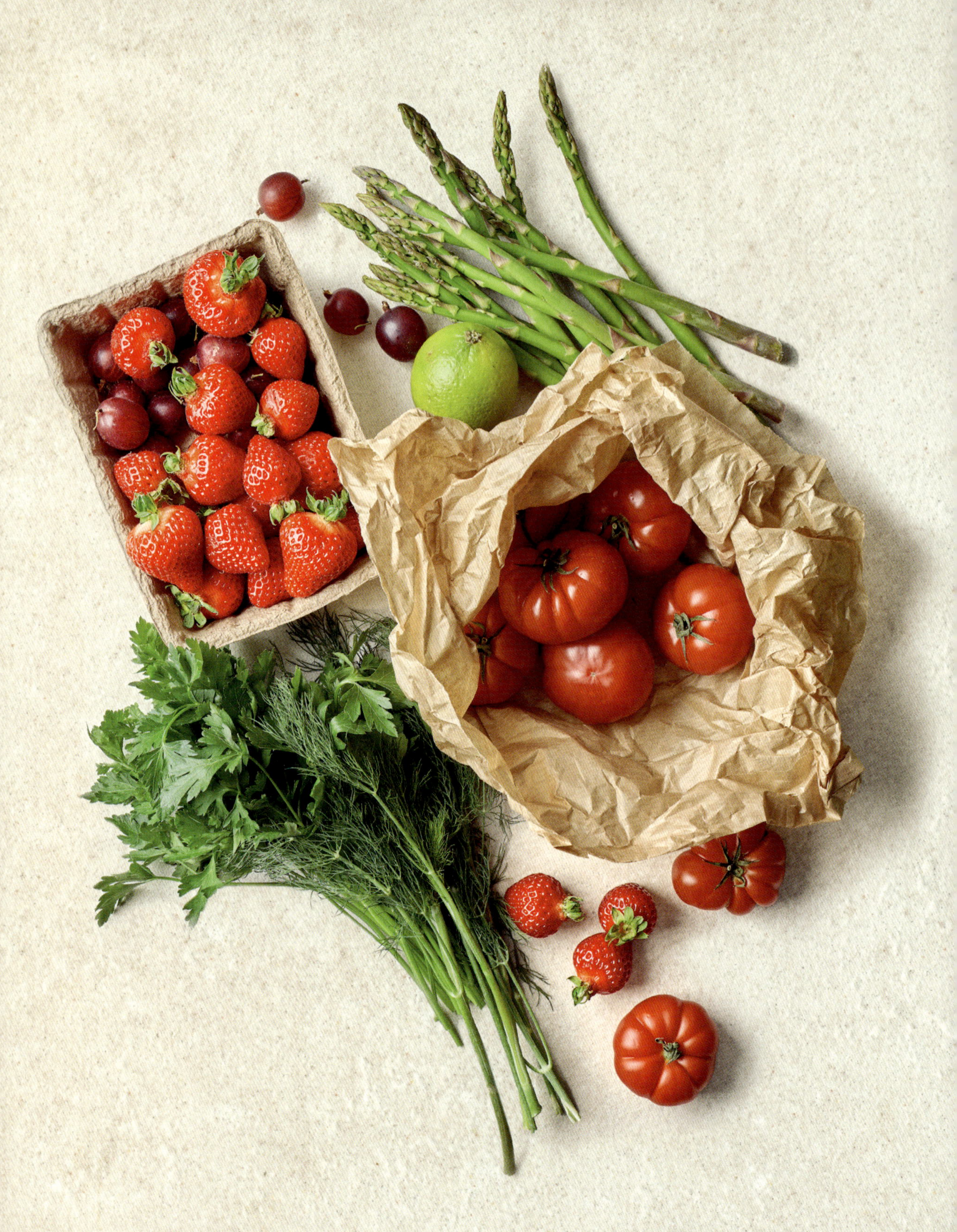

Contents

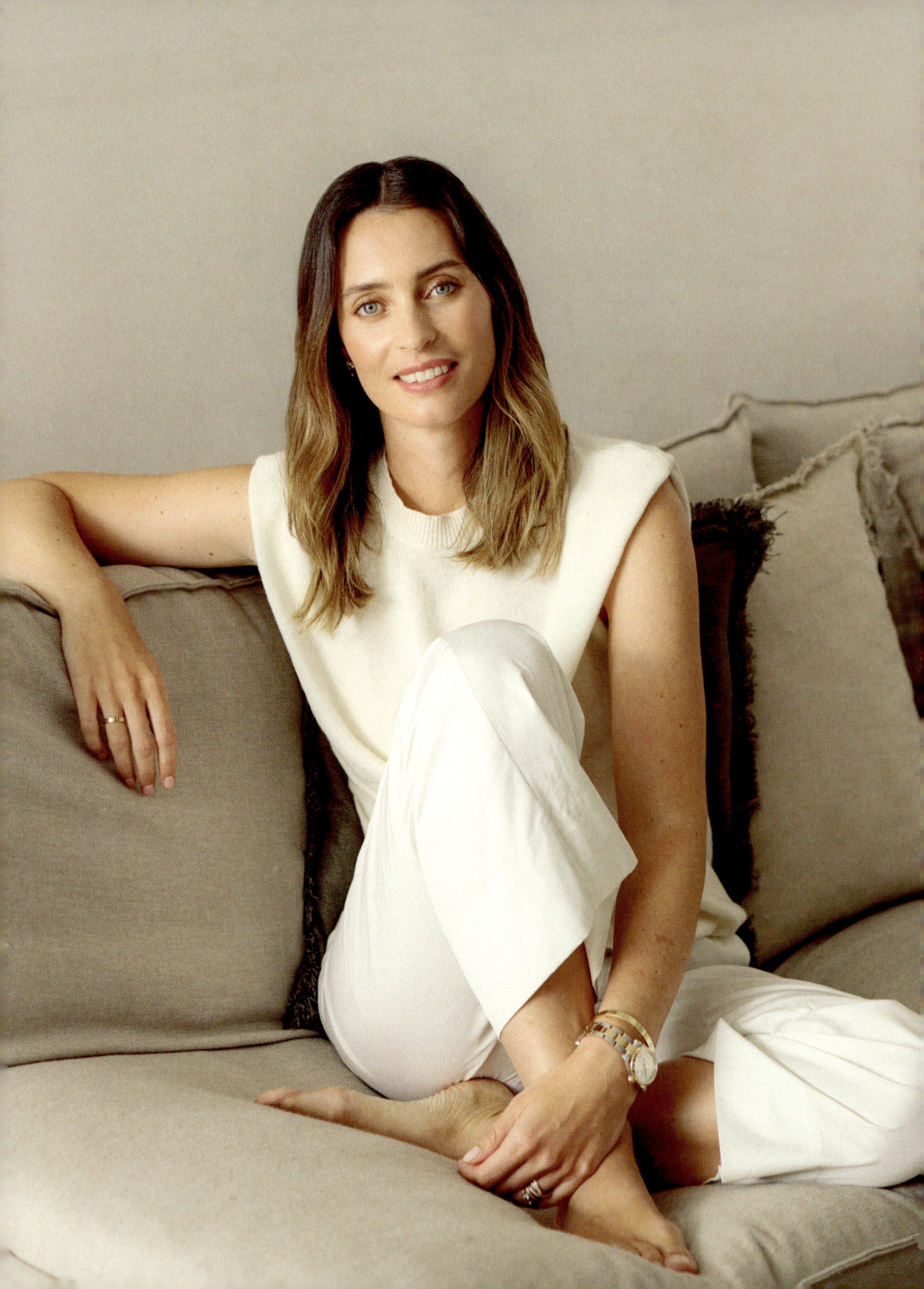

Introduction

This book is your ultimate guide to effortless healthy eating, designed to take the stress out of the nightly 'what's for dinner?' dilemma. By helping you get organized for the week ahead, it supports you in cutting back on ultra-processed foods, hitting your five-a-day, and enjoying 30 different plants each week – all in a way that's simple, practical, and genuinely delicious. With flexible meal plans and fuss-free recipes, it makes nutritious home cooking an easy, seamless part of even the busiest lifestyle.

Where It All Started

Fourteen years ago, I wrote my first blog post for Deliciously Ella. It was a simple recipe for cinnamon-roasted sweet potato wedges with avocado cream that I had made in my parents' kitchen. When I clicked publish, I had no idea that this recipe would go on to change my life entirely.

Since that day in 2012, I've learned so much: I've discovered how to cook delicious, nourishing meals; regained my health; built and sold a business with my husband; navigated loss, grief, and divorce within my family; had two beautiful daughters; written seven cookbooks; launched a podcast; made countless mistakes; burnt out (too many times!);

fallen in and out of love with cooking and the wellness world; tried to make sense of parenting; and been lucky enough to support millions of you with your health and wellbeing. It's been a humbling journey, to say the least – one full of highs and lows, huge lessons, and unexpected adventures.

My life isn't the only thing that's changed beyond recognition during that time. The world of health and wellness has also transformed dramatically, shifting from something incredibly niche to being part of the mainstream. We're now flooded with information, which has brought both greater awareness and overwhelming confusion – a juxtaposition I've found increasingly fascinating over the past year or two. But before exploring where we are today, both as a community and within the broader wellness industry, I'd like to take you back to the beginning – to where my story started. Many of you may already know my story, especially if you've been kind enough to buy one of my other cookbooks, but for those who haven't, I'd love to share why I changed my diet and started eating this way, and why sharing this approach to cooking means so much to me.

This isn't a book about me; it's a book designed to ease the mental load, helping you to get organized for the week so that you eat well every day (or most days). Still, it was my personal challenges that sparked my original interest in wellbeing, and that passion has stayed with me for the past 14 years, continuing to inspire me today. Changing the way I ate changed my life, and if I can help anyone else do the same, it's the most extraordinary privilege.

Growing up, food was, in many ways, an anchor in my life. Amid what became a relatively complex family dynamic, mealtimes were moments of calm; times when we'd sit together and connect. I have vivid memories of devouring my mom's perfect sticky toffee puddings, piping-hot lasagne, chocolate fridge cakes (with extra marshmallows, of course), and her deliciously crispy roast potatoes on Sundays. I had a Barbie cookbook, which I adored, from which I'd whip up endless batches of chocolate chip cookies during the school holidays.

Back then, I wouldn't say I loved food, but I did subconsciously appreciate its emotional importance. As I grew older and went to university, my diet changed. My favorite foods became pick-n-mix candy and cereal. I had absolutely no interest in health and wellness and no understanding of the role food could play in our lives, for better or worse. Aside from an A-level in biology, I had little comprehension of how the body worked or what fueled it. I barely cooked – unless you count boiling pasta – and thought phrases like 'you are what you eat' were meaningless. I didn't even like vegetables!

That all changed in 2011 when my health took a sharp downward turn. In May I was a typical university student; by July I was in and out of hospital, struggling to lead a normal life.

For the rest of that year, I saw countless medical specialists – neurologists, endocrinologists, gastroenterologists, undergoing a barrage of tests: colonoscopies, endoscopies, MRIs, ultrasounds, blood tests. I even swallowed a camera. Yet, time and again, the results came back inconclusive and I was told repeatedly that my symptoms might be psychosomatic.

Eventually, I was diagnosed with Postural Tachycardia Syndrome (PoTS), alongside a few other syndromes. It's a condition affecting the autonomic nervous system, and while its cause wasn't clear, the symptoms were debilitating – chronic fatigue, brain fog, IBS, palpitations, dizziness, chronic pain and headaches, coupled with anxiety and depression. My heart rate would spike to around 180 beats per minute just from standing up, leaving me too dizzy to function. For a year I was largely confined to my house, taking up to 25 different medications a day, none of which seemed to help.

I hit rock bottom about nine months later, when my doctor told me there was nothing more they could do. I sat on the floor of my bedroom feeling hysterical, utterly broken by the thought that this might be my life forever.

But that moment of despair became a turning point. One day, desperate for answers, I began Googling terms like 'natural healing'. What I found was a world of stories – people who had restored their health by swapping ultra-processed foods for a natural, wholefood diet. They focused on simple, holistic approaches: eating more fruit and veg, exercising, prioritizing sleep and practicing mindfulness.

It was a glimmer of hope, and I clung to it. If these changes worked for them, could they work for me too? I had nothing to lose, so I gave up my beloved pick-n-mix and ultra-processed foods, joined a

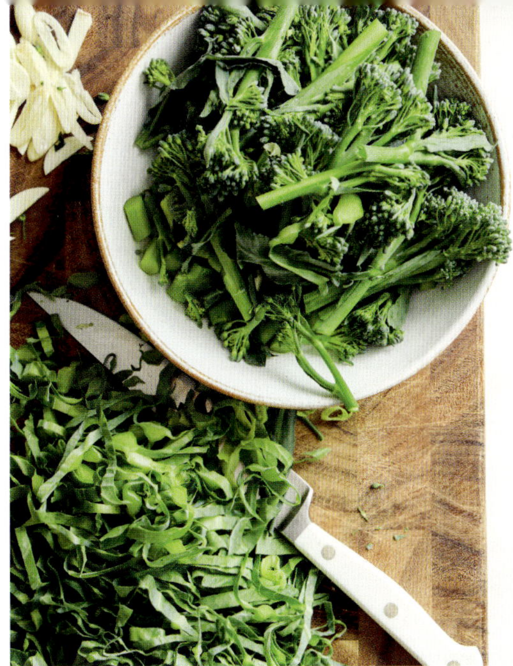

six-month rehabilitation exercise program run by my doctor, and shifted my diet to focus on fresh, nutritious ingredients. My goal was simple: to get my five- (or even ten-) a-day, restore my gut health, support my mental wellbeing and rebuild my life.

There were two major problems, though, as you might remember – I didn't like vegetables and I couldn't cook! Although having spent the last 14 years experimenting with simple home cooking, I now believe everyone can be a good home cook. It's all about building confidence, so don't doubt yourself.

I turned to Google again, but this time I didn't find the inspiration I was looking for. I couldn't find the kinds of recipes I needed – the ones that fill the pages of this book: simple, everyday meals that celebrate humble vegetables, beans, herbs, and spices. Nourishing food that's a joy to make, even during busy weeks. Back then, that type of recipe felt completely novel, but now they're everywhere.

So, I taught myself to cook, sharing the recipes on a simple blog. Slowly but surely my health improved and a community started to form. Two years later, I was off all my medication, and my blog had racked up 150 million hits.

It's fascinating to reflect on how the landscape has shifted over the years. Back in 2012, when I launched Deliciously Ella, the concept of wellness was still relatively novel. By 2015, when my first cookbook was published, it was tipping into the mainstream. Suddenly spiralizers, veg-packed desserts, and NutriBullets were making headlines. Instagram was flooded with colorful smoothie bowls bursting with fruit and veg, and ingredients like almond and cashew butters felt revolutionary. Many of us began experimenting with vegetables in desserts – sweet potato brownies, in my case, spiralizing zucchini and embracing a lifestyle centered on feeling good rather than just dieting.

Was it perfect? Absolutely not. My first attempt at sweet potato brownies would probably now be deemed largely inedible (thankfully, I've since shared a version 2.0 that I promise is delicious!). And while I do still make zucchetti, I think the recipe works better when you toss the zucchetti into hearty salads or it is mixed half-and-half with pasta. But was it well intentioned? Without a doubt. It felt like a movement driven by the desire to feel stronger and healthier – not to chase perfection but to make small, meaningful, positive changes.

By 2022, the global wellness industry had grown to an extraordinary $5.6 trillion, and by 2027 it's expected to reach a staggering $8.5 trillion. While this growth is remarkable, it has also brought with it an overwhelming array of trends and products that can make being 'healthy' feel like an all-consuming, expensive, and unattainable pursuit.

While I have no issue or wish to judge anyone's individual pursuits, I can't help but worry that wellness has become synonymous with endless expensive trends that feel impossible to keep up with. It creates immense pressure. And let's face it, carrots and lentils just don't have the same marketing appeal as biohacking, expensive supplements and wearable devices. But fresh, wholesome foods are so important and our simple, day-to-day healthy habits mustn't be overlooked, especially in today's environment wherein around 55–60% of our calories in the UK come from ultra-processed foods, and only 1 in 4 of us is managing to eat our five-a-day.

Bringing Simplicity Back to Healthy Eating

So, how do we simplify wellness? How do we make eating well on a daily(ish) basis feel realistic and accessible again? I think back to where it all began for me – sharing simple, nourishing meals that worked because they were easy, delicious, and consistent – and that simplicity is what I want to return to today; it's the focus of this cookbook.

When I sat down to write this book, I wasn't entirely sure what kind of book it would be. But I knew one thing: it had to be useful – something that would genuinely help you to eat well on a daily (or almost daily) basis. The inspiration came from your lives and mine. When I asked what you needed, the response was clear: simple, achievable cooking and practical meal plans that make eating well easier. At the same time, I was navigating one of the busiest periods of my life – balancing my role at Deliciously Ella, establishing Plants as its own company, launching the podcast, writing this book, and managing life as a wife and mom of two (including helping one of them with homework for the first time!). With so much going on, I realized I needed exactly the same thing: a way to make cooking healthy, home-cooked meals feel effortless.

Time and mental load are two of the biggest challenges we all face when it comes to making healthier choices. In fact, 78% of the Deliciously Ella community say a lack of time is their biggest barrier to eating well. A recent report found that 73% of home cooks now prefer shorter ingredient lists to save time, reduce food waste, and cut costs, while 42% are cooking more to avoid ultra-processed foods. I feel exactly the same. After a long day, answering the question 'what's for dinner?' can feel overwhelming when you're already stretched thin.

Much of the wellness world seems to demand more – more effort, more ingredients, more perfection. When I launched my podcast, 'The Wellness Scoop', the response was relief: 'Thanks

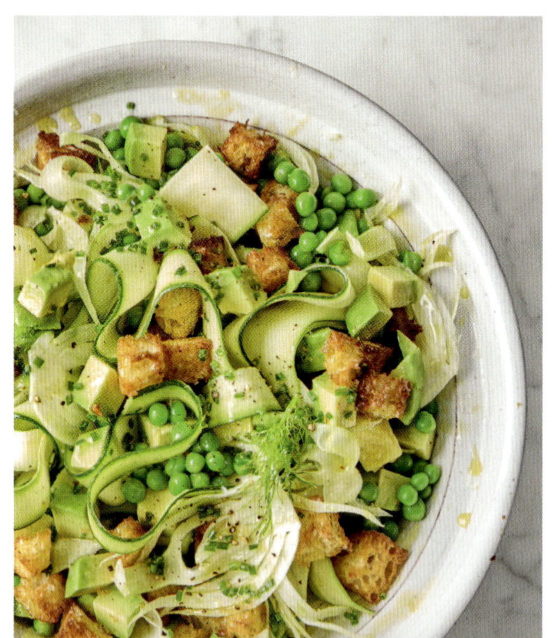

for taking the pressure off!'. That's exactly what I want this book to do too. So, I went back to basics and created easy meal plans to guide me through the week. These plans, full of real, nourishing home-cooked ingredients, have been a lifesaver. They include quick fridge-raid dinners for busy Mondays, big-batch cooks for the weekend, and 15-minute lunches for work-from-home days. This is the food I actually make for my family, and it's made my life so much more manageable.

Over the years, I've learned that eating well isn't about chasing perfection – it's about finding what works for you. And what works is often the simplest solution. These recipes balance deliciousness, nutrition, and ease, so that you can enjoy fresh, wholesome food without the stress. This isn't about adding more to your to-do list – it's about lightening it. The focus is on simple, flexible meal plans that require as few ingredients, steps, pans, and dish-washing as possible. The recipes are adaptable, encouraging creativity without being overwhelming, and include easy swaps so that you can use what's already in your fridge and cupboard.

I've worked to balance variety and practicality, focusing on ingredients we all know and love. In case you're curious, the US favorite, according to Yougov.com vegetables (in order) are: potatoes, sweetcorn, carrots, garlic, Romaine lettuce, green beans, broccoli, bell peppers, tomatoes, cucumbers, white and red onions, avocados. These everyday staples are the building blocks of the recipes in this book –providing wholesome, accessible meals that fit into even the busiest of schedules.

Over the next few pages, you'll find all the recipes you need to eat well on busy weeks, as well as eight weeks of meal plans for when you want the decision of 'what's for dinner?' made for you. If you want to follow the meal plans, each one comes with a shopping list and includes six dinners and two lunches, giving you plenty of flexibility to adapt the plan to your routine. There's no pressure to follow the plans exactly – they're simply a starting point to give you inspiration and make your life easier. Swap recipes to suit your tastes, skip meals if you're out, or freeze the extras from your batch cooking. The goal is to help you enjoy delicious, nourishing meals while effortlessly hitting your five-a-day and cutting down on ultra-processed foods. It's all about real food, real flavor, and a way of eating that feels both satisfying and sustainable. It's all goodness, no fuss.

The chapters are organized to make it easy to find exactly what you need, and if you want to follow the meal plans, each week you'll have:

1. One batch-cook recipe with two different and delicious ways to enjoy it.

2. Three quick fridge-raid or one-pan meals for speedy midweek cooking.

3. One slightly more special dish – for the nights you want to put in a little extra effort (but still keep it simple!).

4. Two speedy, fuss-free lunches that are perfect when you're working from home or having a really busy day.

So, whether you're planning your week or just looking for inspiration, I hope this book brings ease, nourishment, and joy to your kitchen.

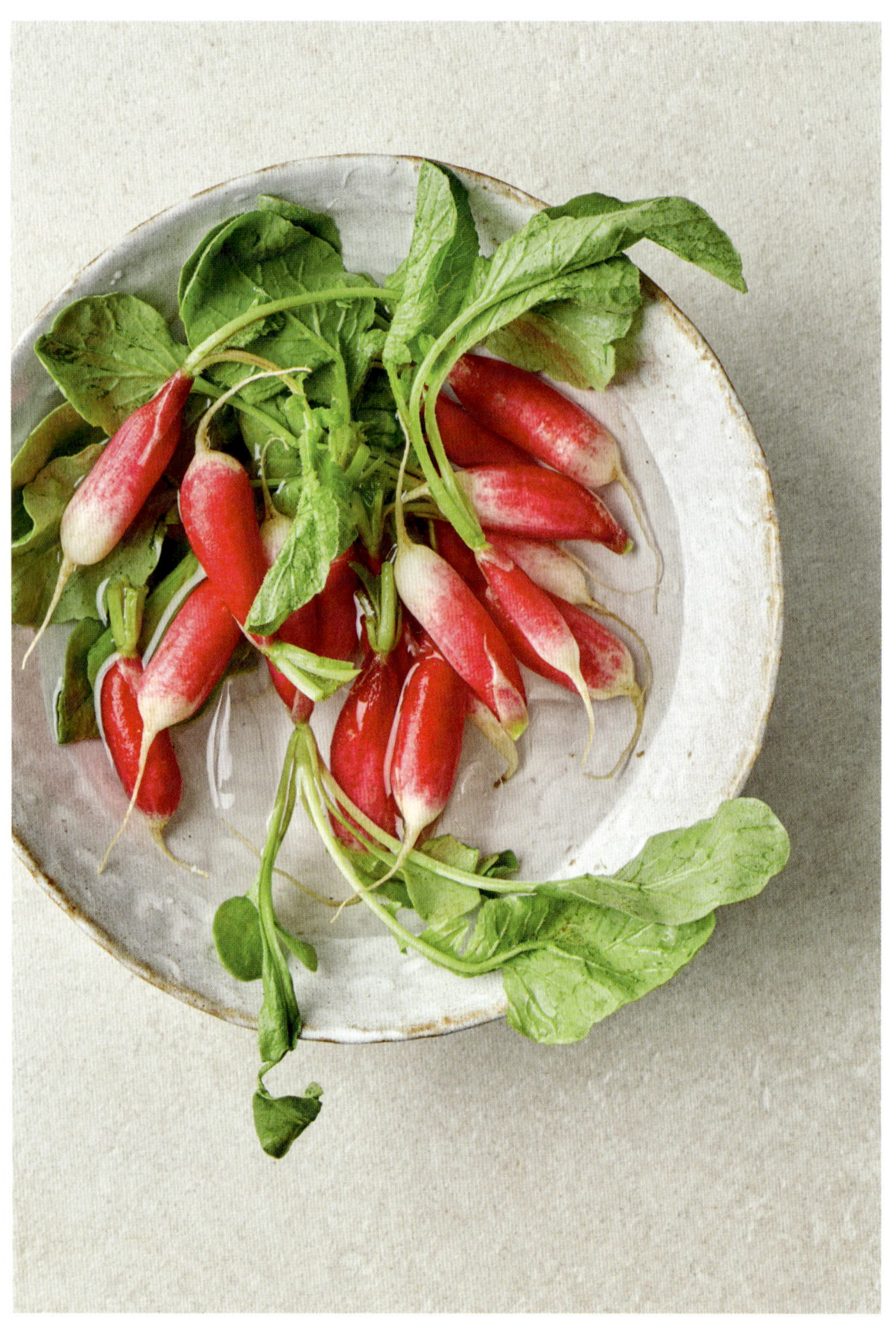

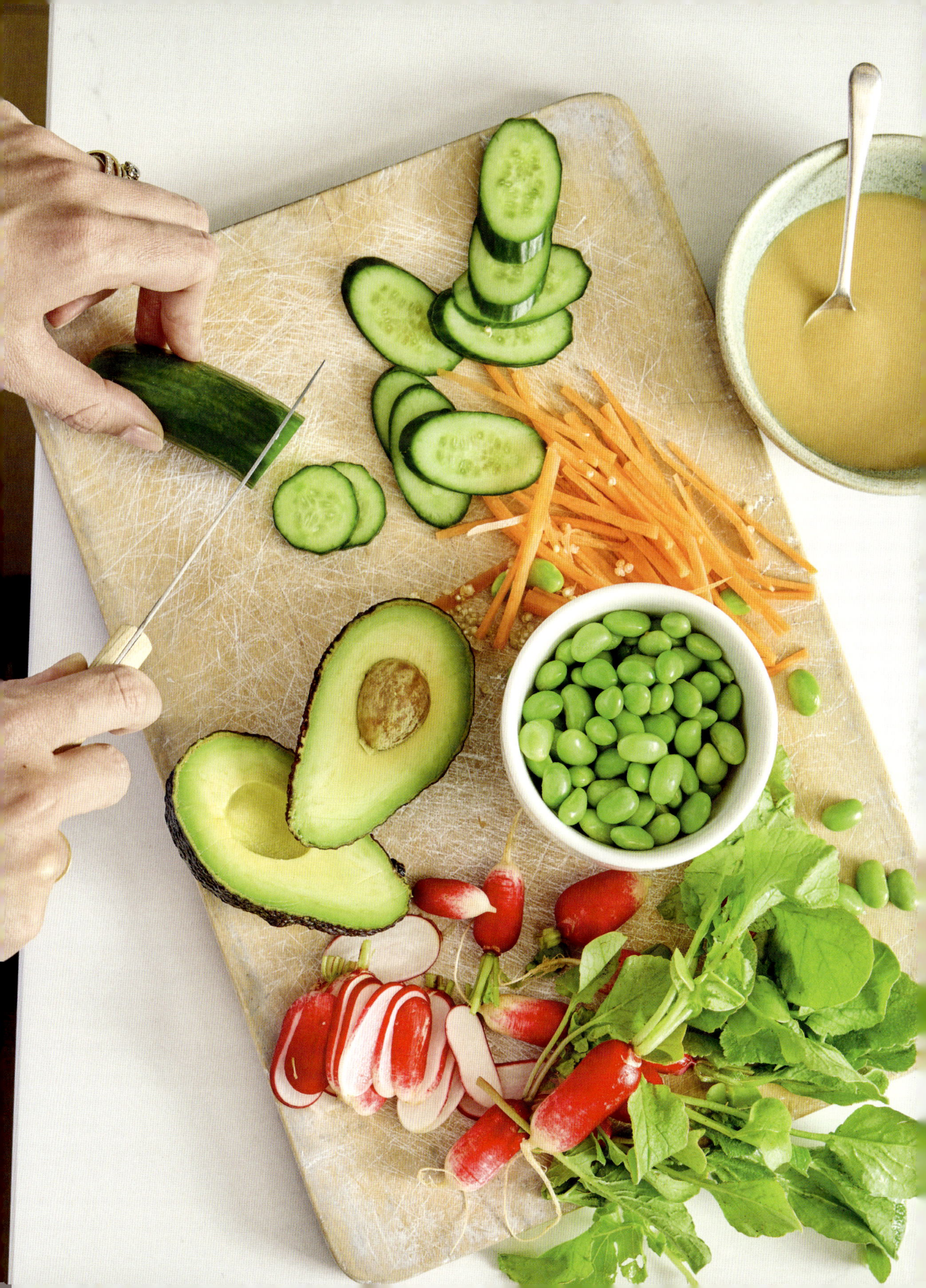

Notes Before You Start Cooking

Before you get going, I wanted to share a few simple notes to explain anything that could be unclear and help make the recipes that little bit easier to follow.

1. **Always read the recipe** from start to finish before you start cooking, so you know what you need and what needs to happen when.

2. **Take a moment to assemble and prep** all your ingredients and tools, so you're not running to the fridge and cupboards.

3. **Keep a mixing bowl** next to your chopping board for trimmings – it saves time and makes the kitchen feel calmer.

4. **Equipment-wise**, other than saucepans, I used a blender (I use a NutriBullet), a mini chopper (I use the Ninja professional chopper), a steaming basket, and a few baking trays.

5. **When it comes to stock**, I've mostly just specified a certain quantity of hot stock, so you can use cubes, powder, or homemade stock, whichever you prefer.

6. **For salt**, I use flaky sea salt and always have a box of Maldon sea salt on my kitchen counter.

7. **I use olive oil** for cooking but for dressings or to finish a dish I've suggested using extra virgin olive oil, as the flavor it brings makes a difference.

8. **Glass jars versus cans of beans** – I know that lots of you now use glass jars of pulses instead of cans. As a general rule you can swap them like for like in any recipe, but in a few recipes I have suggested using a jar as the pulses tend to be higher quality and that makes a big difference to the outcome of the recipe and its flavor. A tin will work just fine if you'd prefer.

9. **Yogurt** – I've specified plain yogurt throughout to give you the choice of using either an unsweetened coconut yogurt for a plant-based option, or Greek yogurt if you're following a more flexible plant-based diet.

10. **Plant counts** are not an exact science and people's definitions as to what counts vary. I have counted each fruit, vegetable, legume, whole grain, nut, and seed as one plant. I've also kept things simple by counting each herb and spice as one, but have left out olive oil, balsamic vinegar and plant milks. Likewise, I've counted things like harissa paste as two plants, but this could be as many as five depending on the brand, same with a tin of mixed beans, which might be three, four or five. Please don't stress about the numbers, the main thing is to use them as a guide to encourage diversity in your diet, which is essential for gut health.

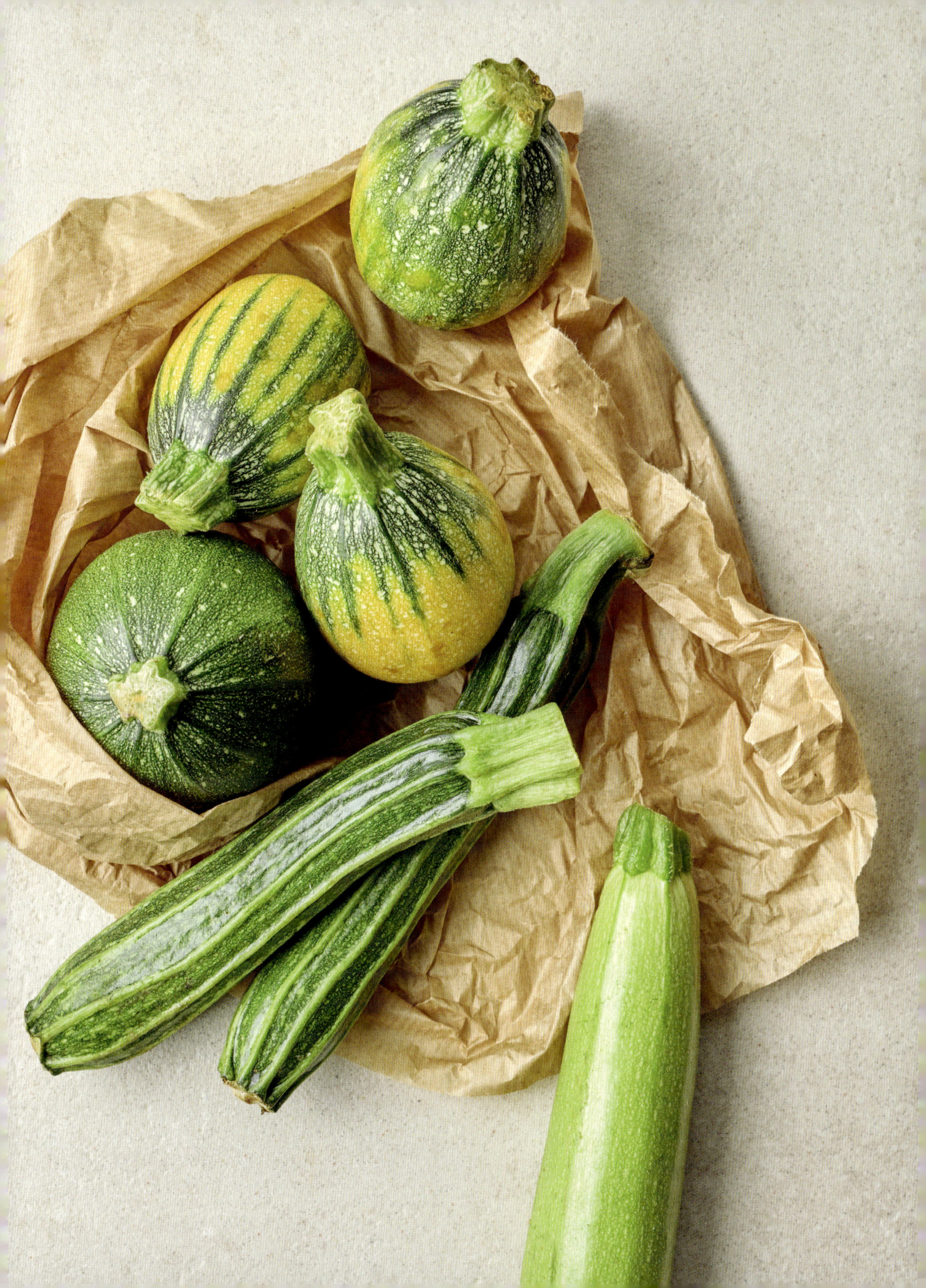

These are the fuss-free dinners we all need on busy weeks.
They're about getting something delicious on the table quickly, without
compromising on flavor or goodness. The recipes can all be made
in 30 minutes or so, with the ingredients coming together in one pan
or tray, which also means that there are hardly any dishes to wash.

ONE PAN

Mushroom Orzo Risotto

Pitta and Cauliflower Salad

Warm Eggplant Salad

Tomato and Spinach Curry

Chickpea and Harissa Orzo

Fajita-Style Tofu Traybake

Miso Tomato Traybake

Cashew Pilau Rice

Lima Bean and Zucchini Orzo

Roasted Carrot Salad

Tortelloni and Bean Broth

Ginger and Tahini Noodles

Walnut and Basil Spaghetti

Miso-Roasted Cabbage

Satay-Style Eggplant Stew

Olive and Tomato Spaghetti

Creamy White Bean and Mushroom Orzo Risotto

7 PLANTS

Serves 2

olive oil
1 small onion, finely chopped
2½ cups mixed mushrooms
    (such as, chestnut and
    shiitake), sliced
3 garlic cloves, crushed or sliced
½ cup orzo
1 teaspoon dried thyme
1 × 14 oz can of white beans,
    drained and rinsed
10 fl oz hot vegetable stock
3½ fl oz oat or almond milk
    (unsweetened)
2 teaspoons white miso paste
1 large handful of baby spinach
    (about 1½ cups), roughly
    chopped
grated zest and juice of 1 lemon
sea salt and black pepper

Make it your own: Add toasted
walnuts for crunch or swap
spinach for cavolo nero or
kale. Add a handful of arugula
on the top for extra greens.
Add nutritional yeast at the
end (with the lemon) for
extra richness, or freshly
grated Parmesan if you're not
plant-based.

When I want something cosy and comforting but super easy, with almost no dish washing, this creamy, zesty white bean and mushroom orzo is my go-to. Everything comes together in one pan, making it the perfect fuss-free meal for busy days. With earthy mushrooms, hearty beans and velvety orzo, it's rich and satisfying, with umami hints of miso in each bite for extra depth and lemon zest for brightness. Doubling the recipe is a great option for quick, delicious lunches too, as the flavor only gets better with time.

1. Heat 1–2 tablespoons of olive oil in a large casserole or saute pan set over a medium heat. Add the onion with a generous pinch of salt and cook for 5 minutes, until softened.

2. Add the mushrooms and cook for another 8–10 minutes until golden. Stir in the garlic for the final 1 minute.

3. Stir in the orzo and thyme, letting them toast for a minute, then add the beans and vegetable stock. Simmer for 7–10 minutes (with the lid off), stirring occasionally, until the orzo is tender and the liquid has been absorbed.

4. Add the milk, miso, spinach, and lemon zest and juice, and let it cook for a final 3–5 minutes, stirring occasionally, until the spinach has wilted and the dish feels thick and creamy. Season to taste (I like lots of pepper in this recipe), then serve and enjoy!

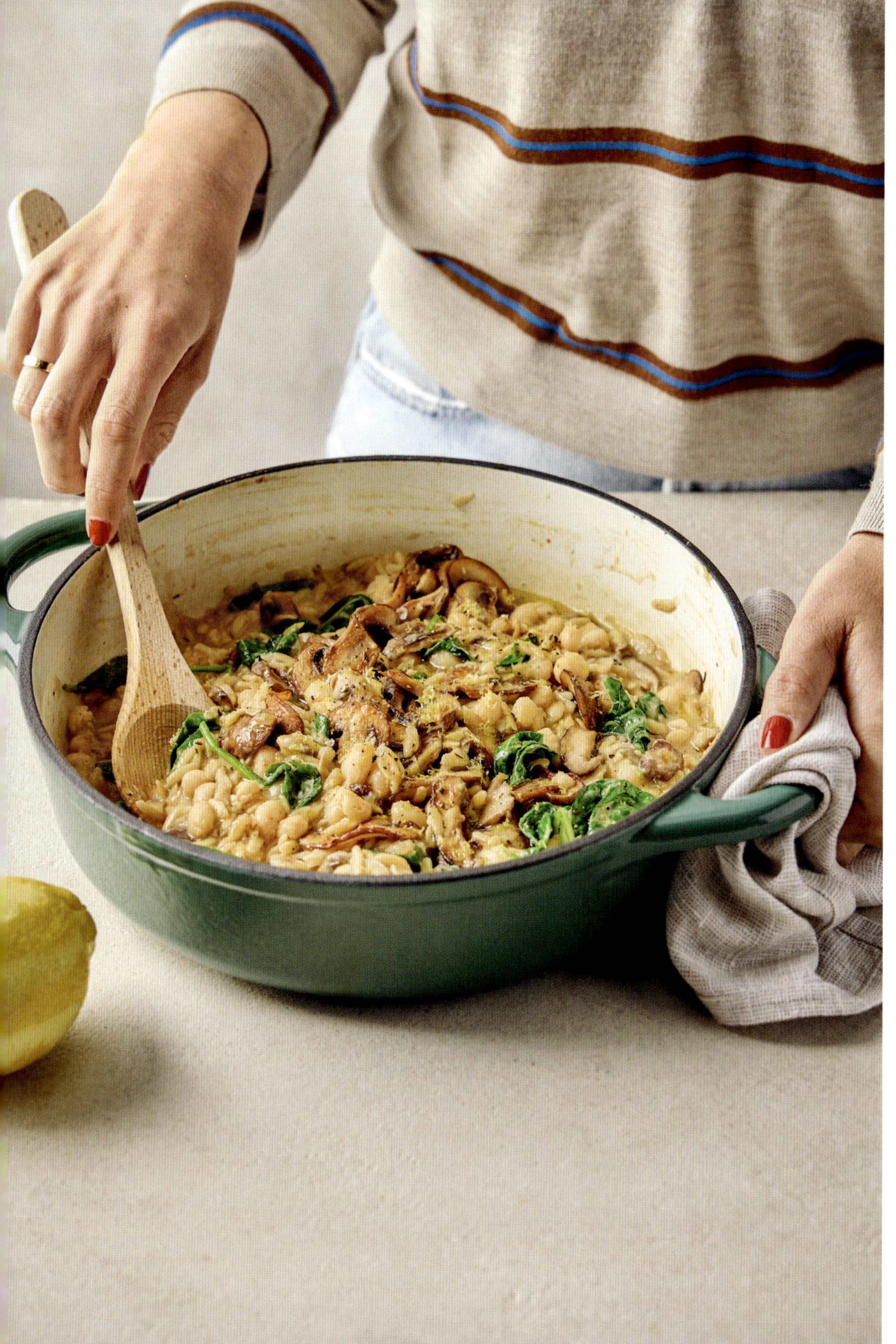

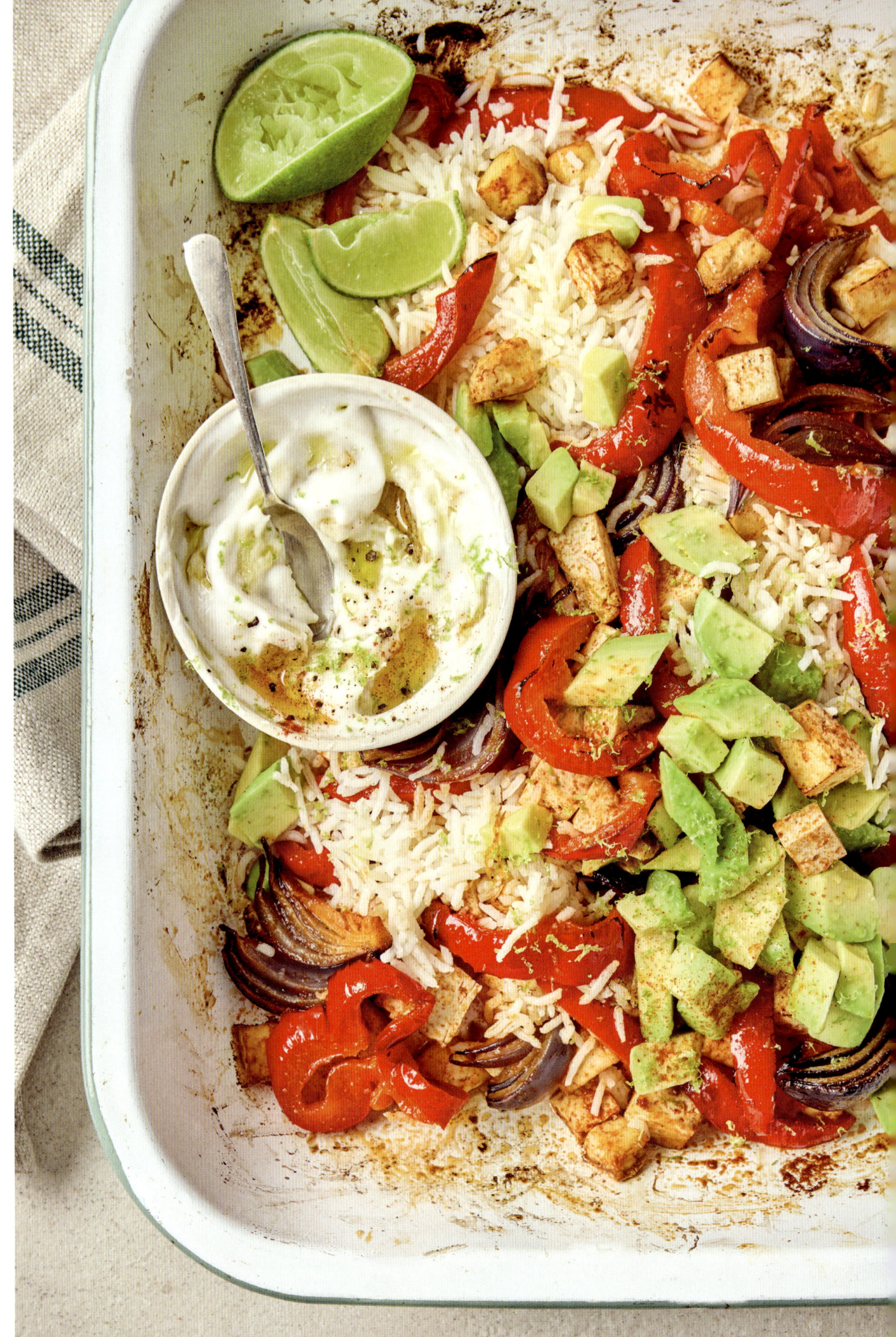

Fajita-Style Tofu Traybake with Garlic Yogurt

8 PLANTS

Serves 2

1 red onion, thinly sliced
2 red bell peppers, thinly sliced
1 × block of firm tofu (about
   10 oz), drained and cut into
   ½ in cubes
olive oil
1 teaspoon ground cumin
1 teaspoon smoked paprika
½ head of garlic, skin on and
   cloves separated
1 × 9 oz pouch of cooked basmati
   rice (or use ½ cup uncooked
   basmati rice)
grated zest and juice of 1–2 limes
4 oz plain yogurt (we use
   unsweetened coconut; about 4
   generous tablespoons)
1 ripe avocado, diced
sea salt

Make it your own: Add things
you already have in your kitchen
like a sprinkle of chili flakes, or a
drizzle of sriracha at the end for
extra spice. A handful of chopped
cilantro is also delicious here.

This is one of my go-to meals after a long day. It's quick, nourishing, and practically cooks itself; just pop everything in the oven and let the bold, smoky flavors of cumin-spiced tofu and paprika-roasted peppers develop. Delicious with broccoli instead of peppers, or for a twist, swap the rice for warm, lightly toasted tortillas and pile them high with the roasted veg, tofu, garlic yogurt, and chunks of avocado.

1. Preheat the oven to 400°F fan. Place the red onion, peppers, and tofu in a large roasting tray. Drizzle with olive oil, then sprinkle over the cumin, smoked paprika, and salt. Toss well to coat and put the garlic cloves in the corner of the tray.

2. Roast for 20–25 minutes, stirring halfway, until the vegetables are soft and slightly charred and the tofu is golden. Remove the tray from the oven.

3. Meanwhile, heat the pouch of rice according to the pouch instructions, then stir it through the tofu and veg along with the lime zest and half of the juice. Alternatively, cook the rice from scratch according to the package instructions while the veg is roasting.

4. Quickly make the garlic yogurt. In a small bowl, mash the roasted garlic (squeezed from the skin), then mix with the yogurt, one tablespoon of olive oil, salt, and the remaining lime juice. Stir well.

5. Serve topped with avocado and the garlic yogurt on the side.

Ginger and Tahini Noodles with Tofu and Edamame

9 PLANTS

Serves 2

olive or sesame oil

small chunk of fresh ginger root (about 1 in long), peeled and grated or finely chopped

1 tablespoon tamari or soy sauce, plus extra to serve

2 tablespoons tahini

1 tablespoon maple syrup

1 teaspoon dried red chili flakes

2 servings of noodles (about 5 oz for two people); rice, soba or wholewheat egg-free noodles work well

½ × block of firm tofu (about 5 oz), drained and cut into ¼ in cubes (you can use the other half in the Five-Bean and Quinoa Chili on page 148)

⅔ cup frozen edamame

juice of ½ lime

handful of sesame seeds, plus extra for garnish

2 green onions, finely sliced

1 avocado, cubed

Make it your own: Add frozen sweetcorn kernals, small florets of broccoli, peas or sugar snap peas in step 3 for extra plant points. For extra flavor, stir through harissa for a little spice, crushed peanuts for crunch, or fresh cilantro for freshness at the end.

A creamy noodle bowl packed with umami from the tamari, peanut butter, and warming fresh ginger root. This is a fast, flavorful meal with minimal effort – just what you need as a midweek meal!

1. Warm 1 tablespoon of oil in a large frying pan or sauté pan set over a medium–high heat. Add the ginger and cook for 2–3 minutes until crispy.

2. Meanwhile, boil the kettle and measure out 17 fl oz of water. Then stir 1 tablespoon of oil, the tamari, tahini, maple syrup, and chili flakes together in a small bowl, until smooth. Carefully pour the sauce into the pan, followed by the boiled water and stir until combined.

3. Add the noodles, tofu, and edamame to the pan. Reduce the heat to medium–low and simmer for 3–5 minutes, stirring every so often, until the noodles are just cooked.

4. Remove from the heat, add the lime juice and stir in the sesame seeds. To serve, divide the noodles into bowls, then top with the green onions, avocado, and extra sesame seeds, adding some extra tamari to taste if wished.

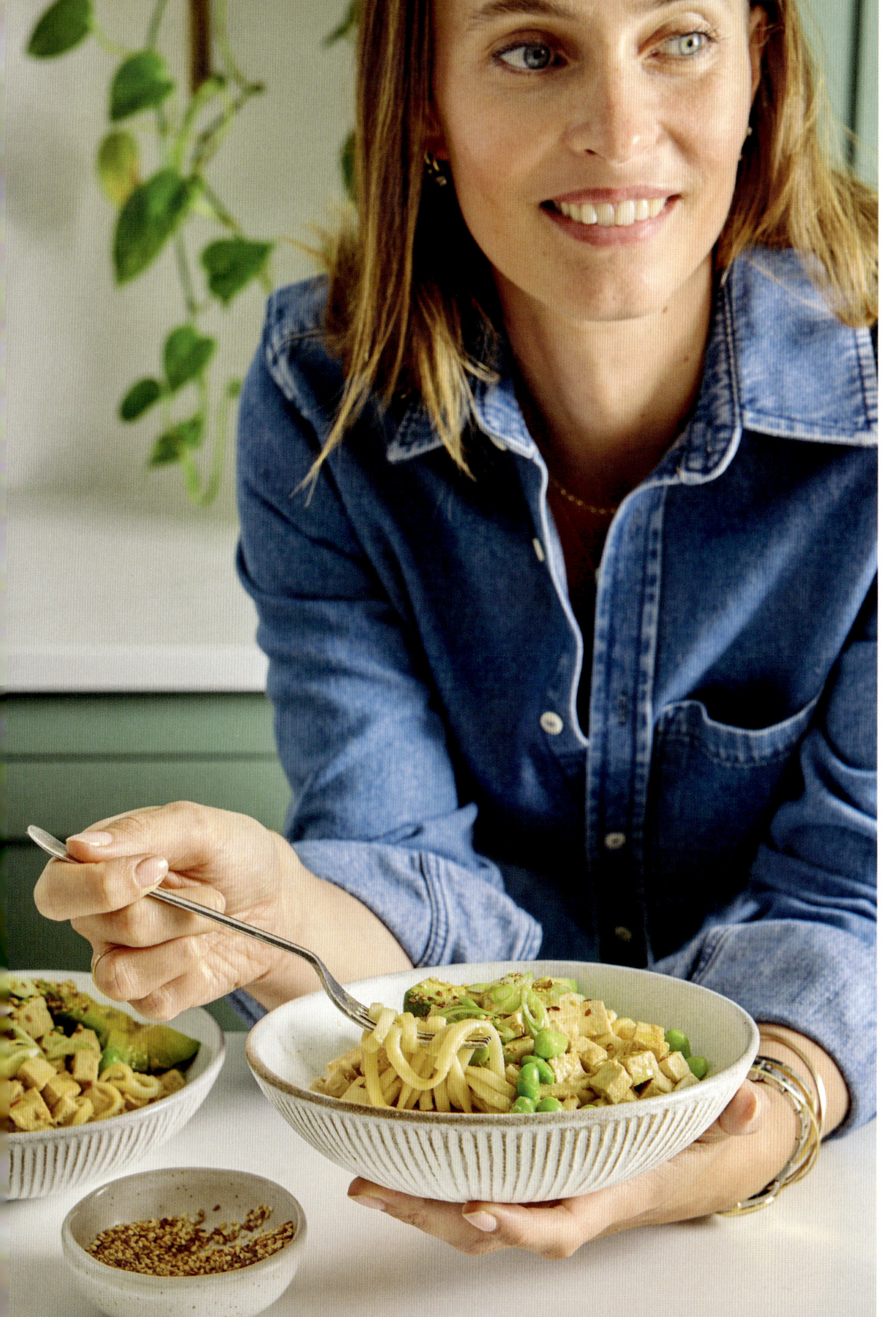

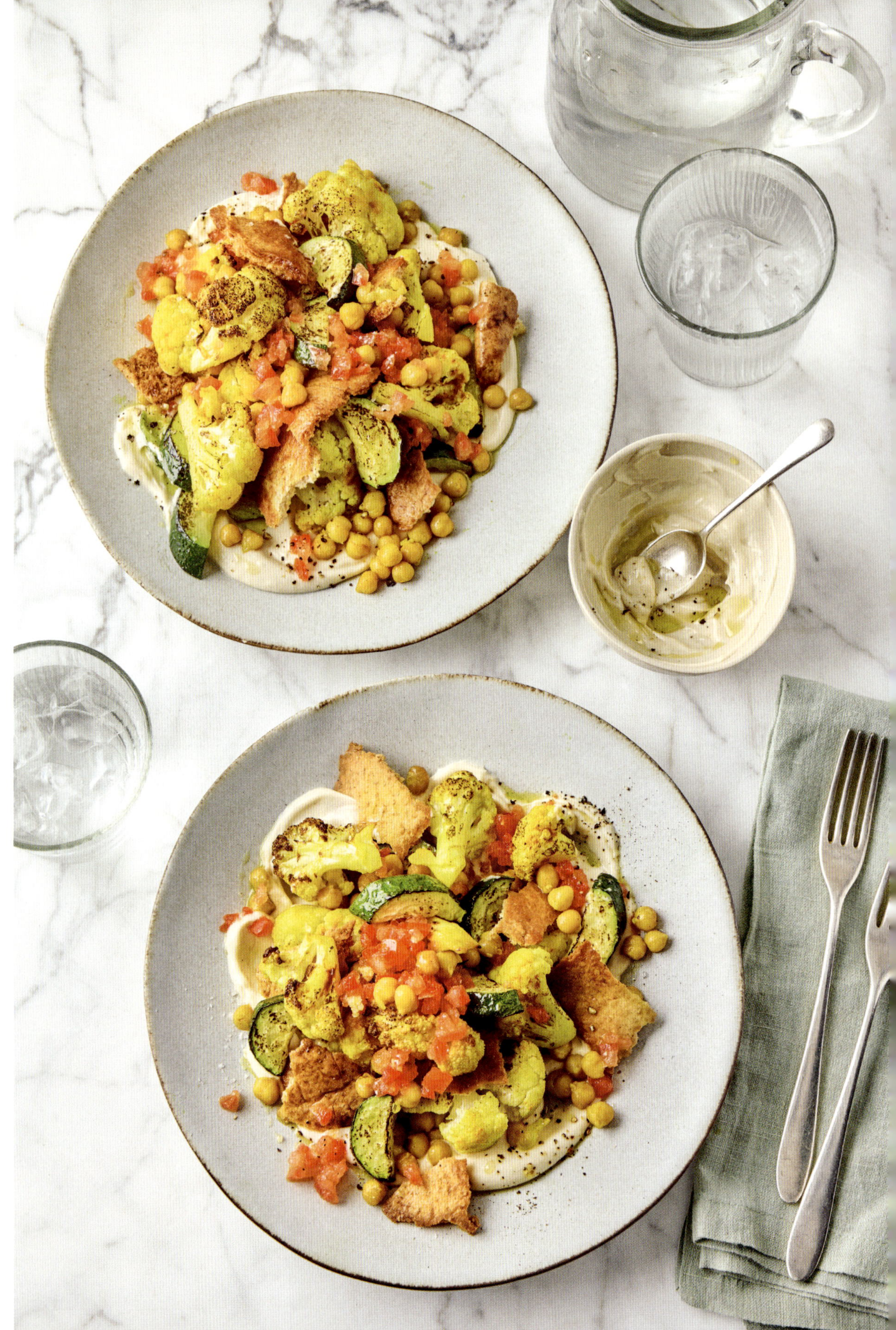

Crunchy Pitta and Cauliflower Salad with Tahini Yogurt

8 PLANTS

Serves 2

1 small cauliflower (about 8
  cups), chopped into small
  florets
1 × 14 oz can of chickpeas,
  drained and rinsed
olive oil
1 teaspoon ground turmeric
1 zucchini, sliced into half moons
2 wholewheat pitta breads, torn
  into pieces or cut into triangles
¾ cup plain yogurt
5 tablespoons tahini
grated zest and juice of 1 lemon
1 tomato, deseeded and chopped
sea salt and black pepper
extra virgin olive oil, to finish

This warm, crunchy, flavor-packed salad is one of my favorite recipes in the book; I've been making it on repeat for the last year. With roasted spiced cauliflower, crispy chickpeas, and toasted pitta all piled on a creamy tahini yogurt base, it's a huge hit with everyone I've cooked it for.

1. Preheat the oven to 400°F fan. Place the cauliflower and chickpeas on a large, flat baking tray, drizzle with 1 tablespoon of olive oil, and toss with the turmeric, 1 teaspoon of salt, and some black pepper. Roast for 10 minutes.

2. Add the zucchini and pitta to the tray (or use a second tray if you don't have enough space), drizzle with a little more olive oil and cook for a further 10–15 minutes, until the pitta is crisp and golden.

3. Meanwhile, mix the yogurt with the tahini, lemon zest and juice, 1 tablespoon of olive oil, and a generous sprinkling of salt and pepper in a small bowl.

4. Once everything is golden and crisp, remove the tray from the oven and leave to cool a little. To serve, spread the yogurt on two plates, then top with the roasted veg, tomato, and a little extra virgin olive oil.

Make it your own: Add a sprinkle of toasted sesame seeds for extra crunch. Swap zucchini for eggplant or asparagus. Stir in a handful of cooked quinoa for extra protein. Add 2 crushed garlic cloves, some sumac or a sprinkling of dried red chili flakes to the tahini yogurt, or stir a handful of fresh cilantro through the salad for extra flavor.

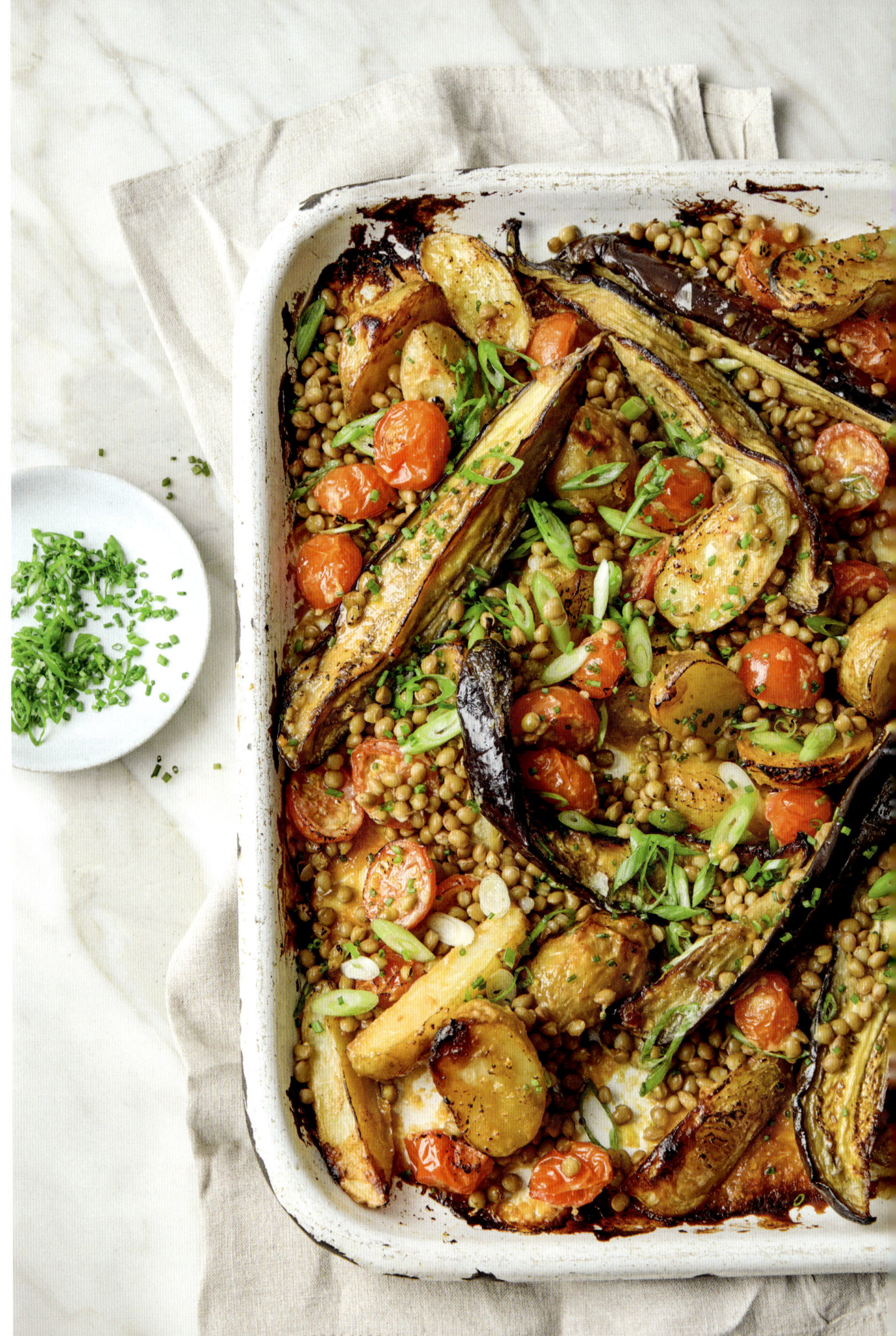

Miso-Blistered Tomato Traybake with Potatoes and Lentils

9 PLANTS

1 large eggplant
¾ lb baby potatoes, halved or
    quartered
olive oil
2 tablespoons white miso paste
1 garlic clove, finely chopped or
    crushed
small chunk of fresh ginger root
    (about 1 in), peeled and finely
    chopped
1 tablespoon maple syrup
pinch of dried red chili flakes
1 cup cherry tomatoes, halved
1 × 14 oz can of brown lentils,
    drained and rinsed
2 green onions, thinly sliced
about 1–2 tablespoons finely
    chopped chives
sea salt

Make it your own: Swap the lentils for chickpeas or white beans. Use cauliflower instead of potatoes, or serve everything with quinoa, rice, or warm pitta breads to make it even heartier. If you've got leftover yogurt, mix a couple of tablespoons with some sliced green onions, extra chopped chives, and a pinch of chili flakes, then finish with a drizzle of olive oil before serving with the traybake.

This is the kind of dish that feels much more impressive than the minimal effort involved – everything roasts together on one tray, creating layers of flavor through the juicy miso-blistered tomatoes, silky eggplant, and golden baby potatoes. The lentils soak up the sticky, garlicky marinade and turn deliciously crispy around the edges, while a spoonful of herby yogurt brings it all together. It's hearty, colorful, and incredibly satisfying – ideal for a simple weeknight dinner.

1. Preheat the oven to 400°F fan. Slice the eggplant in half lengthways, keeping the stem intact. Cut each half lengthways twice more to create three long wedges per side.

2. Add the eggplant and potatoes to a large roasting tray. Drizzle over 2 tablespoons of olive oil, season with salt, and roast for 25–30 minutes, until the potatoes are nearly tender and the eggplant is golden.

3. Meanwhile, in a bowl stir together the miso, garlic, ginger, maple syrup, chili flakes and tomatoes with another tablespoon of olive oil.

4. Once ready, remove the tray from the oven and spoon the miso-tomato mixture generously over the vegetables. Return to the oven for 15 minutes, until the tomatoes are blistered and everything is golden and caramelized.

5. Scatter the lentils over the tray and gently mix everything so the lentils soak up the marinade. Roast for a final 5 minutes to warm the lentils through.

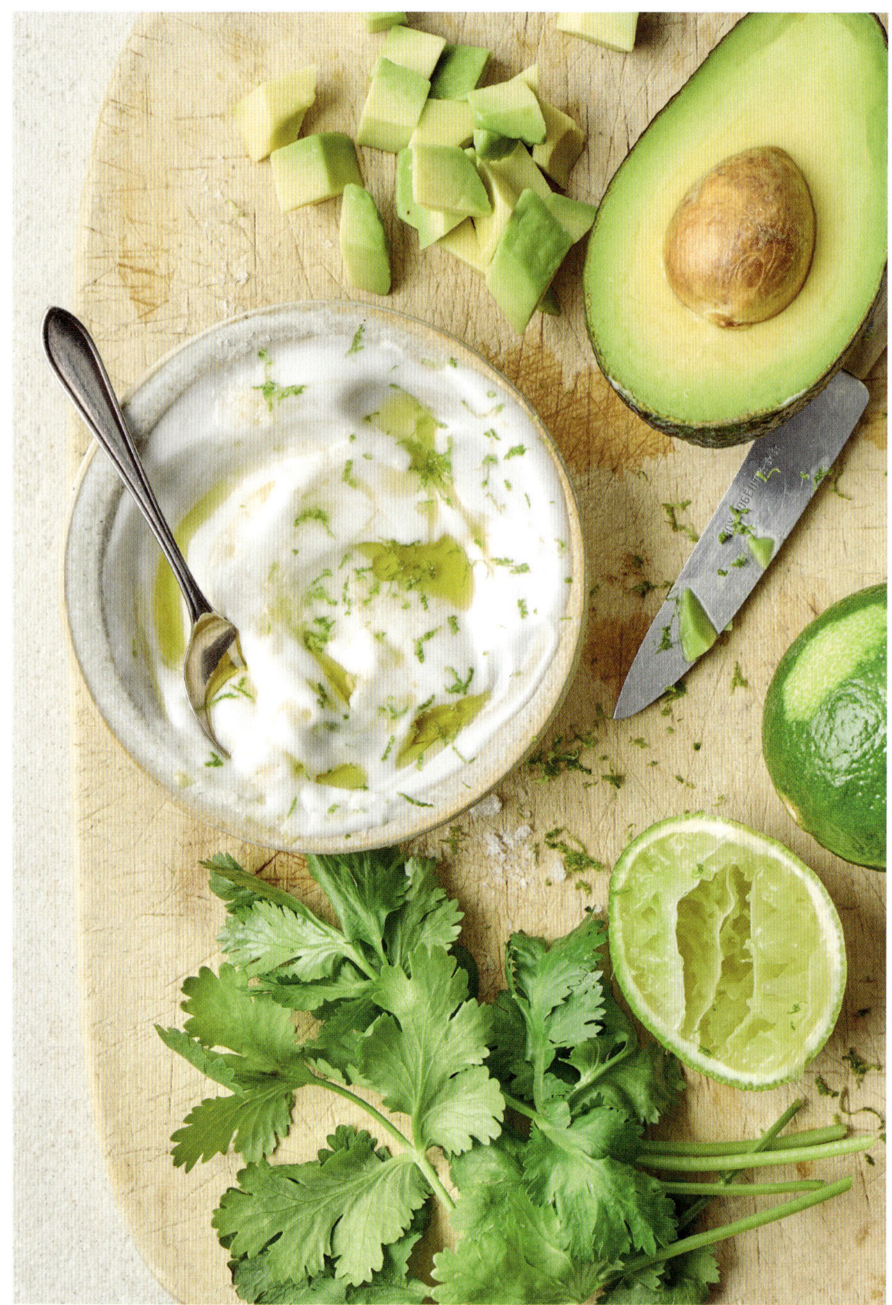

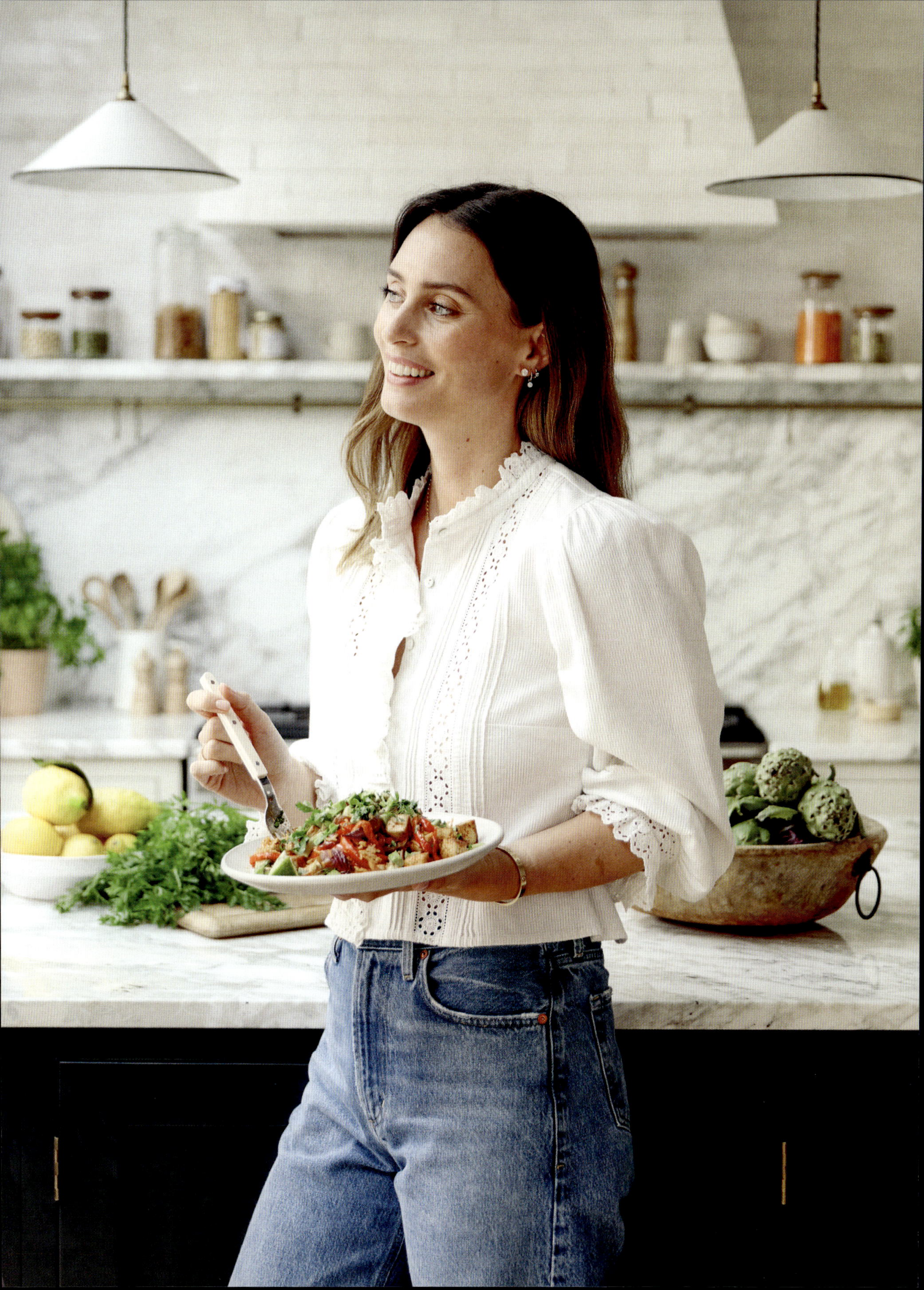

Creamy Walnut and Basil Spaghetti with Peas

7 PLANTS

Serves 2

2 handfuls of spinach (about
  3 cups)
⅔ cup frozen peas, defrosted
1 garlic clove, crushed or finely
  chopped
6 oz pasta (for two people)
1 bunch of asparagus (about
  ¾ cup), trimmed and cut into
  1 inch pieces
handful of walnuts (about ½ cup)
1 bunch of basil (about 1 cup),
  plus extra to serve
about 2–3 tablespoons finely
  chopped chives
2 tablespoons nutritional yeast
4 tablespoons extra virgin
  olive oil
sea salt and black pepper

This recipe comes together with minimal mess and maximum flavor. It's a vibrant, creamy pasta dish that's as comforting as it is fresh, with peas and spinach blended into a silky sauce, crunchy walnuts for texture, and tender asparagus stirred through at the end. It's quick, wholesome, and packed with green goodness.

1. Bring a large saucepan of salted water to the boil, add the spinach, peas, and garlic and cook for 2–3 minutes. Lift out the veg using a slotted spoon and transfer to a high-speed blender. If you find this is tricky or if you don't have a slotted spoon, drain the vegetables and catch the cooking water in a jug or in another pan, then carefully pour it back into the pan.

2. Bring the water back to the boil, add the pasta and cook according to the package instructions, adding the asparagus for the final 2 minutes. Drain, reserving a mugful of cooking water.

3. While the pasta is cooking, add the walnuts, basil, chives, nutritional yeast, and extra virgin olive oil to the blender full of blanched greens. Blitz until smooth, adding a splash of pasta water to loosen as needed, and season to taste.

4. Add the sauce to the pan of drained pasta and asparagus and stir, adding a splash of the reserved cooking water to loosen as needed. Divide into bowls and scatter over the reserved basil.

Make it your own: Swap the walnuts for pine nuts, pistachios, or pumpkin seeds. Swap the asparagus for green beans. Swap the peas for frozen edamame.

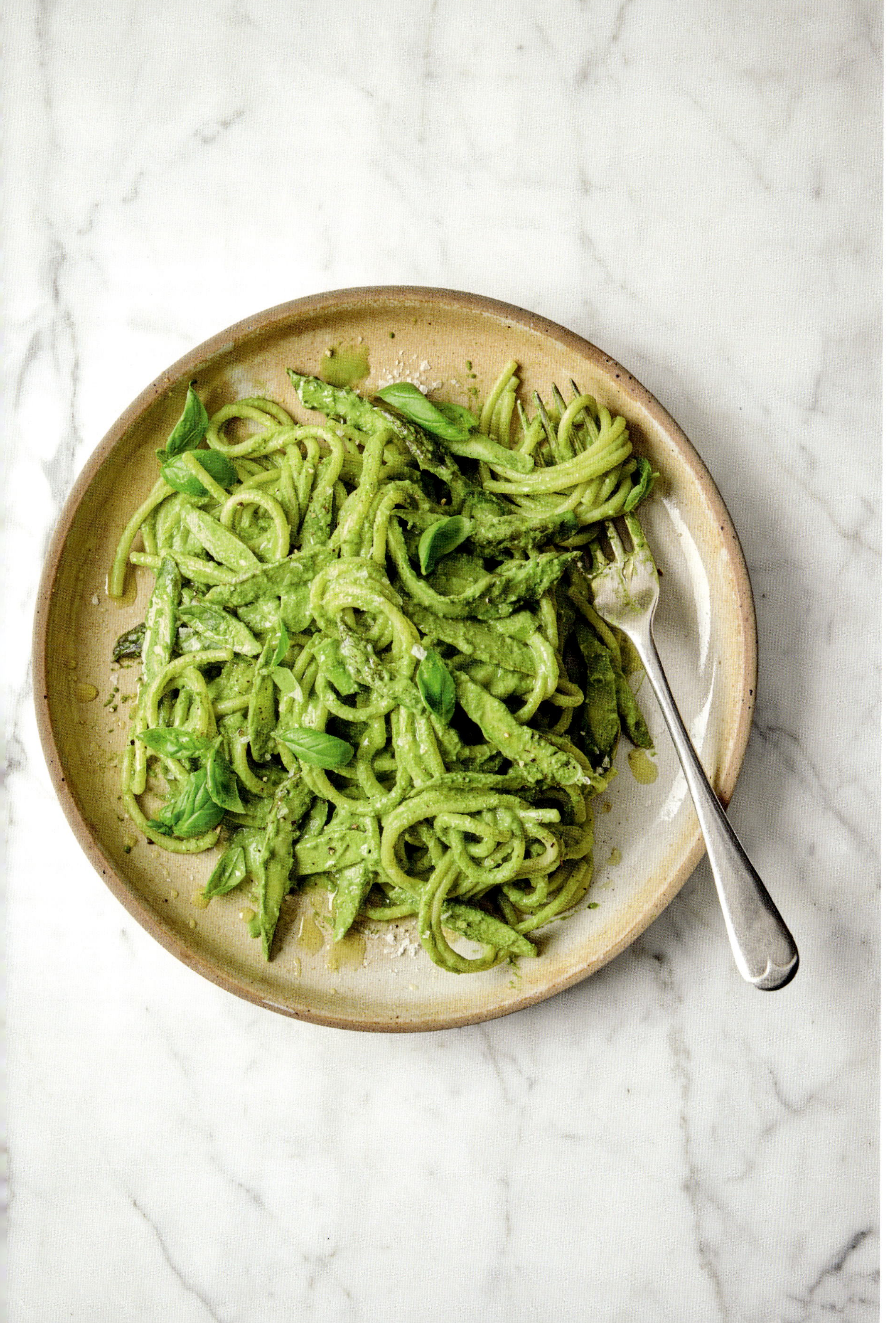

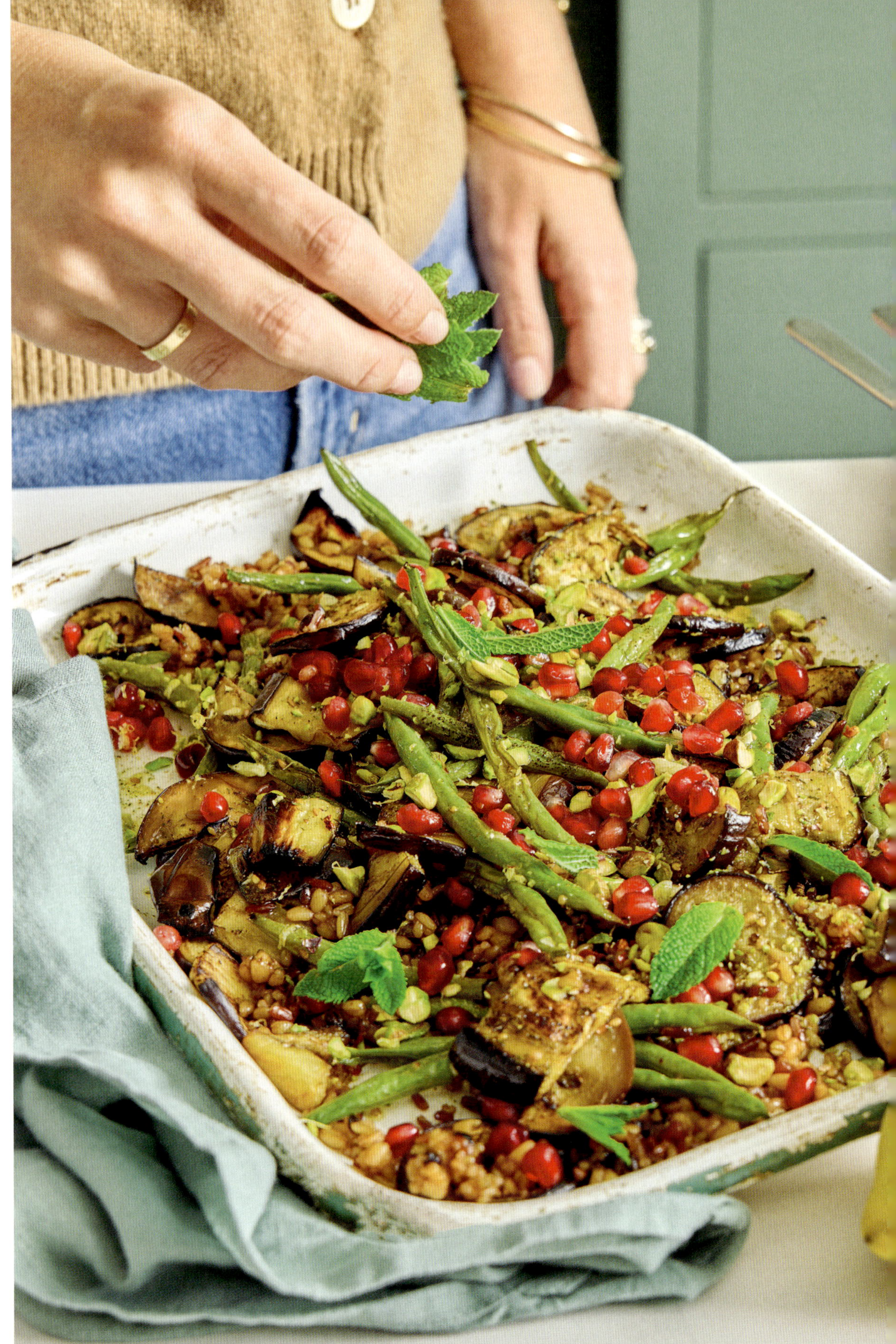

Warm Eggplant, Pistachio, and Pomegranate Salad

9 PLANTS

Serves 2

2 small eggplants, halved
lengthways and cut into ¼ inch
slices
1½ cups green beans, trimmed
olive oil
1 large garlic clove, crushed
1 tablespoon za'atar, plus extra to
serve (optional)
pinch of dried red chili flakes
(optional)
1 × 9 oz pouch of cooked mixed
grains (we like to use one that
has quinoa in it for protein)
handful of pistachios (about
⅙ cup), toasted (see below)
and roughly chopped
grated zest of 1 lemon
handful of pomegranate seeds
(about ½ cup)
handful of mint (about ½ cup),
roughly chopped
sea salt and black pepper

This is one of those dinners that feels like so much more than the sum of its parts. It's brilliantly vibrant and packed with nine different plants.

1. Preheat the oven to 350°F fan. Place the eggplant and green beans on a large baking tray. Drizzle over 1 tablespoon of the olive oil and add a pinch of salt. Cook for 20 minutes, tossing halfway through, until tender and golden.

2. Remove the tray from the oven, add the garlic, za'atar, and chili flakes (if using), and 1 tablespoon of olive oil, along with the grains, and toss well. Scatter the pistachios over the top and return the tray to the oven for 5 minutes until everything is just golden.

3. Before serving, toss through the lemon zest, pomegranate seeds, and mint. Season to taste and scatter over an extra pinch of za'atar, if you like.

Tip: To toast any type of nut or seed, preheat the oven to 350°F fan. Place the nuts/seeds in a baking tray and roast for 10 minutes until golden, then remove and leave to cool.

Turmeric and Cashew Pilau Rice

8 PLANTS

Serves 2

olive oil
2 cardamom pods, gently crushed
½ teaspoon cilantro seeds
1 bay leaf
handful of cashews (about ⅙ cup)
½ cup of basmati rice (for two servings), rinsed
½ teaspoon ground turmeric
1 cup cherry tomatoes, halved
sea salt
small handful of cilantro (about ½ cup), roughly chopped, to garnish
dried red chili flakes, to finish (optional)

After a long day, we all want dinner on the table with minimum fuss and maximum flavor, and this really delivers! Ready in 20 minutes, this simple, faff-free supper feels deliciously comforting. For extra flavor, add a little ground ginger into step one or for more protein, stir through some chickpeas or pan-fried tofu at the end.

1. Warm 1 tablespoon of olive oil in a medium saucepan set over a medium heat. Add the cardamom, cilantro, bay leaf and cashews. Cook for 2–3 minutes until fragrant.

2. Stir in the rice and cook for 1 minute.

3. Next, add the turmeric, tomatoes, 7 fl oz of water and a pinch of salt. Bring to the boil, then reduce the heat to low and simmer with the lid on for 10 minutes, until all the water has been absorbed.

4. Remove the pan from the heat and let it stand with the lid on for 5–10 minutes, then fluff the rice through with a fork.

5. To serve, season with salt to taste. Divide into bowls and garnish with the cilantro and a pinch of chili flakes, if using.

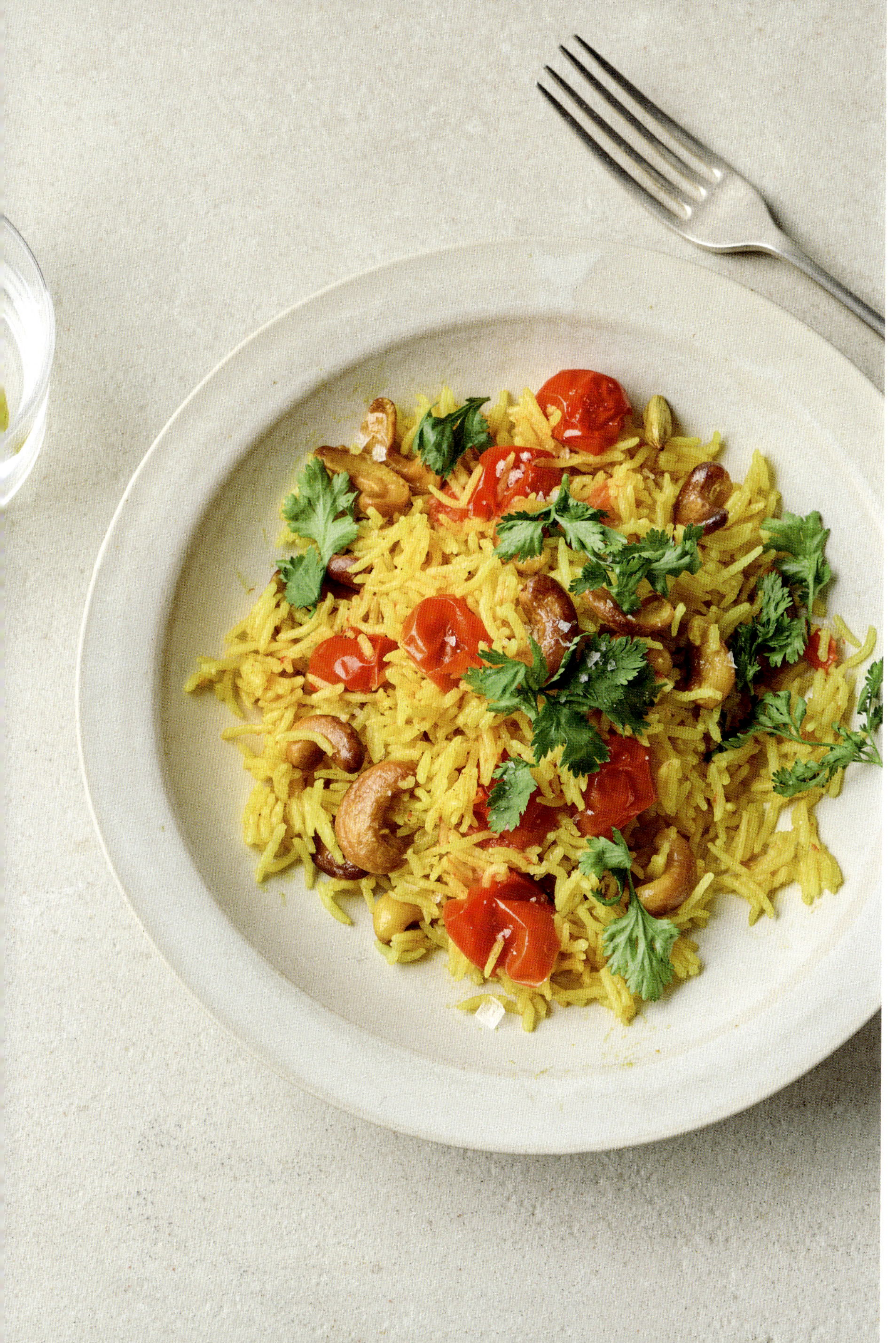

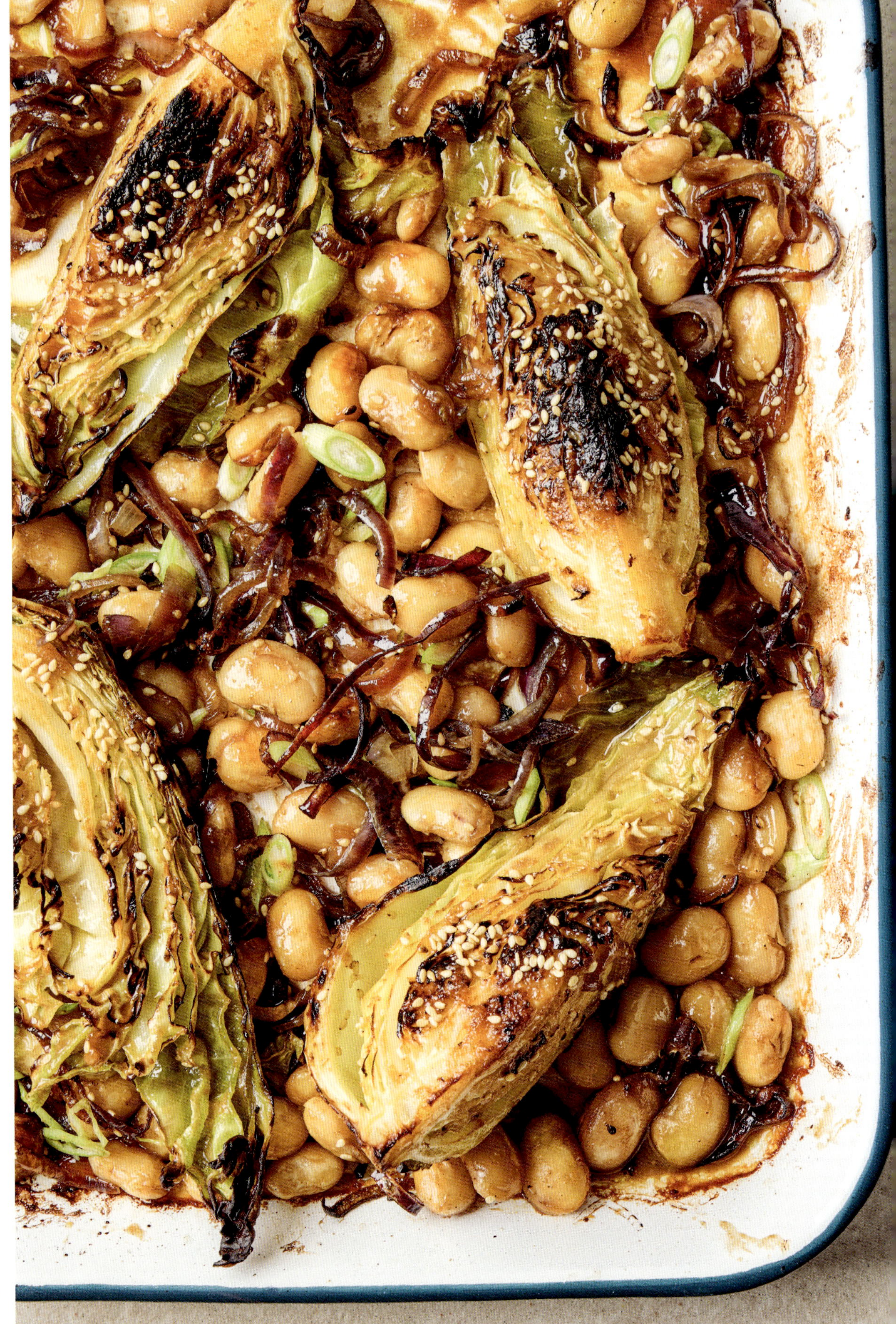

Miso-Roasted Cabbage with Lima Beans and Red Onion

7 PLANTS

Serves 2

1 small hispi cabbage (about
   16 oz in weight), quartered
   lengthways
olive oil
2 tablespoons tamari or soy
   sauce
1 tablespoon maple syrup
3 tablespoons white miso paste
1 × 14 oz can of lima beans,
   drained and rinsed
1 red onion, finely sliced
2–3 green onions, thinly sliced
sprinkle of sesame seeds, to
   finish
handful of cilantro (about ½ cup),
   finely chopped

Make it your own: This is
delicious served with noodles,
rice, grains, garlic yogurt, a crisp
salad or simply with some hot
pitta breads. Add a little pickled
ginger for a kick too!

It's so easy to fall into the habit of cooking the same few vegetables on repeat, but aiming for 30 different plants a week is all about bringing more variety to the table. This cosy one-pan dish is a perfect example, making cabbage (a veg most of us don't turn to enough) the star of the show. Roasted until golden and caramelised with a sweet, savory miso glaze, it's simple, yet full of flavor, especially when scattered with fresh herbs and sesame seeds to finish.

1. Preheat the oven to 400°F fan.

2. Put a large oven-proof casserole or frying pan over a high heat and add a tablespoon of olive oil. When hot, add the cabbage and fry for 8–10 minutes, turning often, until charred and softened at the edges.

3. Meanwhile mix the tamari, maple syrup, and miso with 2 tablespoons of olive oil.

4. Once the cabbage is ready, remove the pan from the heat and temporarily transfer the cabbage on to a plate. Put the lima beans and red onion into the pan and toss through half of the tamari mixture. Put the cabbage back on top of the beans, cut side up and brush the remaining tamari mixture over the cabbage so it's all coated.

5. Finally, place the pan in the oven and cook for 15–20 minutes, until the beans are crisp and the cabbage is tender and golden. Finish by sprinkling over the green onions, sesame seeds, and cilantro.

Sticky Shallot, Tomato, and Spinach Curry

9 PLANTS

Serves 2

olive oil
2 garlic cloves, grated or finely
    chopped
small chunk of fresh ginger root
    (about 1 in), peeled and grated
    or finely chopped
1 bird's eye chili, thinly sliced
    (or use 1 teaspoon/a pinch of
    dried red chili flakes)
2 teaspoons cumin seeds
2 teaspoons cilantro seeds
3 thinly sliced banana shallots
    (about 1⅓ cups)
1½ cherry tomatoes, halved
handful of green beans (about
    ¾ cup cups), trimmed
2 large handfuls of spinach
    (about 3 cups)
3 tablespoons plain yogurt
sea salt

On the table in under 30 minutes, this simple curry is perfect for a midweek supper. It's light, fresh, and full of flavor, without the heaviness of a rich sauce. Add a little more yogurt if you'd like it extra creamy, and serve with whatever you've got to hand – rice, flatbreads, crispy chickpeas, or a scoop of lentils mixed with olive oil, all work brilliantly.

1. Warm a large frying pan or shallow casserole over a medium–low heat. Add 1 tablespoon of olive oil, then the garlic, ginger, chili, cumin, and cilantro seeds. Cook for 1–2 minutes, until fragrant.

2. Next, add the shallots and a pinch of salt. Cook for 10 minutes, stirring occasionally, until softened and glossy.

3. Increase the heat, then add the cherry tomatoes and green beans. Cook for 5–7 minutes until the beans are just tender.

4. Add the spinach and stir until wilted, then remove the pan from the heat and mix in the yogurt. Season to taste with salt.

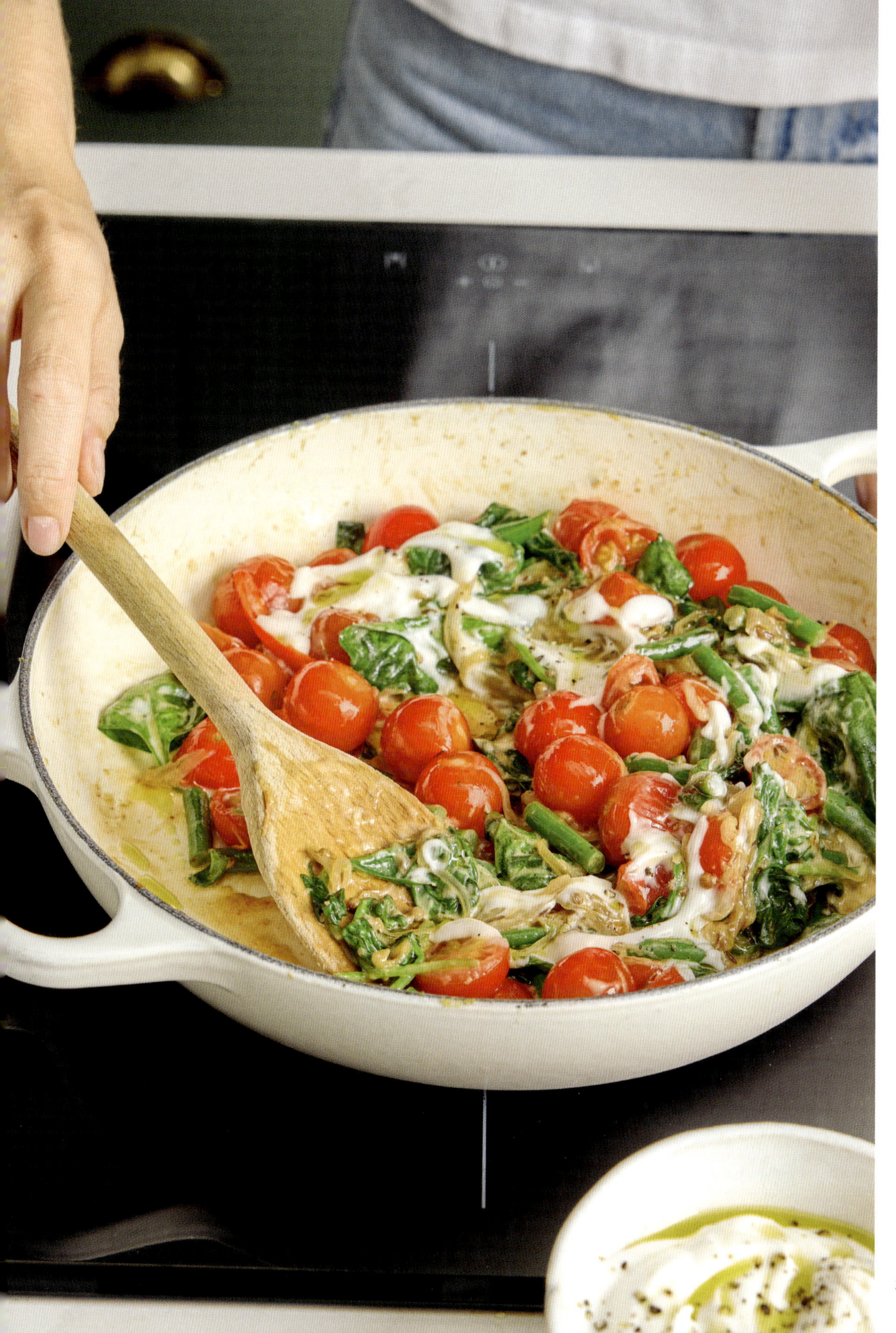

Creamy Lima Bean and Zucchini Orzo

6 PLANTS

Serves 2

olive oil
2–3 garlic cloves, crushed
2 zucchini, coarsely grated
1 × 18 oz jar of lima beans, plus
   the stock from the jar
¾ cup of orzo
11 fl oz water
2 tablespoons plain yogurt
grated zest of 1 lemon
handful of basil (about 1 cup),
   roughly chopped, plus extra to
   garnish
extra virgin olive oil, to finish
   (optional)
large handful of arugula (about
   2 cups)
sea salt and black pepper

This is one of my go-to dinners when I want something comforting but light and fresh. The zucchini melts into the orzo, giving it a risotto-like creaminess without any of the stirring, and the lima beans make it filling enough to feel substantial. Finished with lemon zest, basil, and arugula, it's vibrant, cosy and ready in 20 minutes.

1. Warm 1 tablespoon of olive oil in a large frying pan or shallow casserole set over a medium heat. Add the garlic and cook for 2–3 minutes, until just golden.

2. Add the zucchini and cook, stirring frequently, for 5 minutes until most of the liquid has bubbled away.

3. Pour in the lima beans, along with the stock from the jar, the orzo, and 11 fl oz of water. Bring to a simmer and cook for 6–8 minutes, stirring every so often to prevent it sticking to the pan, until the orzo is al dente. Don't worry if it seems a little under-done, it will carry on cooking in the residual heat of the pan.

4. Remove from the heat and stir in the yogurt, lemon zest, and basil. Season to taste.

5. To serve, divide into bowls, drizzle with a little extra virgin olive oil (if using), then scatter over the arugula and remaining basil.

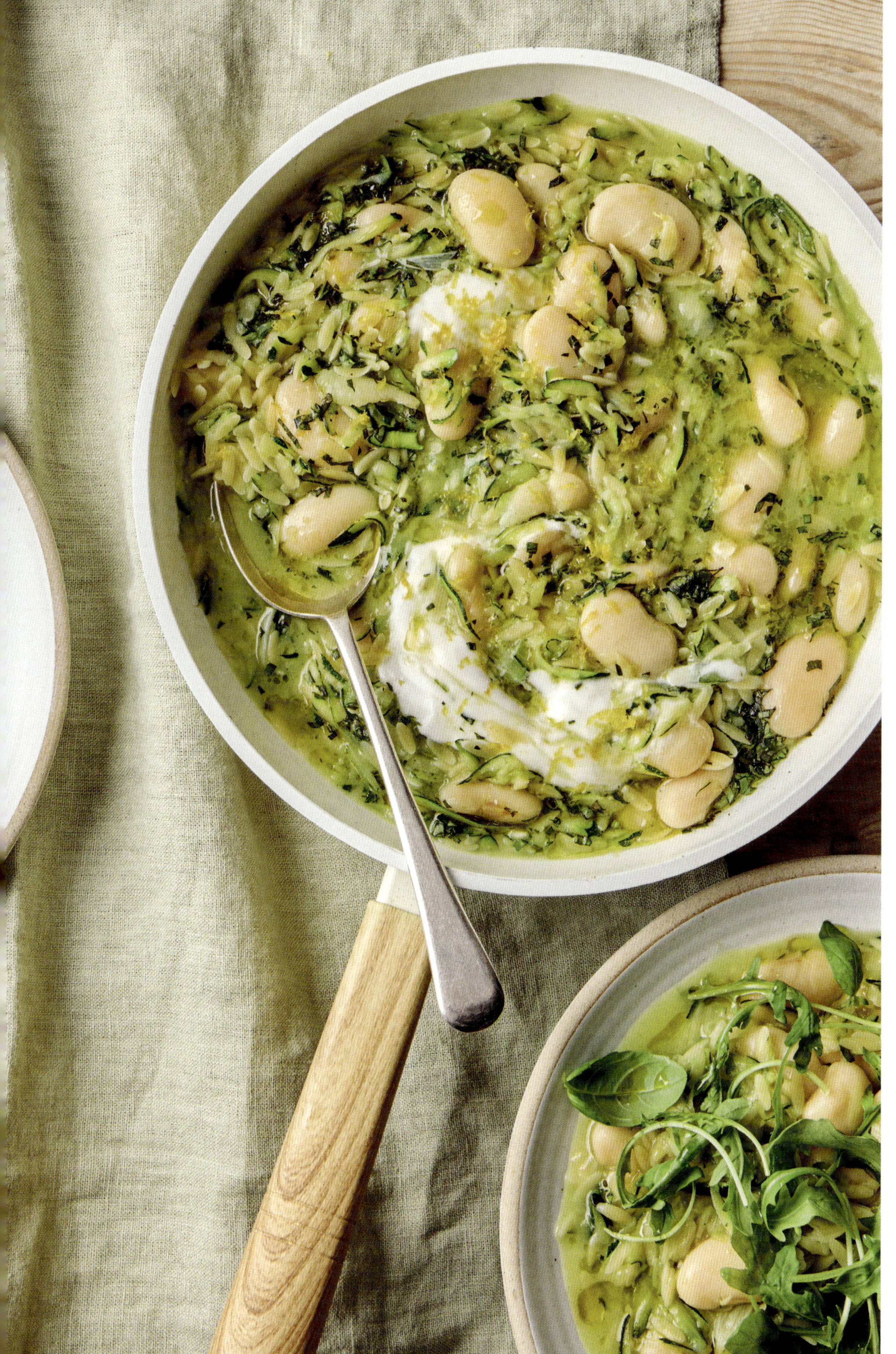

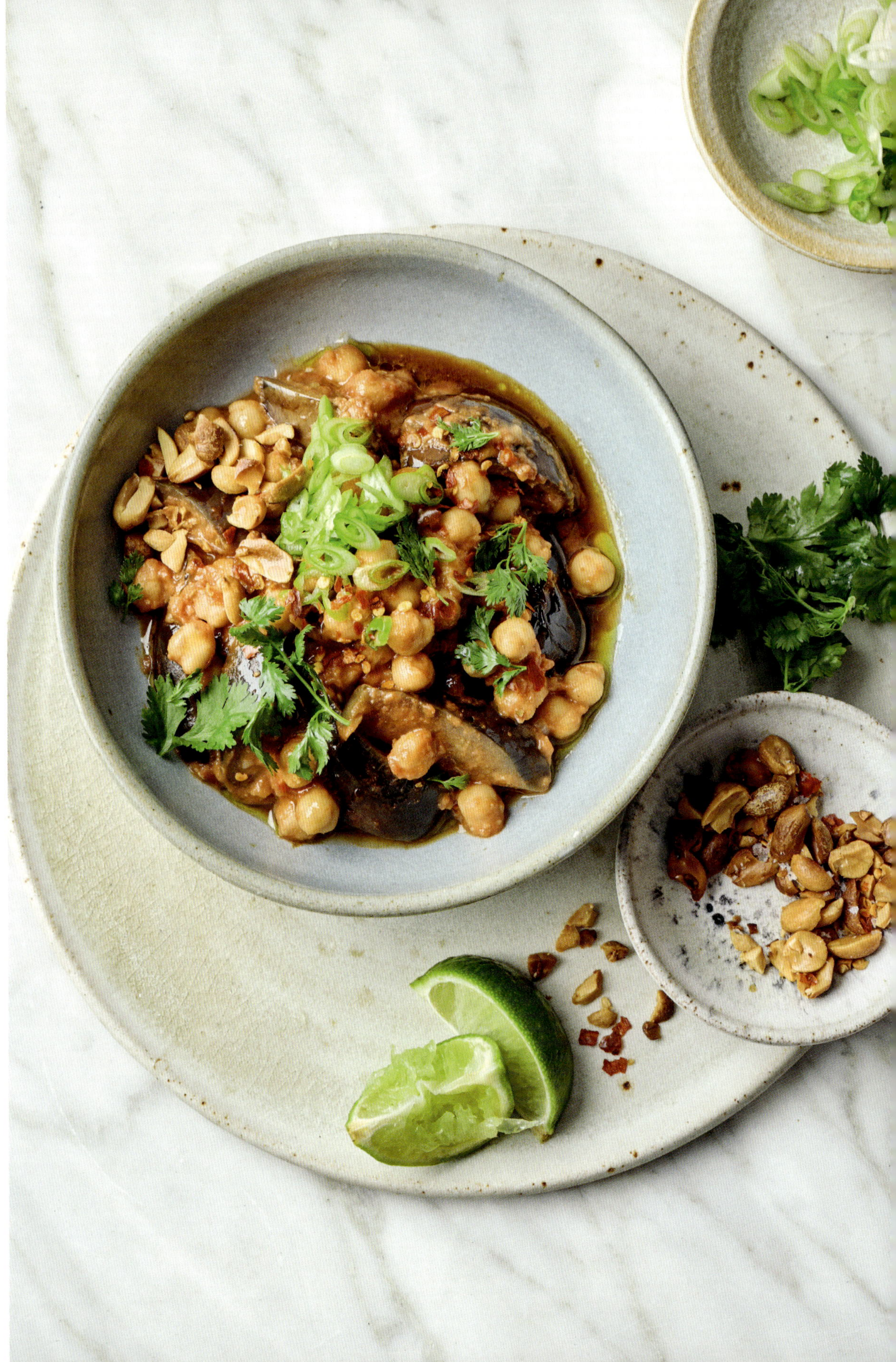

Satay-Style Eggplant Stew

Serves 2

olive oil
1 red onion, thinly sliced
1 eggplant, quartered lengthways
   and cut into large chunks
3 garlic cloves, crushed/grated
1 × 14 oz can of chickpeas or
   white beans, drained and
   rinsed
1 × 14 oz can of chopped
   tomatoes
4 tablespoons smooth peanut
   butter
2 tablespoons tamari or soy
   sauce
2 teaspoons maple syrup
14 fl oz boiling water
sea salt

To serve

2–3 green onions, finely sliced
handful of cilantro (about ½ cup),
   roughly chopped
handful of roasted peanuts,
   roughly chopped
dried red chili flakes (optional)

When I want something rich and comforting, I turn to this peanut butter, chickpea, eggplant and tomato stew. Simmered with red onions, soy and maple syrup and topped with green onions, cilantro, chili, and crunchy roasted peanuts, it's packed with plants. Plus there's very little prep or chopping, making it the quick win you need on busy weeks!

1. Warm 2 tablespoons of olive oil in a large saucepan or casserole set over a medium–high heat. Add the onion, eggplant, and a pinch of salt and cook for 8–10 minutes, stirring occasionally, until softened.

2. Add the garlic and cook for 1–2 minutes, until fragrant.

3. Stir in the chickpeas, tinned tomatoes, peanut butter, tamari, maple syrup, and boiling water. Bring to a simmer and cook for 10–12 minutes until you have a thick, luscious sauce. Taste and adjust the seasoning as needed.

4. Serve with a sprinkling of green onions, cilantro, roasted peanuts, and a pinch of chili flakes (if using).

Simple Harissa Orzo and Basil Bake

8 PLANTS

Serves 2

2 shallots, finely diced
3 garlic cloves, crushed or
  minced
1¼ cups cherry tomatoes, halved
olive oil
¾ cup orzo
1 × 14 oz can of chickpeas,
  drained and rinsed
14 fl oz boiling water
1 tablespoon white miso paste
1–2 tablespoons of harissa paste
  (use chili or rose harissa and
  adjust the quantity to your
  taste)
1–2 tablespoons balsamic
  vinegar, to taste
large handful of basil (about
  1 cup), roughly chopped
sea salt and black pepper

One-pan meals are a lifesaver on busy weeks. This is one of those recipes that basically cooks itself – you just chop a few shallots, garlic, and tomatoes, then let the oven do the rest. Orzo cooks fast, soaking up all the smoky and slightly sweet flavors from the harissa, balsamic vinegar, and miso. The chickpeas add heartiness, while the cherry tomatoes and fresh basil keep it light and vibrant.

1. Preheat the oven to 350°F fan. In a large baking dish or shallow casserole, mix the shallots, garlic, and cherry tomatoes with 2 tablespoons of olive oil and season generously.

2. Roast for 10–15 minutes, then add the orzo, chickpeas, boiling water, miso, and harissa. Stir well, making sure everything is evenly coated.

3. Bake for 12–14 minutes, until the orzo is tender and all of the liquid has been absorbed.

4. Remove from the oven, stir in the balsamic vinegar, two-thirds of the basil, and season to taste. Scatter over the remaining basil and drizzle over a little olive oil to serve.

Make it your own: Use canned cherry tomatoes if you can't find fresh tomatoes or they're not in season. Swap harissa paste for dried chili flakes, add roasted red bell peppers for extra sweetness, or top with toasted pine nuts or mixed nuts for crunch. For more greens, scatter over a big handful of arugula to serve.

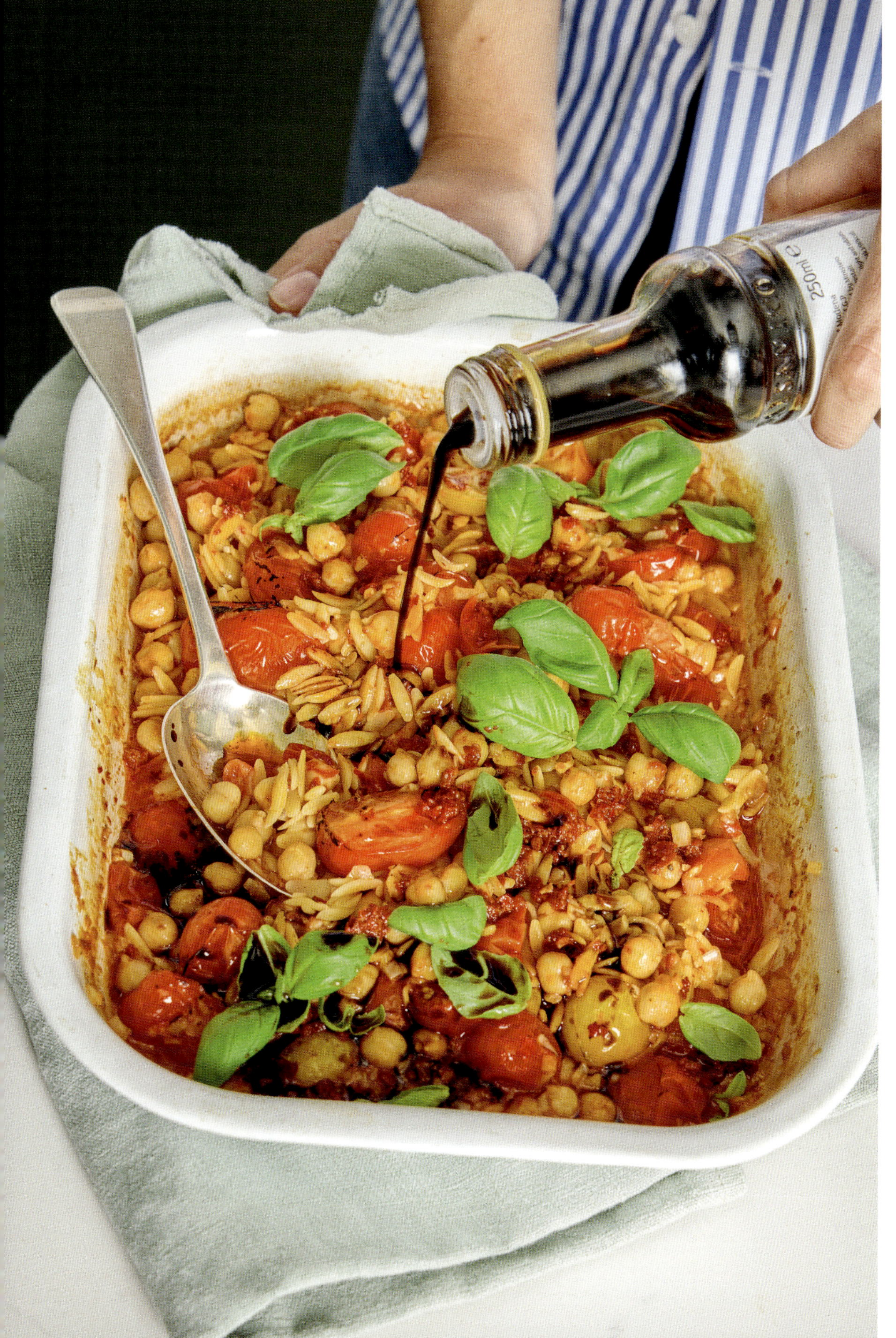

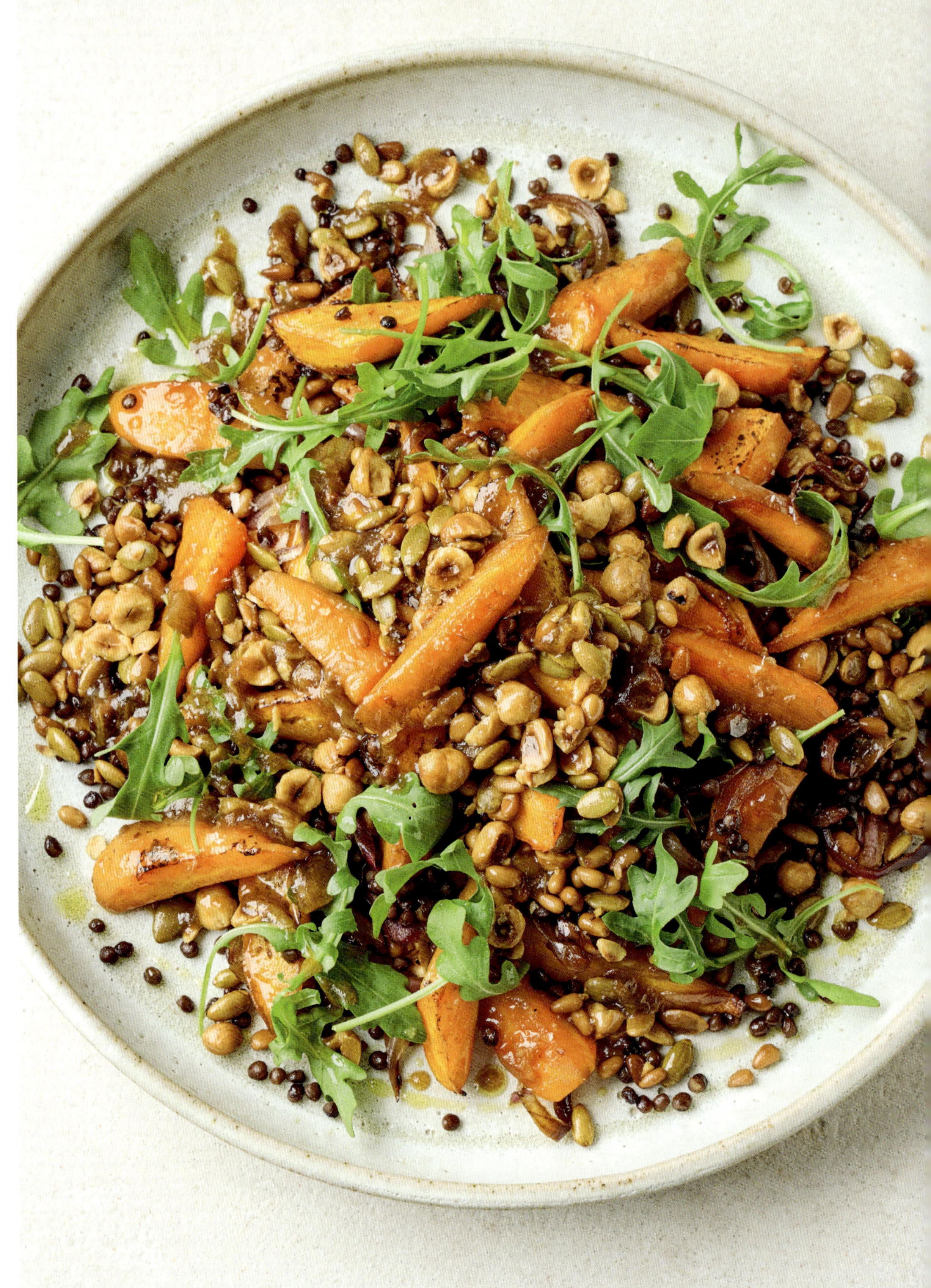

Roasted Carrot and Hazelnut Salad with Garlic and Balsamic

10 PLANTS

Serves 2

3 carrots (about 11 oz), peeled
    and cut lengthways into ½ inch
    wedges
2 red onions, thinly sliced
olive oil
2 tablespoons balsamic vinegar
2 tablespoons maple syrup
4 garlic cloves, unpeeled
1 × 14 oz can of lentils (I like
    beluga lentils), drained and
    rinsed
handful of pine nuts (about
    ⅓ cup)
handful of hazelnuts (about
    ⅓ cup)
handful of pumpkin seeds
    (about 50g)
handful of cilantro (about ½ cup),
    roughly chopped
large handful of arugula
    (about 1 cup)
sea salt and black pepper

With a roasted garlic and balsamic dressing, toasted hazelnuts, crispy lentils, pine nuts, and cilantro, this simple roasted veggie warm salad brings a huge amount of flavor with very little effort. It's a great simple supper, or an amazing addition to a big spread when you've got friends coming over.

1. Preheat the oven to 350°F fan. On a large, shallow baking tray, toss together the carrot, onion, 2 tablespoons of olive oil, 1 tablespoon of the balsamic vinegar, 1 tablespoon of the maple syrup, and a good pinch of salt. Pop the garlic cloves in the corner of the tray.

2. Roast for 20 minutes then remove the tray from the oven and lift out the garlic cloves – they should be soft and squashy.

3. Stir in the lentils, pine nuts, hazelnuts, and pumpkin seeds. Roast for another 15 minutes, until everything is tender and golden.

4. Meanwhile, make the dressing. Squeeze the roasted garlic cloves out of their skins, add to a small bowl and mash with a fork, then whisk in 2 tablespoons of olive oil, the remaining tablespoon of balsamic vinegar and maple syrup, a pinch of salt and some black pepper.

5. Tip the roasted vegetables and lentil mixture into a large salad bowl, followed by the cilantro and arugula. Drizzle over the dressing, toss gently to combine and season to taste. Serve warm or at room temperature.

Quick Olive and Tomato Spaghetti with Capers and Parsley

6 PLANTS

Serves 2

olive oil
2 garlic cloves, crushed or grated
pinch of dried red chili flakes
1 teaspoon dried oregano
2 tablespoons Kalamata olives,
  pitted
1 tablespoon capers, drained
1 × 14 oz can of cherry tomatoes
17 fl oz boiling water
6 oz uncooked spaghetti,
handful of flat-leaf parsley (about
  ½ cup), roughly chopped
sea salt and black pepper

Rich, and deeply flavorsome, this easy puttanesca-inspired spaghetti comes together in just 20 minutes. Packed with chili, garlic, olives, capers, parsley, and tomatoes, it's great for plant diversity too. For extra fiber and protein, stir in a can of brown lentils in step two. This is delicious served with a fresh green salad and a zingy vinaigrette.

1. Warm 1 tablespoon of olive oil in a large casserole or sauté pan (large enough to fit the spaghetti without breaking it up) set over a medium–low heat. Add the garlic and chili and cook for 1–2 minutes until fragrant.

2. Stir in the oregano, olives, capers, cherry tomatoes, and boiling water. Bring to a vigorous simmer, then add the pasta, making sure it's mostly covered by the sauce.

3. Simmer for 10–12 minutes, until the spaghetti is al dente stirring every now and again as the pasta softens; this will help it cook evenly.

4. Season generously, then stir in the parsley and a drizzle of olive oil.

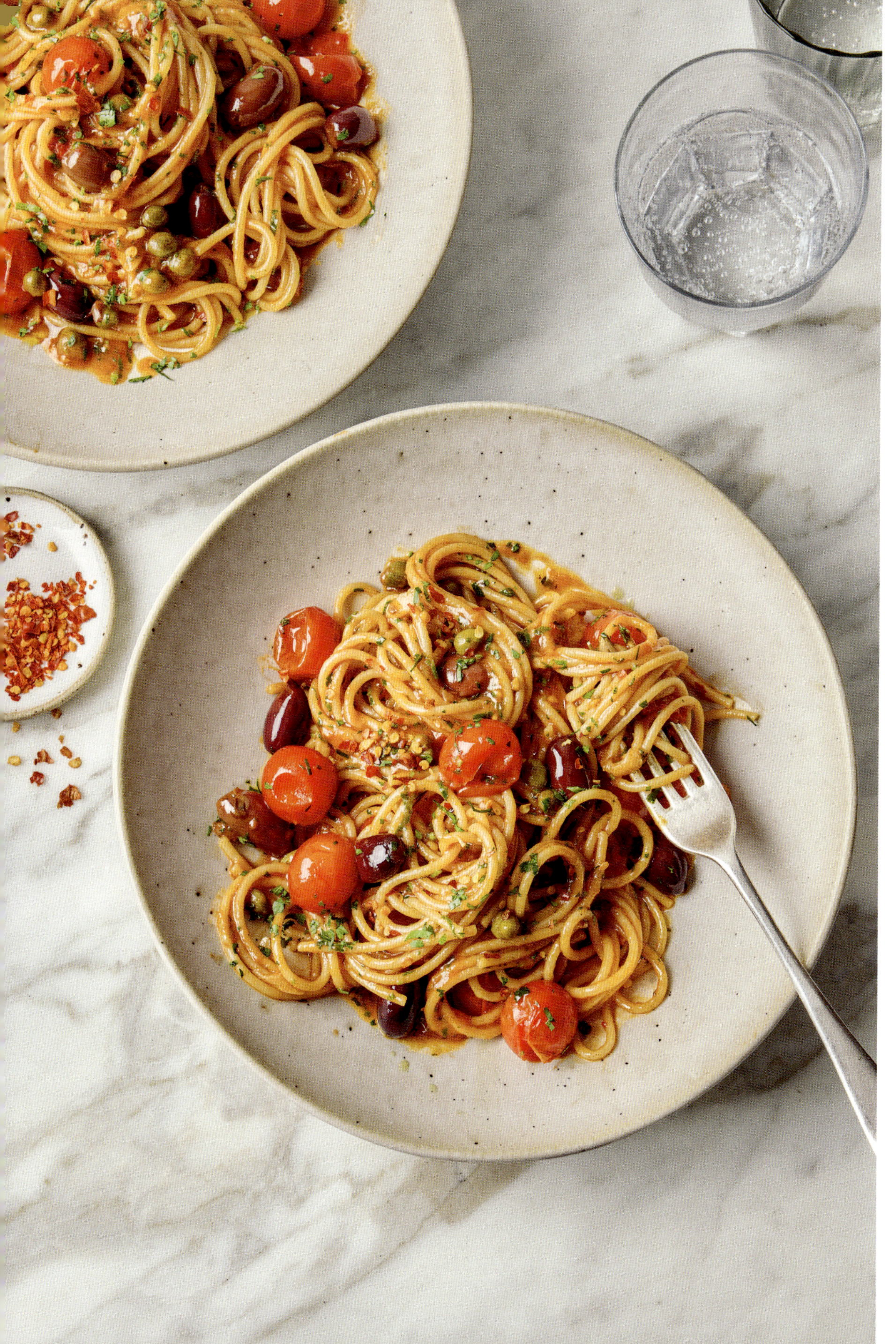

Tortelloni and Bean Broth

7 PLANTS

Serves 2

olive oil
2 garlic cloves, grated or crushed
1 leek, thinly sliced
2 celery sticks, thinly sliced
1 × 14 fl oz can of coconut milk
14 fl oz hot vegetable stock
1 × 9 oz package of tortelloni
1 × 14 oz can of borlotti beans (or
   use cannellini or lima beans),
   drained and rinsed
¾ cup frozen peas, defrosted
handful of basil (about ¾ cup),
   chopped, plus extra leaves for
   garnish
grated zest of 1 lemon
pinch of dried red chili flakes
   (optional)
sea salt and black pepper
extra virgin olive oil, to finish

I love a bowl of this soothing tortelloni soup; it's one of those comforting meals I come back to again and again. It's creamy and full of flavor, with leeks, beans, peas, coconut milk, and stuffed pasta all simmered in one pan, then finished with lemon and basil to keep it fresh. On the table in 30 minutes, it's a really quick win for busy evenings.

1. Warm 1 tablespoon of olive oil in a shallow casserole or sauté pan set over a medium heat. Add the garlic and cook for 1–2 minutes until just golden.

2. Next, add the leek, celery, and a pinch of salt. Cook for 8–10 minutes, stirring often, until softened.

3. Stir in the coconut milk and vegetable stock. Bring to a gentle boil, then add the tortelloni, beans, and peas. Cook for 3–4 minutes until everything is just tender.

4. Remove from the heat and stir in the chopped basil, lemon zest, and chili flakes, if using. Taste to check the seasoning and adjust as needed.

5. To serve, divide into bowls, drizzle over a little extra virgin olive oil, then add the remaining basil and a generous grind of black pepper.

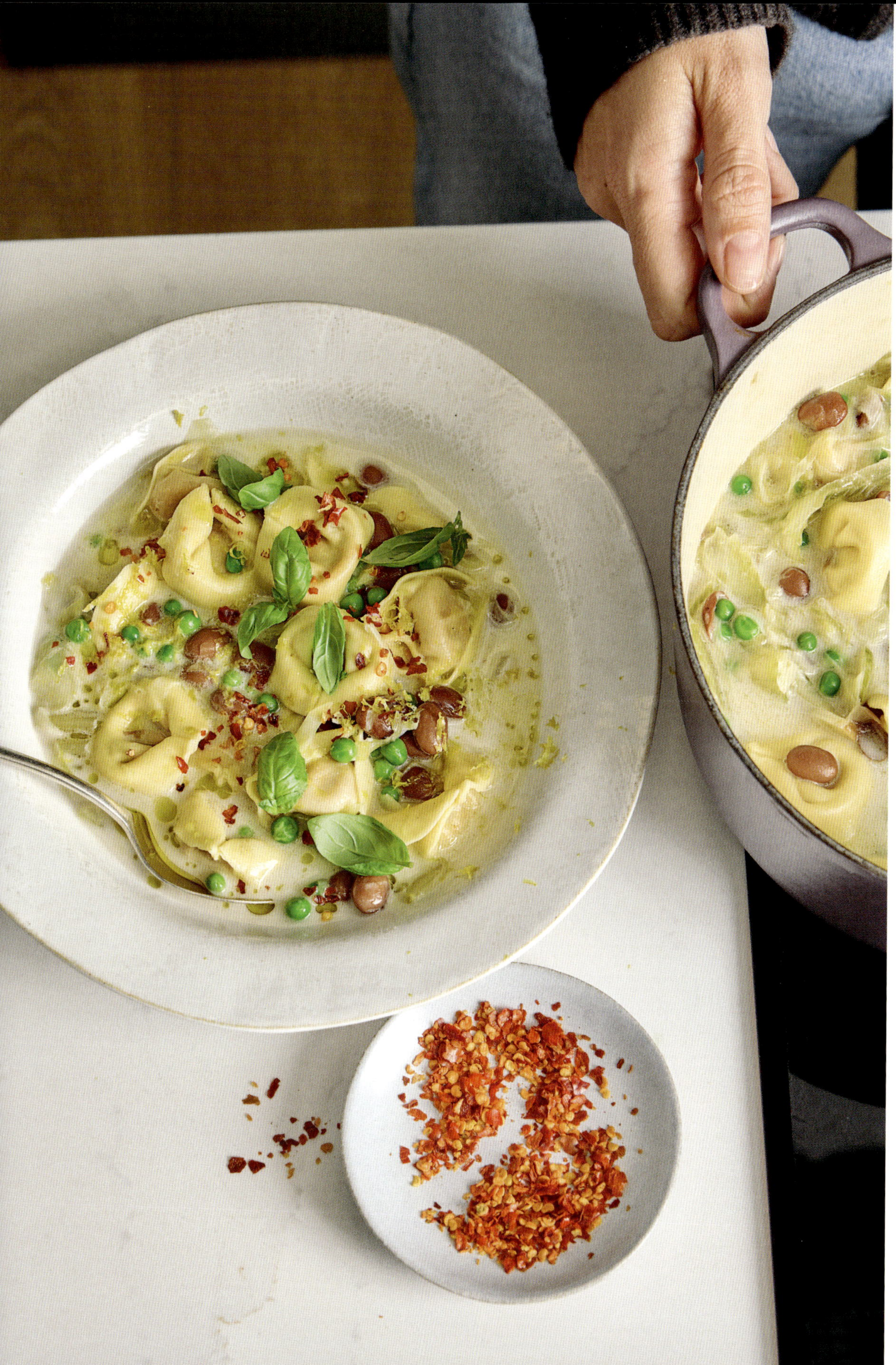

These quick, no-faff lunches are ready in under 15 minutes and use no more than one pan. Easy salads, cosy bowls, delicious sandwiches, and speedy dips for spreading on toast are perfect for days when you need to get something on the table fast or for a quick packed lunch, and will keep you nourished and energised all afternoon.

EASY LUNCHES

Cucumber, Edamame, and Tofu Bowls with Soy and Sesame

5 PLANTS

Serves 2

1 small cucumber, deseeded and
    cut into thin quarter moons
2 tablespoons rice vinegar
2 tablespoons maple syrup
4–6 tablespoons tamari or soy
    sauce
½ cup jasmine rice
1 × block of firm tofu (about
    10 oz), drained and cut into
    cubes
⅔ cup frozen edamame
1 tablespoon sesame seeds, plus
    extra to serve
1 avocado, sliced

I am completely obsessed with this lunch! Ready in under 15 minutes, it is so easy to throw together yet incredibly delicious. It is deeply flavorful, wonderfully light, and so satisfying. For a lighter option, simply skip the rice, or swap it for noodles.

1. In a large bowl, toss the cucumber with the rice vinegar, maple syrup, and soy sauce. Let it sit for 10 minutes, stirring occasionally, to lightly pickle while you prepare the rest.

2. Put the rice on to cook according to the package instructions. Pat the tofu dry with a clean kitchen towel or paper towel to remove excess moisture. Put the tofu and edamame into a steamer basket set over the rice and steam for the final 5 minutes of the cooking time.

3. Once cooked, add the tofu, edamame, and sesame seeds to the cucumber bowl, tossing everything together.

4. If using, spoon the rice into bowls, top with the pickled cucumber mix, then add the avocado slices. Sprinkle extra sesame seeds over the top to finish.

Make it your own: Swap the rice for noodles, add a drizzle of chili oil for a little heat, or freshly chopped chili and green onion for more flavor.

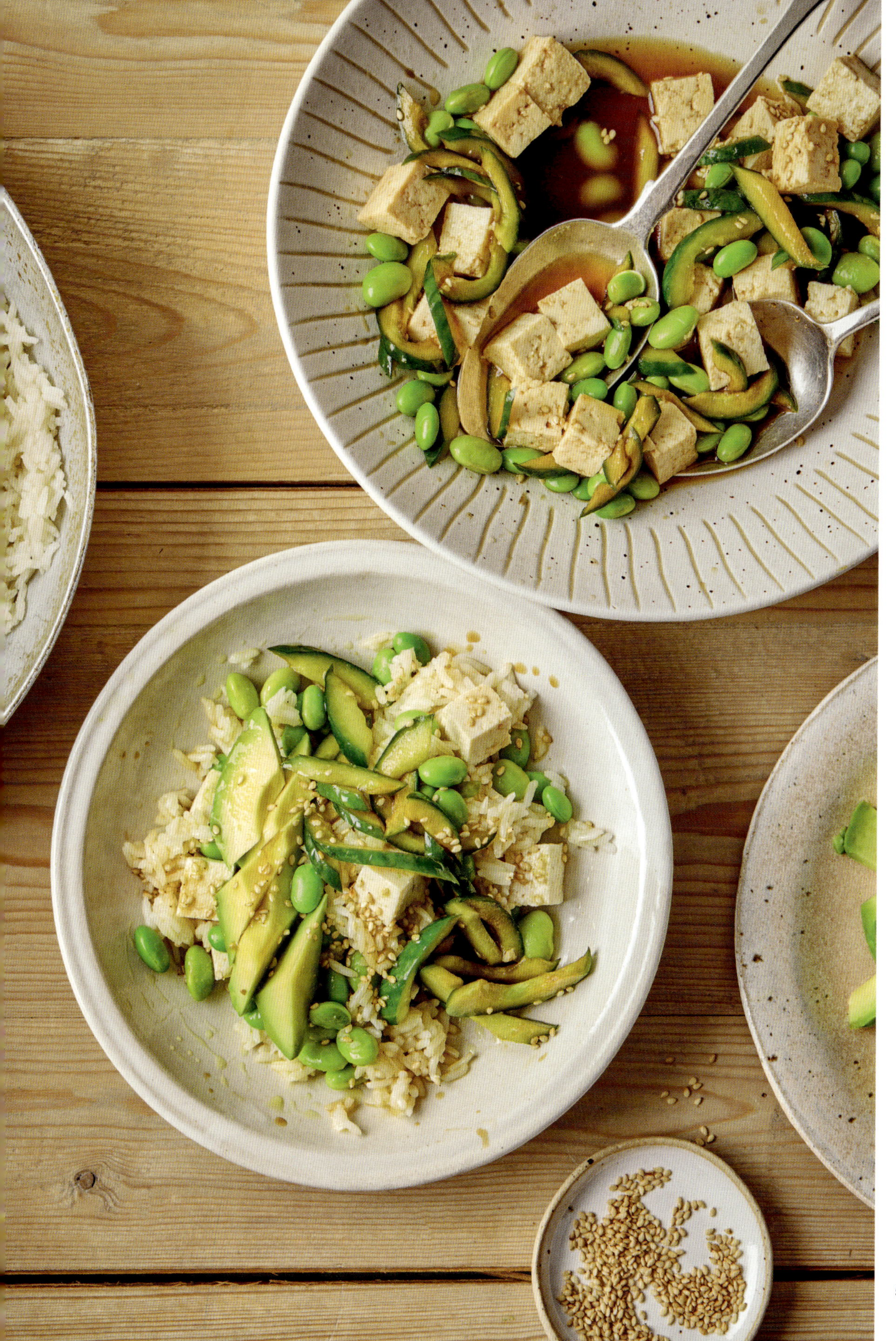

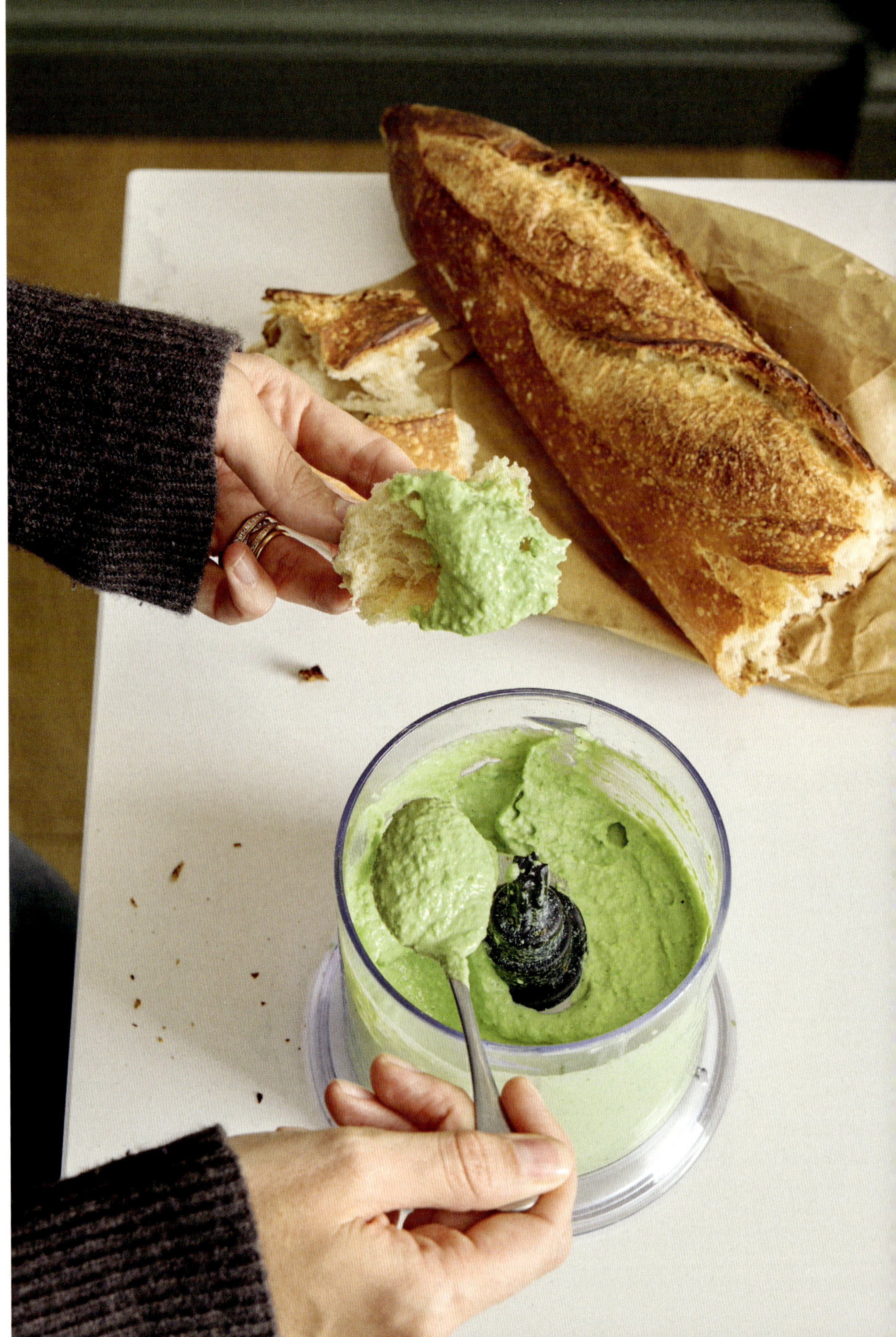

Protein-Packed Whipped Greens

7 PLANTS

Serves 2

⅔ cup frozen peas
⅔ cup frozen edamame
extra virgin olive oil
2 garlic cloves, thinly sliced
½ × block of silken tofu (about
   5 oz), drained
handful of basil (about ¾ cup)
1 heaped tablespoon plain yogurt
juice of ½ lemon
sea salt and black pepper

To serve
2 slices of sourdough

This super-speedy lunch has quickly become a staple in my house. With seven different plants, it's an upgrade on avocado toast and comes together in minutes to create a delicious, velvety spread or dip with hints of tahini, garlic, and basil. I love it with crusty bread, in a sandwich, or even used as a dressing. If you're following the meal plan for this week, you can use your leftover cucumber from the Herby Avocado Noodle Salad (see page 95) as crudites with this too!

1. Bring a small saucepan of salted water to the boil. Add the peas and edamame and cook for 3–4 minutes, until just tender. Drain and refresh in cold water, then transfer to a high-speed blender.

2. Return the pan to a low heat and warm 2 tablespoons of extra virgin olive oil. Add the garlic and cook for 3–4 minutes, until crisp and golden. Remove from the heat, leave to cool briefly then add the garlic and its oil to the blender.

3. Add the tofu, basil, yogurt, and lemon juice to the blender and season generously. Blitz until smooth and creamy – the mix should be thick and spreadable.

4. To serve, toast the bread, spoon over the whipped greens and finish with a drizzle of extra virgin olive oil and a pinch of salt.

Make it your own: Serve in toasted pitta with crunchy cucumber rounds, a handful of arugula, and slices of tomato. The mix also works brilliantly as a dip or spread over wraps.

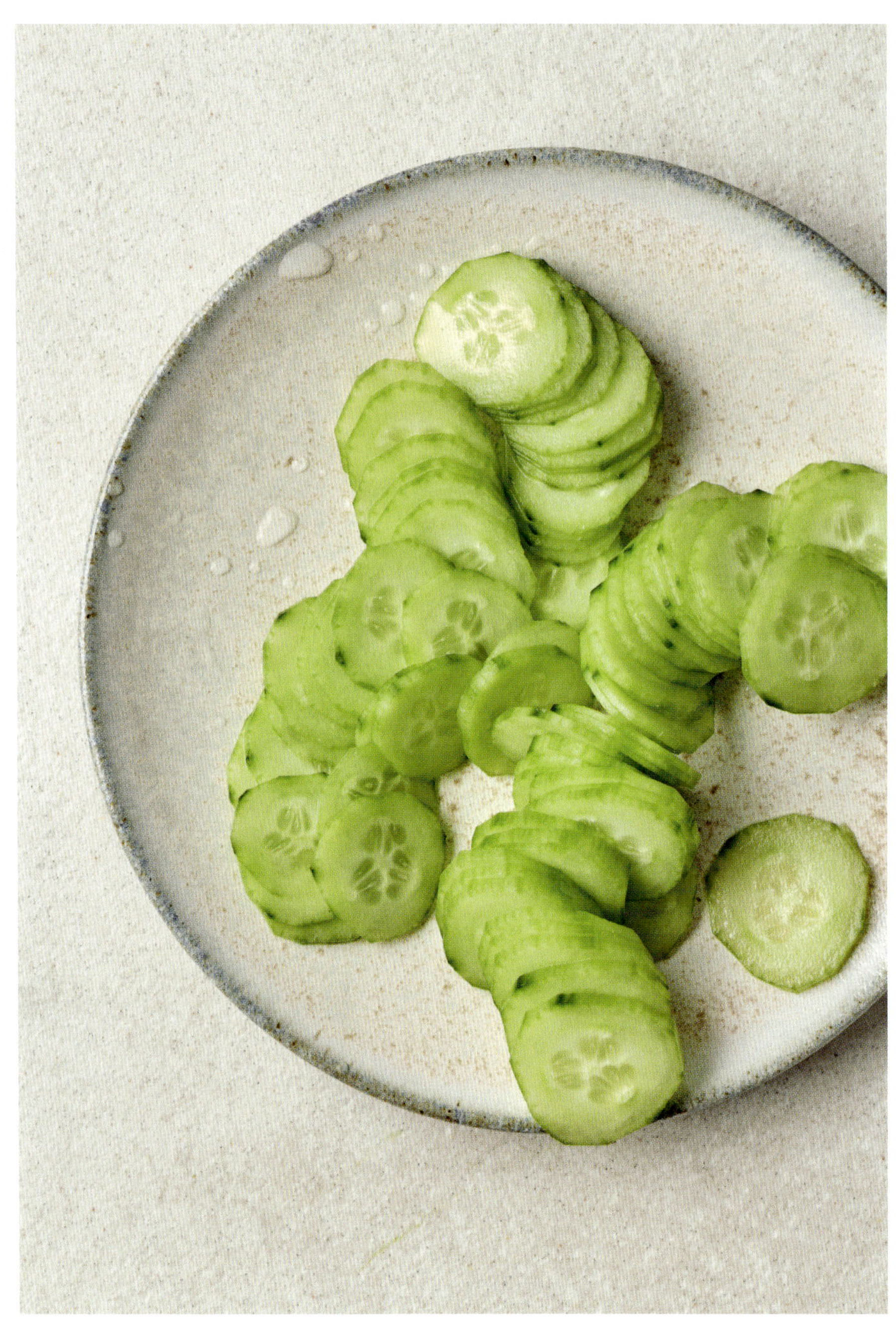

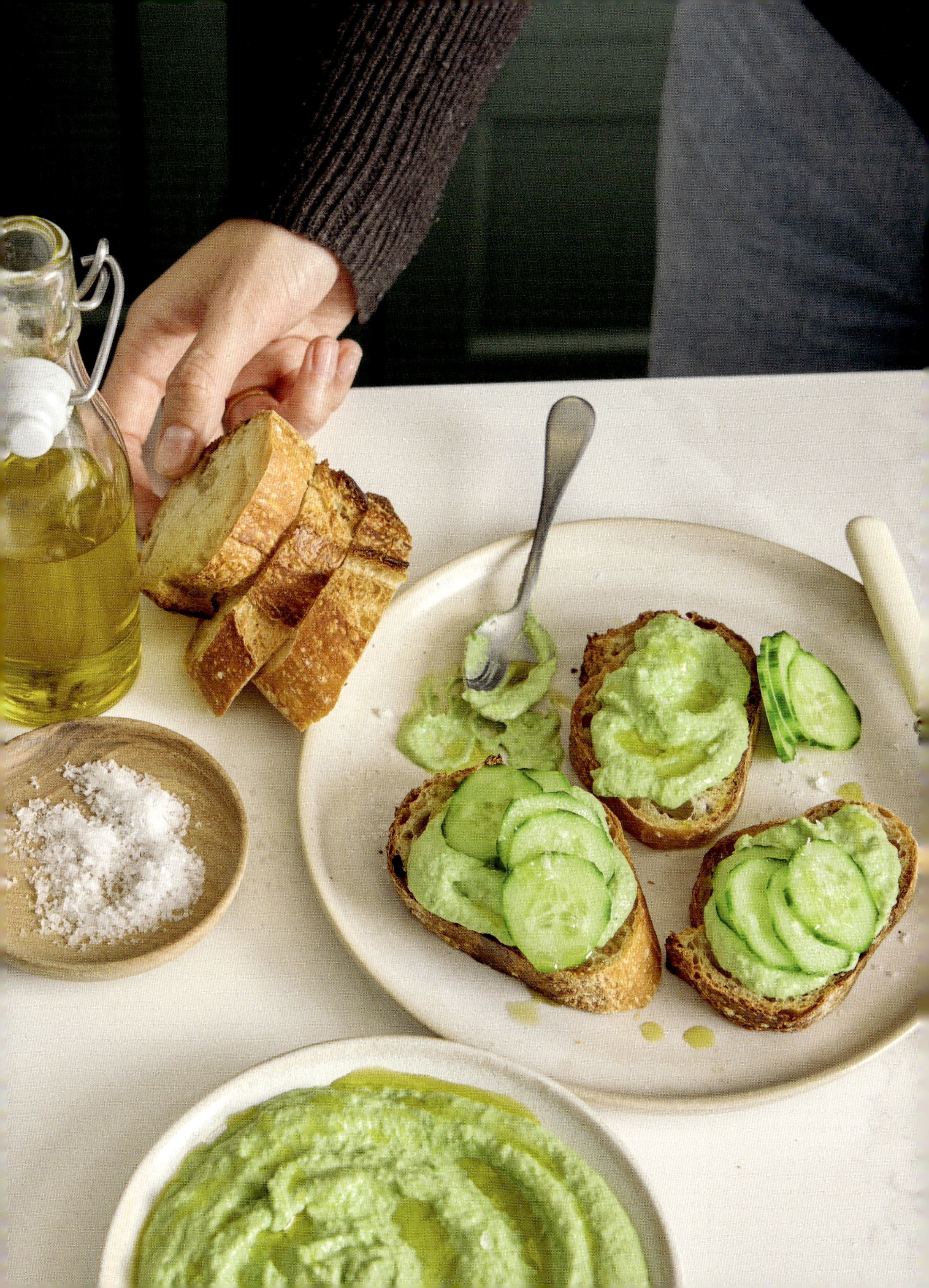

Hazelnut and Lentil Salad with Sweet Peanut Dressing

6 PLANTS

Serves 2

½ small red cabbage (about
   3 cups when finely sliced),
   core removed and finely sliced
   (use the other half in the Beet,
   Dill, and Green Bean Salad
   with Mustard on page 76)
2 carrots, coarsely grated
1 × 9 oz pouch of cooked puy
   lentils
½ bunch of cilantro (about ½
   cup), roughly chopped, plus
   extra to serve
⅓ cup hazelnuts or peanuts,
   toasted (see page 33) and
   roughly chopped
sea salt

For the dressing
⅕ cup smooth peanut butter
grated zest and juice of 2 limes
2 tablespoons maple syrup
3 tablespoons olive oil

This no-cook salad is everything you need on busy days. It's crunchy, vibrant, and full of texture, with lentils, hazelnuts, heaps of veg, and the most delicious sweet peanut dressing. I'd recommend making a double batch of the dressing – it's brilliant drizzled over grain bowls or roasted veg later in the week (or simply eaten with a spoon!).

1. To make the dressing, whisk together all of the ingredients, along with 2 tablespoons of water in a bowl, until smooth.

2. Put the cabbage, carrots, lentils, cilantro, nuts, and a pinch of salt into a large bowl and toss with the dressing. Serve with a little extra cilantro on top.

Make it your own: Swap the toasted hazelnuts or peanuts for almonds.

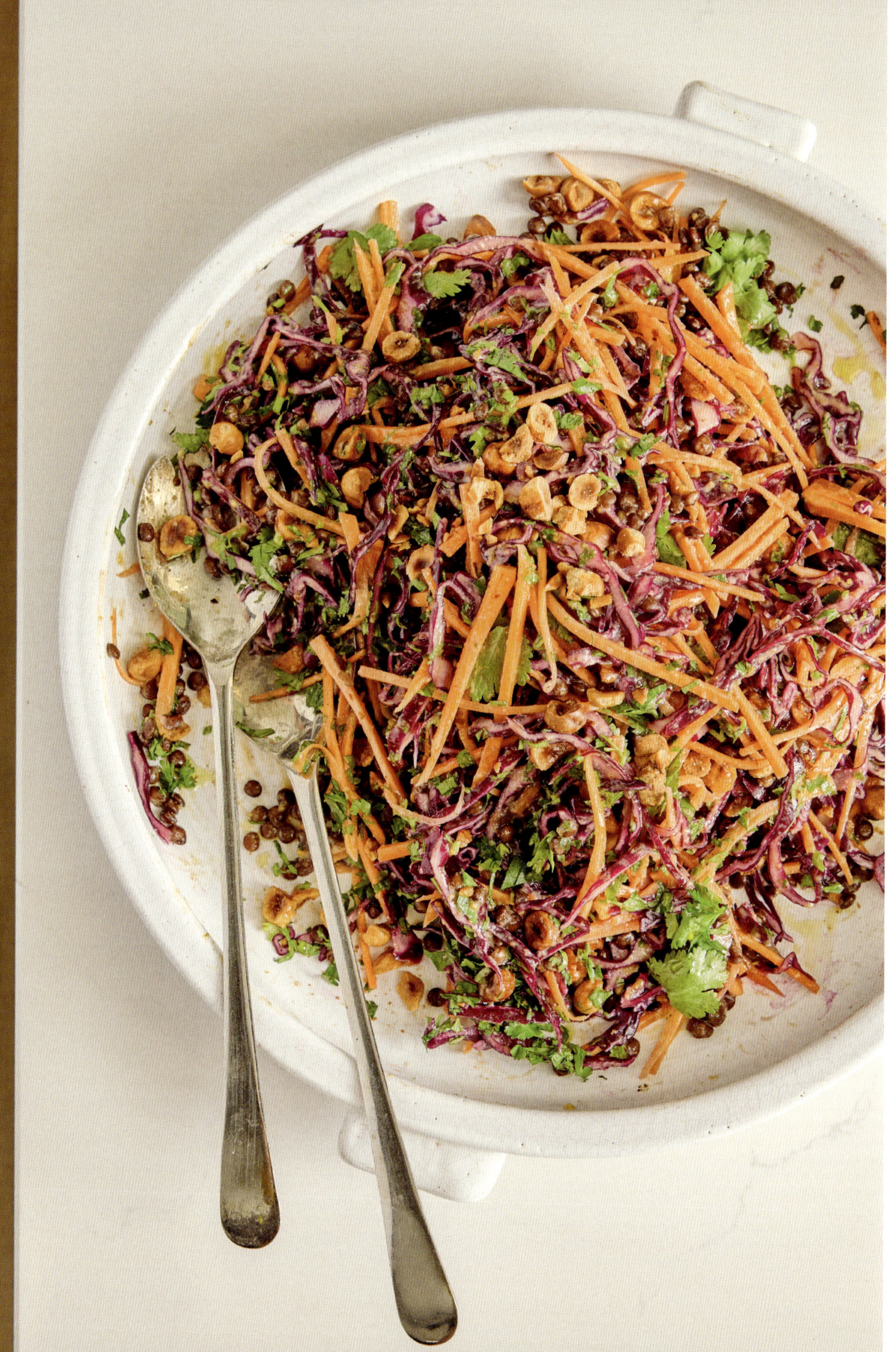

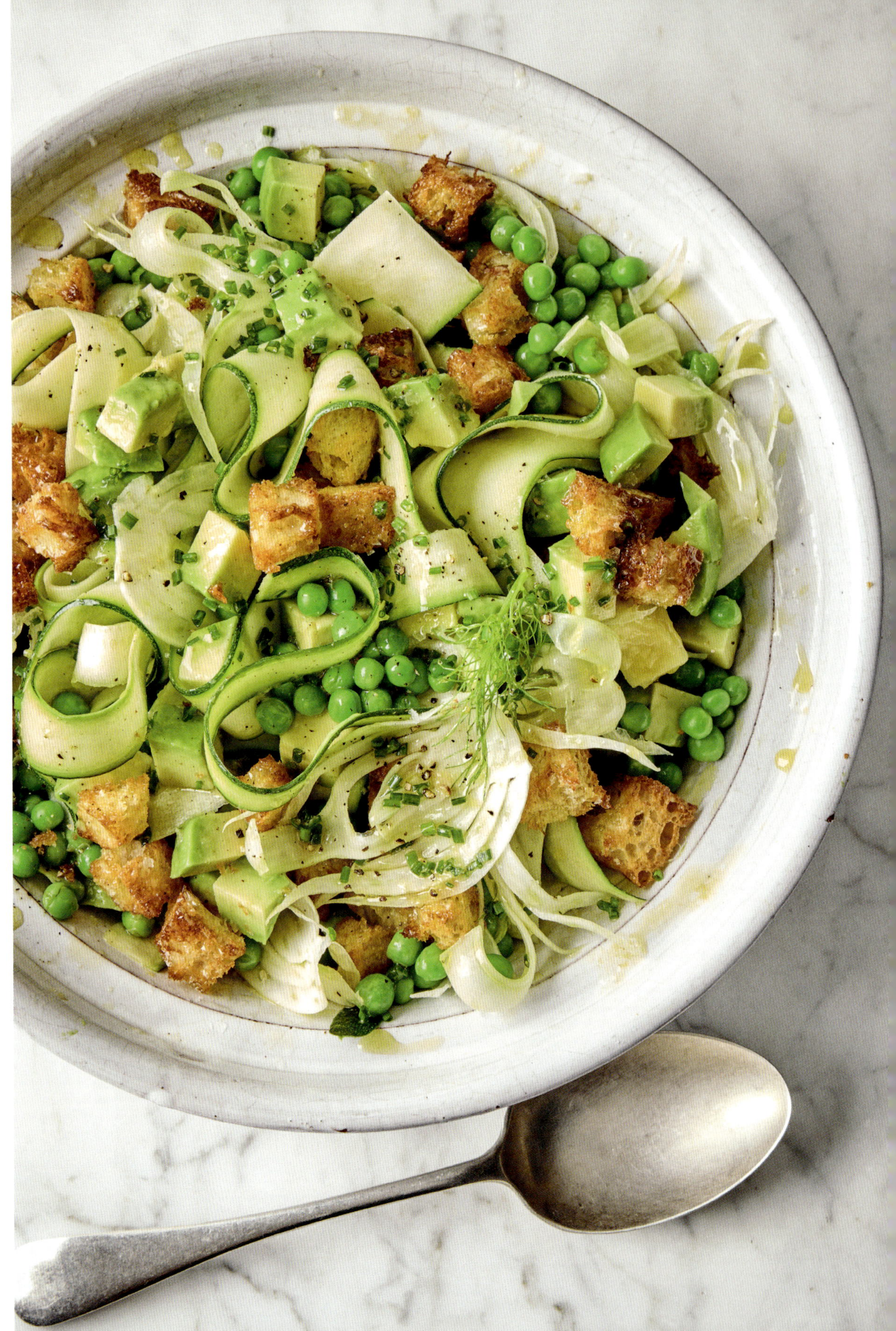

Plant-Packed Avocado Salad with Zucchini Ribbons and Croutons

7 PLANTS

Serves 2

1 small fennel bulb, finely sliced into thick match sticks (you can also thinly slice it using a mandoline)

1 zucchini, shaved into ribbons (leaving the inner part with seeds)

⅔ cup frozen peas

2 slices of bread (I love this with sourdough)

1 garlic clove, peeled

1 avocado, diced

about 2–3 tablespoons chives, finely chopped

For the dressing

2 tablespoons apple cider vinegar

grated zest and juice of ½ lemon

extra virgin olive oil

sea salt and black pepper

This is one of my favorite meals! I make it whenever I want something light, crunchy, and tangy. It comes together in just 15 minutes, and it's packed with vibrant greens. If you're unsure about fennel, definitely give it a try – the apple cider vinegar and lemon really bring it to life, softening the aniseed flavor. Its crunch balances perfectly with the creamy avocado, sweet peas, and garlicky croutons for the most delicious mix of textures.

1. To make the dressing, in a large salad bowl, whisk together the apple cider vinegar, lemon zest, and juice, 2 tablespoons of extra virgin olive oil, a pinch of salt, and lots of black pepper. Add the fennel and zucchini, and set aside to marinate while you prep the rest of the salad.

2. To defrost the peas, simply put them into a small saucepan of boiling water and cook for 1–2 minutes, then drain and let them cool while you make the croutons.

3. Toast the bread, then rub the slices with the garlic clove for extra flavor. Tear into bite-sized croutons.

4. Finally add the peas, avocado, chives, and croutons to your salad bowl and gently mix.

Make it your own: Swap the fennel for thinly sliced celery if preferred for a milder crunch. Capers are such a great addition for more tang! Leave out the croutons for a light salad, or swap them for canned beans, lentils, or chickpeas.

Spicy Lima Bean Sandwich

6 PLANTS

Serves 2

olive oil
2 garlic cloves, finely chopped
1 × 14 oz can of lima beans,
    drained and rinsed
grated zest and juice of ½ lemon
½ tablespoon harissa paste
4 tablespoons plain yogurt
4 slices of bread, toasted
handful of arugula (or any other
    salad leaf)
1 avocado, sliced
sea salt and pepper

When I'm working from home and need something quick but deeply satisfying, this sandwich is one I often come back to. The lima beans are pan-fried until golden, then mashed with harissa, lemon, and yogurt to make the creamiest, punchiest filling. Piled on to toasted bread with avocado and arugula, it's such an easy way to pack in plants – and it tastes every bit as good as it sounds.

1. Add 1 tablespoon of olive oil to a large frying pan over a medium heat, add the garlic and fry for 1 minute, until fragrant. Stir in the lima beans and cook for about 4–5 minutes, until they're starting to crisp around the outside.

2. Remove the pan from the heat and stir in the lemon zest and juice, harissa, and yogurt, along with some salt and pepper. Mash the mix slightly with a potato masher (or a fork), so that about two thirds of the beans are broken down.

3. To assemble your sandwiches, simply drizzle a little oil over 2 slices of the toast and pile each with half of the beans, arugula, and avocado, before placing the second slice of toast on top.

Make it your own: The lima beans also make a great baked potato filling!

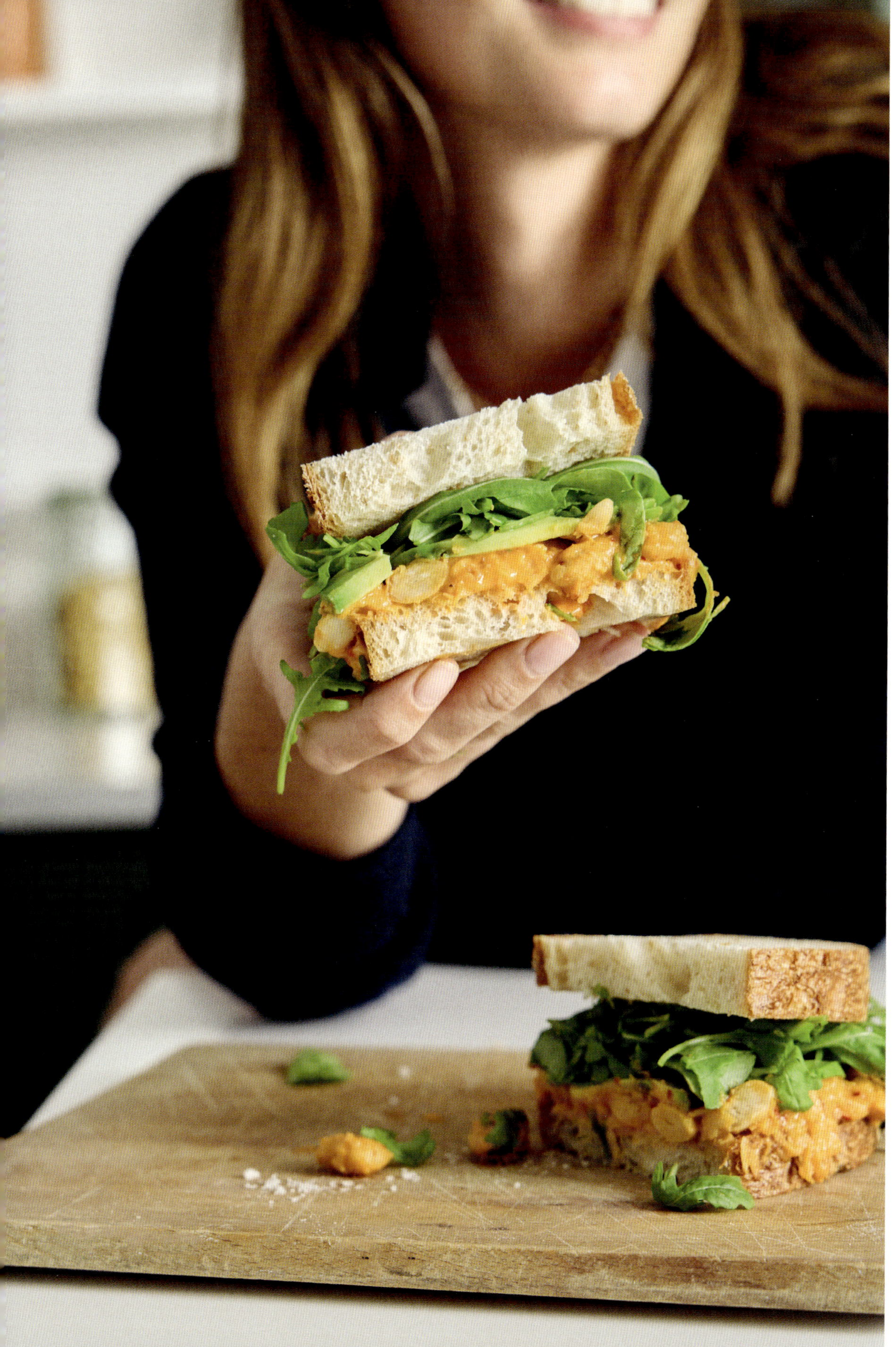

Miso and Tahini Quinoa Salad

Serves 2

⅔ cup quinoa
⅔ cup frozen edamame
olive oil
2 × servings of no-cook fresh
   veg (fresh tomatoes, sliced
   radishes, avocado, half moons
   of cucumber, or zucchini,
   pre-roasted beets, thinly sliced
   matchstick carrots – whatever
   you have)
1 handful of salad greens
   (about ⅔ cup)
sea salt and black pepper

For the dressing
2 tablespoons olive oil
2 teaspoons white miso paste
2 tablespoons tahini
1 tablespoon apple cider vinegar
1 tablespoon maple syrup
3 tablespoons water
1 garlic clove, crushed

This salad is all about the rich, creamy dressing, which is so flavorsome. I use the quinoa and dressing as a base, then switch up the veg with whatever's in season or lingering at the back of my fridge! It's endlessly adaptable, always satisfying, and is the kind of lunch that keeps you feeling energized and full all afternoon.

1. Place the quinoa in a small saucepan with double the volume of salted water (about 1⅓ cups) and bring to a boil. Simmer for 12–15 minutes until the water is absorbed and the quinoa is fluffy, adding the frozen edamame for the last 2 minutes of cooking.

2. Once cooked, drain, then drizzle with 1 tablespoon of olive oil and a sprinkle of salt and set aside to cool slightly.

3. While the quinoa cooks, whisk the dressing ingredients together in a small bowl.

4. In two serving bowls, assemble sections of veggies, quinoa, and greens, then drizzle over the dressing.

Make it your own: Adding a can of chickpeas is delicious – I just add it to the quinoa at the same time as the edamame.

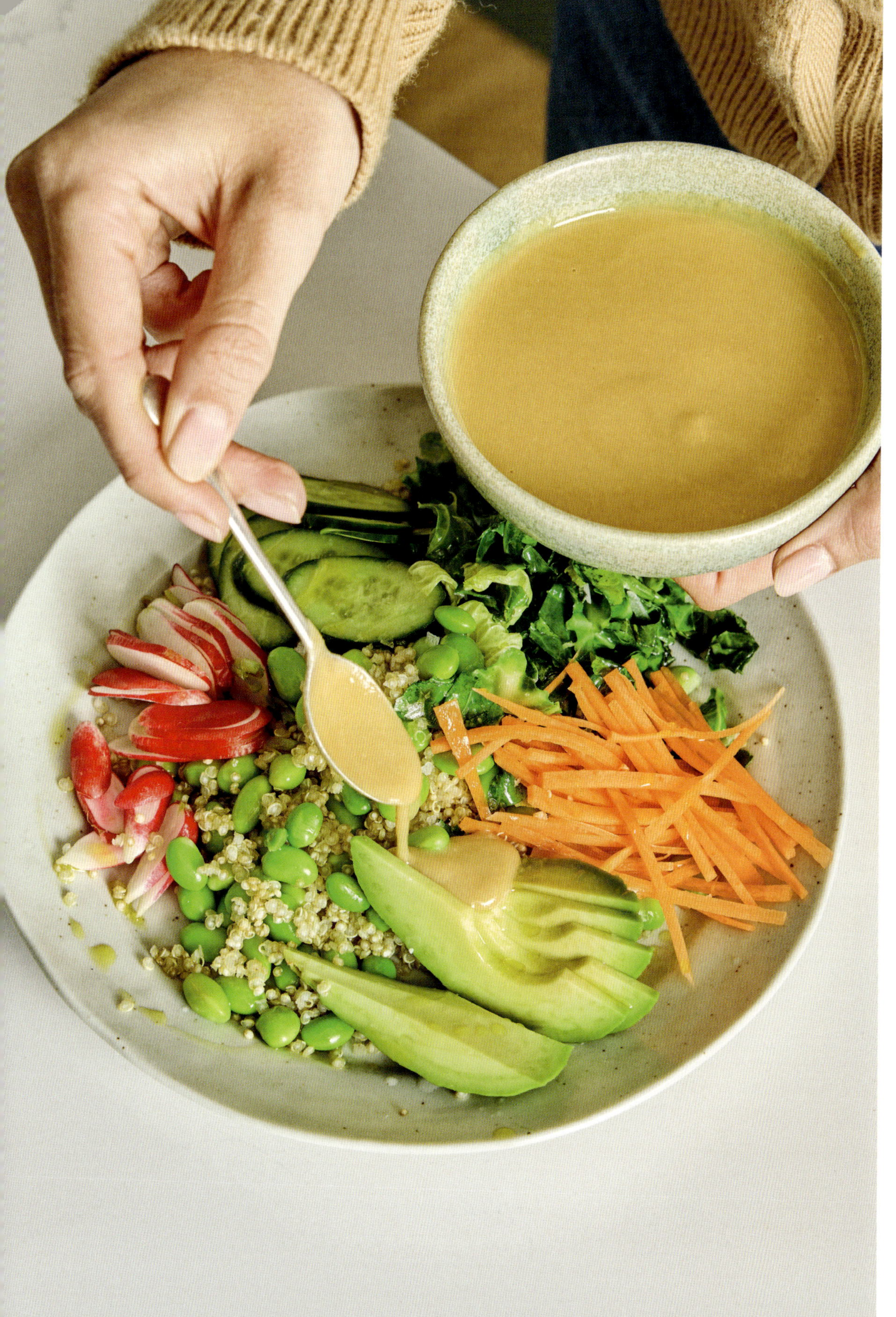

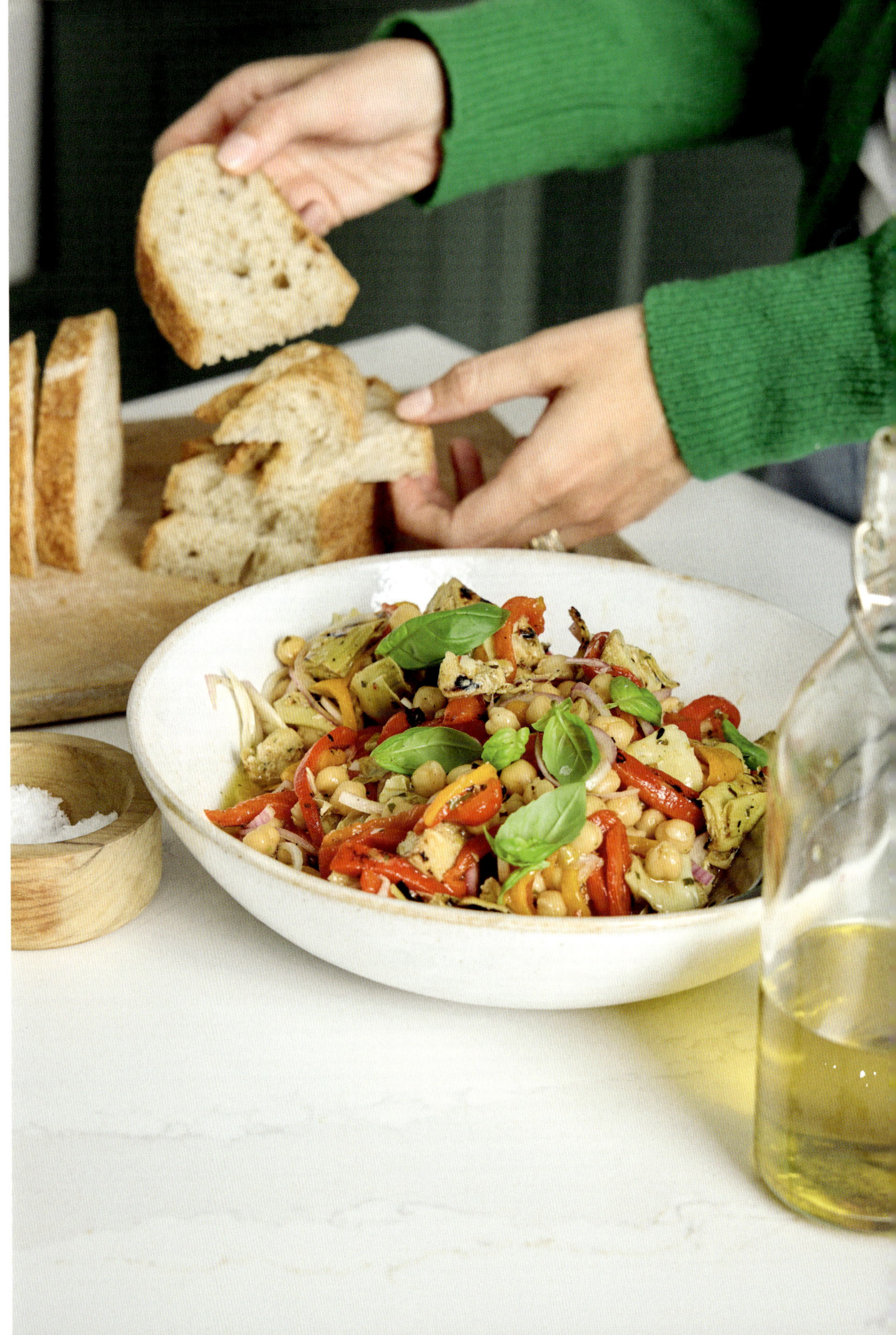

No-Fuss Artichoke and Red Bell Pepper Salad

6 PLANTS

Serves 2

1 × 14 oz can of chickpeas, drained and rinsed
1 × 9 oz jar of marinated artichokes, drained and cut into quarters
1 × 9 oz jar of flame-roasted red bell peppers, drained and sliced into 1cm strips
1 red onion, finely sliced
1–2 tablespoons of apple cider vinegar, to taste (I like it quite tangy)
3 tablespoons olive oil (use the oil from the jar of artichokes if yours are stored in olive oil)
2 teaspoons maple syrup
pinch of cayenne pepper or dried red chili flakes (more if you like a little heat)
handful of basil leaves (about ¾ cup), roughly torn
grated zest of 1 lemon
sea salt and black pepper

It's easy to get stuck in a loop with the same lunches each week, but adding just one or two new ingredients can make all the difference – both in terms of flavor and variety. This no-cook salad is a brilliant example, bringing jarred artichokes and roasted red peppers into the mix for something a little different. Tossed with chickpeas, lemon zest, and a quick maple and apple cider vinegar dressing, it's bold, fresh and full of plant diversity, and ready in under 10 minutes. It also gets better over time, so save the second serving for lunch later in the week, if you like.

1. Place the chickpeas, artichokes, red pepper, and red onion in a large mixing bowl.

2. To make the dressing, in a small bowl, whisk together the apple cider vinegar, olive oil, maple syrup, cayenne pepper, and a pinch of salt and pepper.

3. Pour the dressing over the salad ingredients and toss well to coat evenly.

4. Toss through the basil and lemon zest and finish with a pinch of salt and a generous crack of black pepper.

Tip: This is lovely spooned over the Sun-Dried Tomato and White Bean Dip (see page 184), or served with toasted sourdough, pitta, or flatbread for an easy, satisfying lunch. You can also add avocado, arugula, or lots of croutons (see page 102).

Garlic and Chive Cream Cheese

4 PLANTS

1 × block of firm tofu (about 10 oz), drained
about 3–4 tablespoons chopped chives
4 tablespoons extra virgin olive oil
2 tablespoons apple cider vinegar
1 teaspoon white miso paste
1 small garlic clove (or half for a milder flavor)
sea salt

If you're feeling a little skeptical about this one, I really don't blame you. I was genuinely shocked by the results the first time I made it. Most store-bought cream cheeses – plant-based or not – tend to use various gums and preservatives, so this is a great swap for something more nourishing. It's super creamy, takes just a couple of minutes to make, and tastes unbelievably good spread thickly on toasted bagels topped with sliced tomatoes and flaky sea salt.

1. Squeeze as much water as you can from the tofu. I wrap it in kitchen paper or paper towels and press it firmly to get it really dry.

2. Add everything to a high-speed blender or food processor and blend until completely smooth, scraping down the sides as needed. The mixture should be thick, creamy, and spreadable.

3. Keep in the fridge and use within 4–5 days.

Make it your own: This version is flavored with garlic and chives, but you can easily mix it up. Try dried red chili flakes, sun-dried tomatoes, capers, or your favorite fresh herbs.

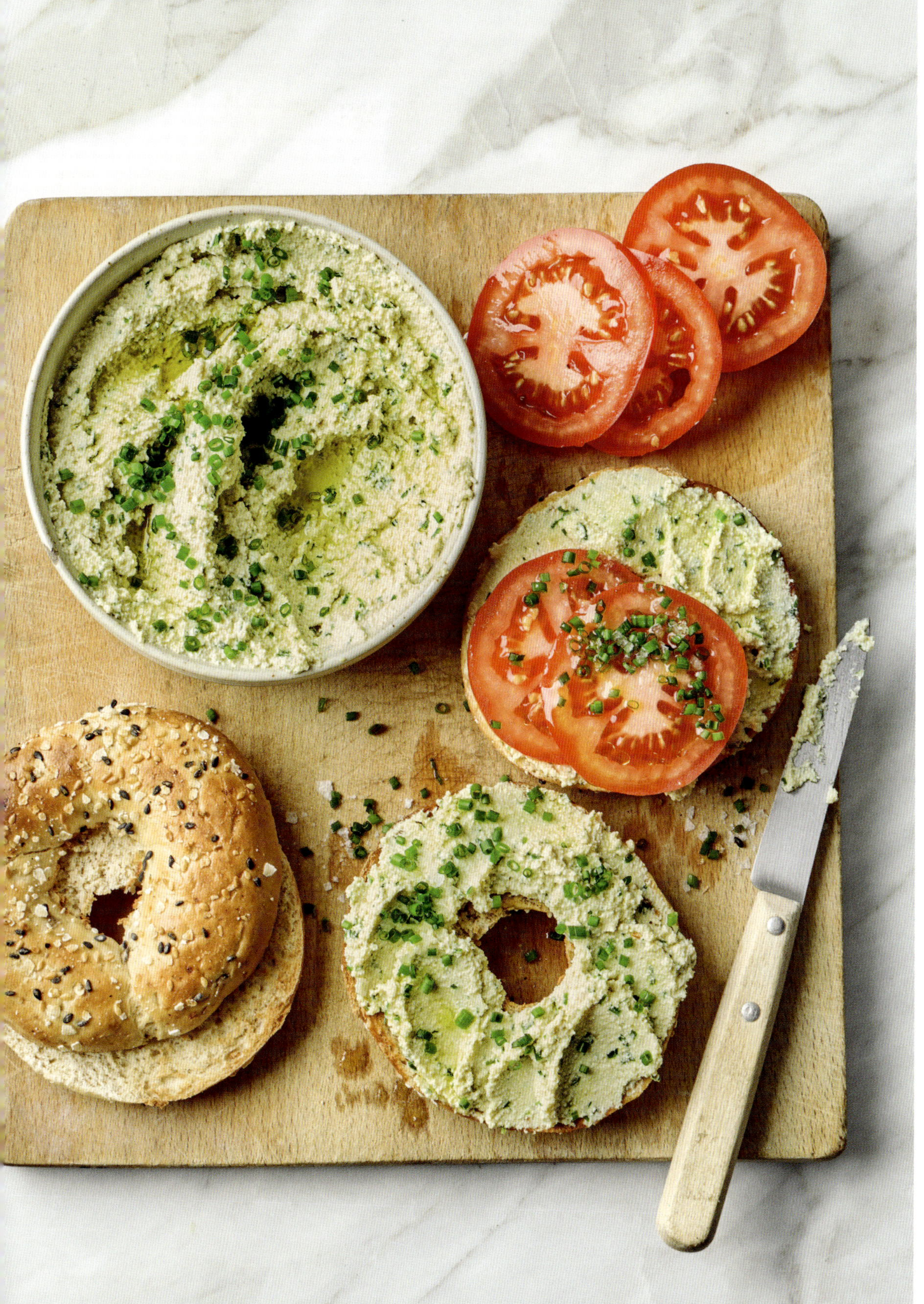

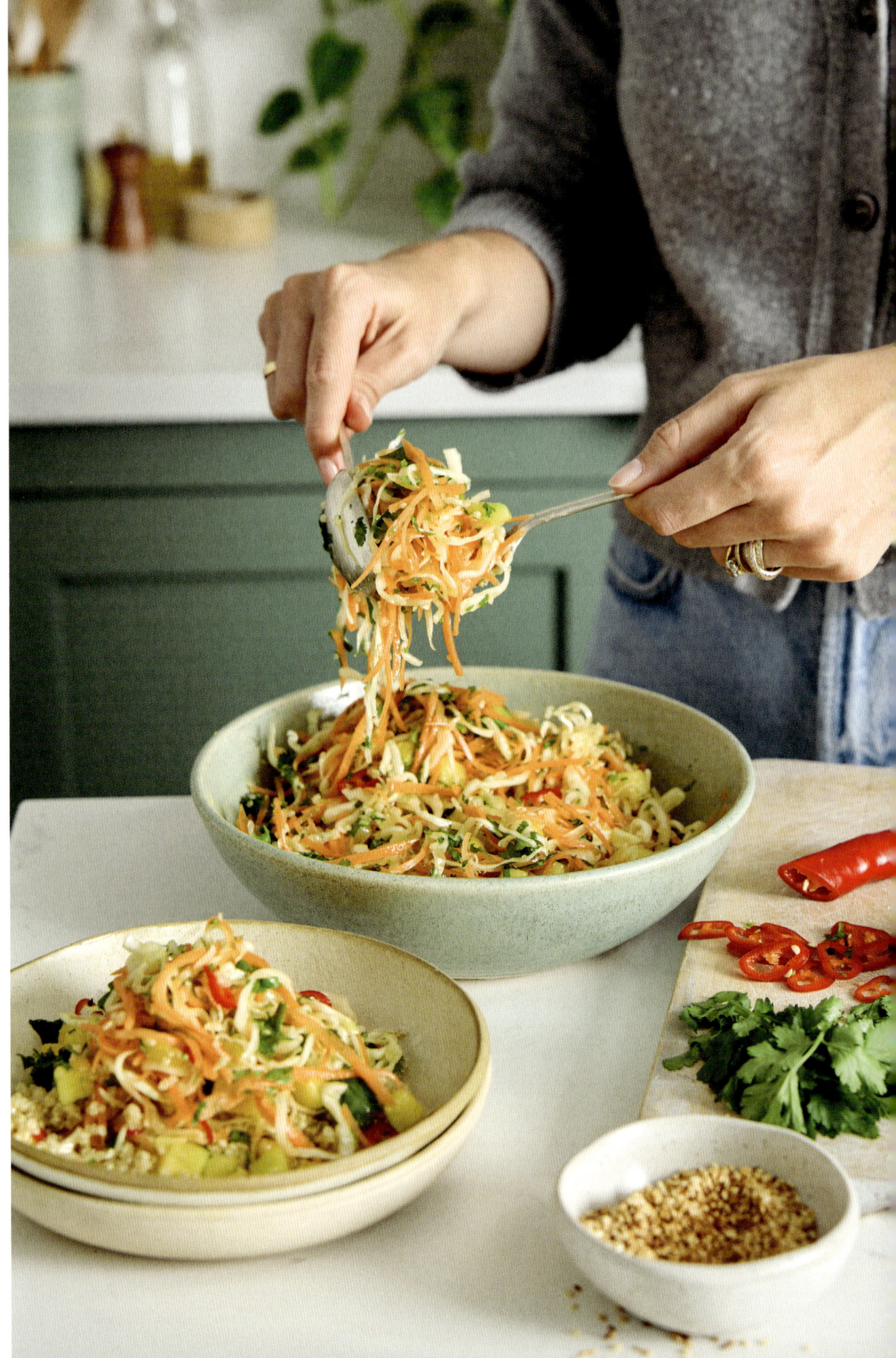

Crunchy Cabbage, Sesame, and Mango Salad with Quinoa

8 PLANTS

Serves 2

2 tablespoons apple cider or rice
   vinegar
1 tablespoon maple syrup
1 garlic clove, crushed
olive oil
⅓ small white cabbage, shredded
   (see recipe introduction)
½ cup quinoa
about 160ml hot vegetable stock
1 ripe mango, peeled and cubed
2 carrots, peeled and grated
handful of cilantro (about
   ¾ cup), stalks finely chopped
   and leaves roughly chopped
sea salt
2 tablespoons sesame seeds,
   toasted (see page 33), to serve
1 red chili, finely chopped, to
   serve

This vibrant salad is exactly the kind of lunch I love – fresh, colorful, and ready in minutes. Note that you want the cabbage to be really finely shredded or chopped so that it will soften in its marinade and not be too crunchy. If you're following the meal plan you'll use the rest of the cabbage to make the Pulled Eggplant Tortillas with Crispy Roasted Cabbage (see page 133).

1. In a large salad bowl, mix the vinegar, maple syrup, garlic, and 2 tablespoons of olive oil with a generous sprinkling of salt. Add the cabbage and leave to gently marinate while the quinoa cooks.

2. Cook the quinoa in the vegetable stock, according to the package instructions. Drain, then return it to the pan and set aside to steam dry while you prepare the salad.

3. Gently toss the mango, carrot, and cilantro through the cabbage.

4. Transfer the quinoa to two serving bowls and top with the salad, then sprinkle with toasted sesame seeds and chili to finish.

Make it your own: For extra protein, add chickpeas, toasted almonds, or edamame. You can also swap quinoa for brown rice or couscous for a different texture. Add dried red chili flakes or a drizzle of sriracha for extra heat if you like, or avocado for extra creaminess.

Creamy Garlic and Parsley Chickpeas with Spinach

6 PLANTS

Serves 2

olive oil
4 garlic cloves, finely sliced
½ teaspoon dried red chili flakes
1 × 18 oz jar of chickpeas, plus
   the stock from the jar
2 handfuls of spinach (about
   3 cups), roughly chopped
grated zest of ½ lemon
2 tablespoons plain yogurt
handful of flat-leaf parsley (about
   ¾ cup), roughly chopped
sea salt and black pepper
crusty bread, to serve (optional)

A simple and deeply satisfying dish that comes together in minutes. The chickpeas simmer in a rich, garlicky oil with chili, thickening into a silky, creamy sauce. Fresh spinach and parsley add brightness, while lemon zest lifts the flavors. Perfect on its own, or served with crusty bread to soak up every last bit.

1. Warm 4 tablespoons of olive oil in a frying pan set over a low heat. Add the garlic and chili flakes and cook for 2–4 minutes until fragrant and just golden.

2. Pour the chickpeas into the pan along with their stock, mix well, and simmer gently for 5 minutes.

3. Once the sauce has thickened, stir in the spinach, lemon zest, yogurt and most of the chopped parsley, reserving some for garnish. Simmer for 2–3 minutes until the spinach has wilted then season generously.

4. Spoon into bowls, finish with the reserved parsley, a drizzle of olive oil, and black pepper. Serve with crusty bread.

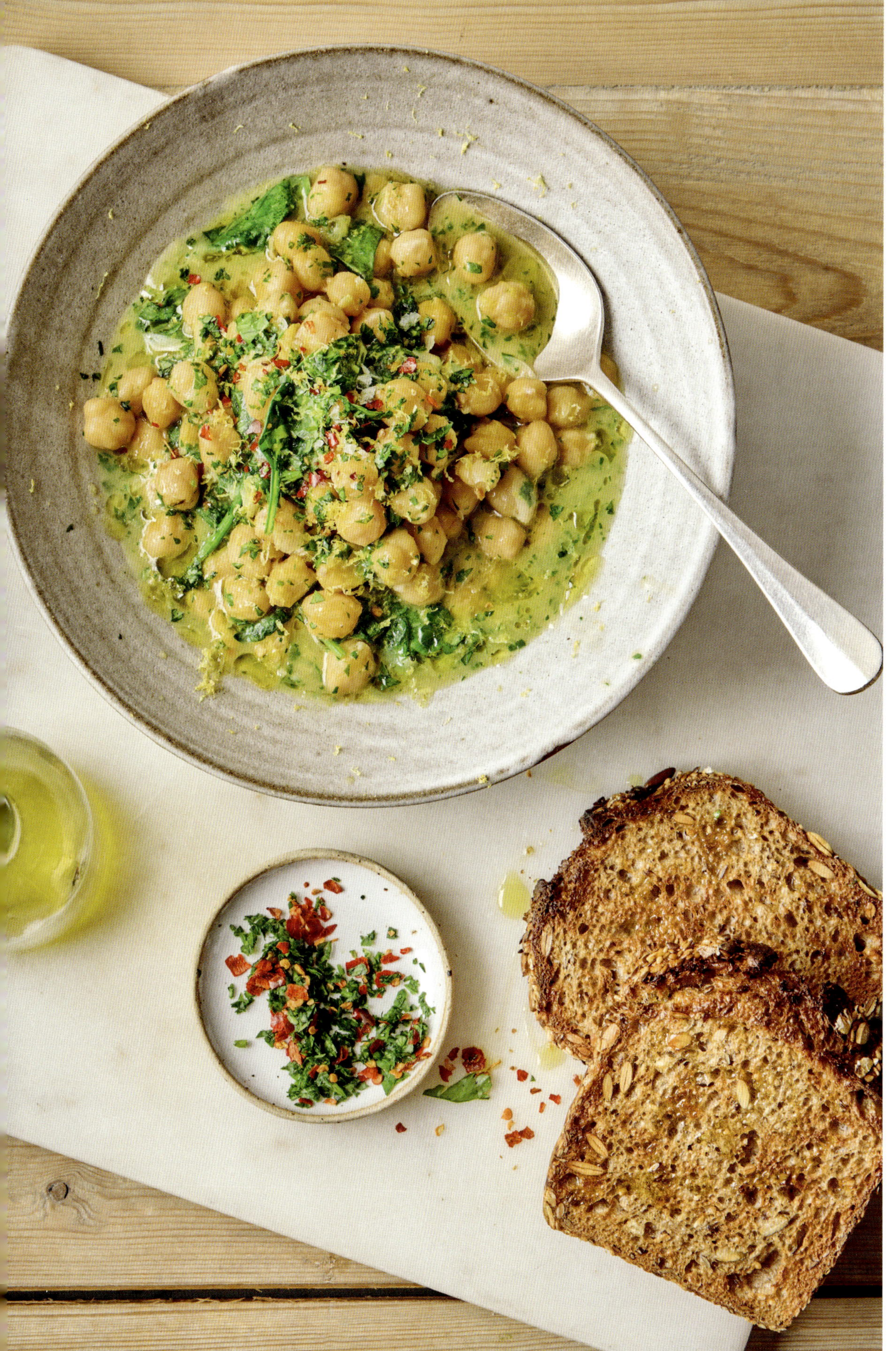

Beet, Dill, and Green Bean Salad with Mustard

7 PLANTS

Serves 2

⅔ cup green beans, trimmed
2 small or 1 large beet (about
   2 cups), peeled and coarsely
   grated or cut into matchsticks
½ red cabbage, shredded
   (you can use the rest in the
   Hazelnut and Lentil Salad with
   Sweet Peanut Dressing on
   page 60)
1 × 9 oz pouch or 1 × 14 oz can
   of lentils (puy or beluga work
   well)
2 handfuls of walnuts (about
   ½ cup), roughly chopped
½ bunch of dill (about 1–2
   tablespoons) roughly chopped
2 tablespoons dukkah (optional)
sea salt and black pepper

For the dressing

1 teaspoon wholegrain mustard
1 teaspoon apple cider vinegar
squeeze of lemon juice
4 tablespoons extra virgin
   olive oil

This crunchy, colorful salad is packed with texture, flavor, and plenty of goodness. The zingy mustard and lemon dressing ties it all together and really brings the veg to life. It holds up well for lunch the next day (just keep the dressing separate) and works just as nicely served as part of a meal for sharing or for a quick solo lunch.

1. Bring a small saucepan of salted water to the boil, add the green beans and cook for 3–5 minutes, until just tender. Drain and refresh under cold water until cool to touch.

2. Tip the green beans into a large salad bowl and toss together with the grated beets, red cabbage, lentils, walnuts, dill, and dukkah, if using.

3. To make the dressing, simply whisk together all of the dressing ingredients. Pour over the salad and season generously.

4. Serve as it is, for a light lunch or with sourdough, baguette, pitta bread, or mixed grains for something a little heartier.

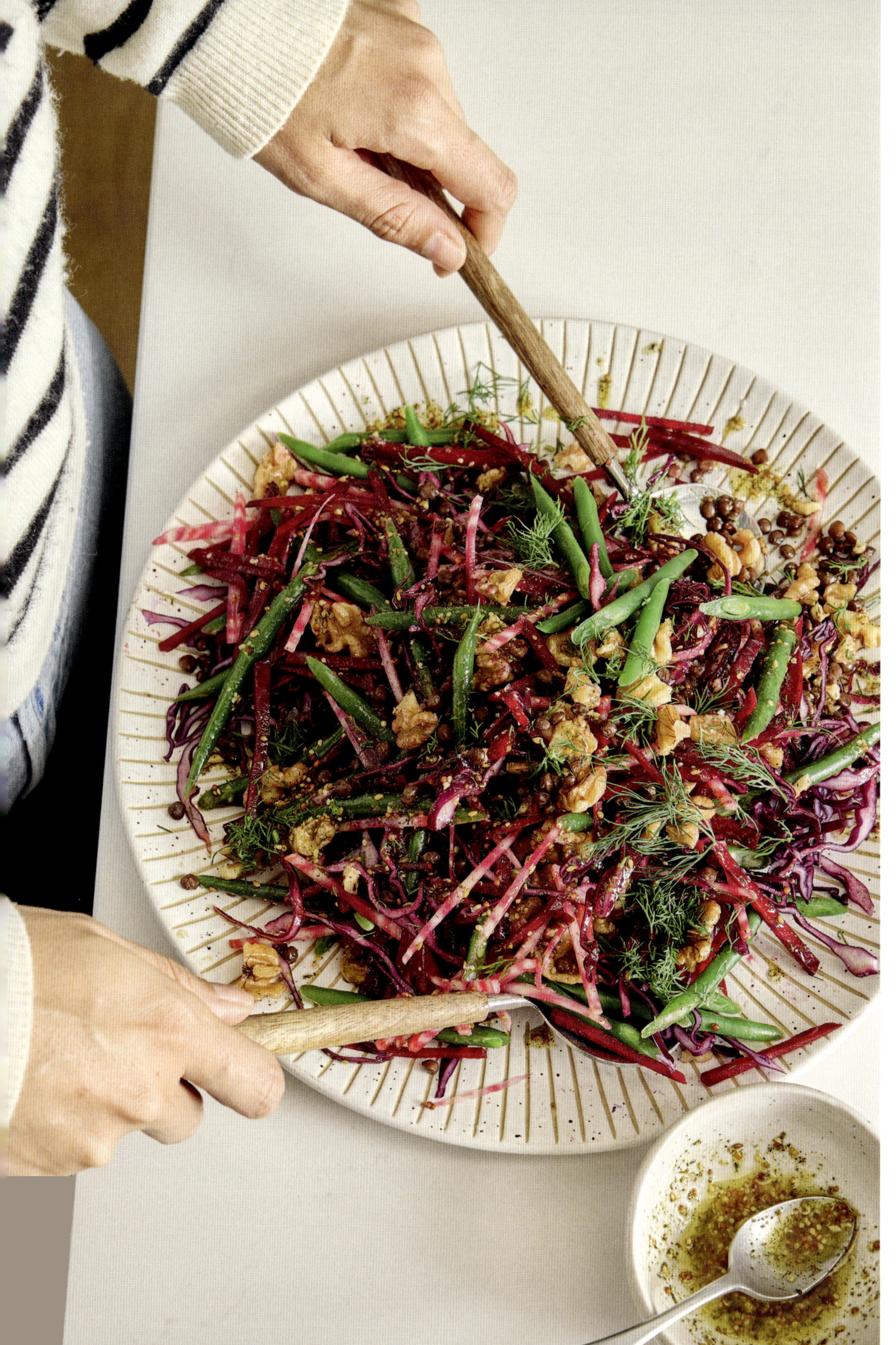

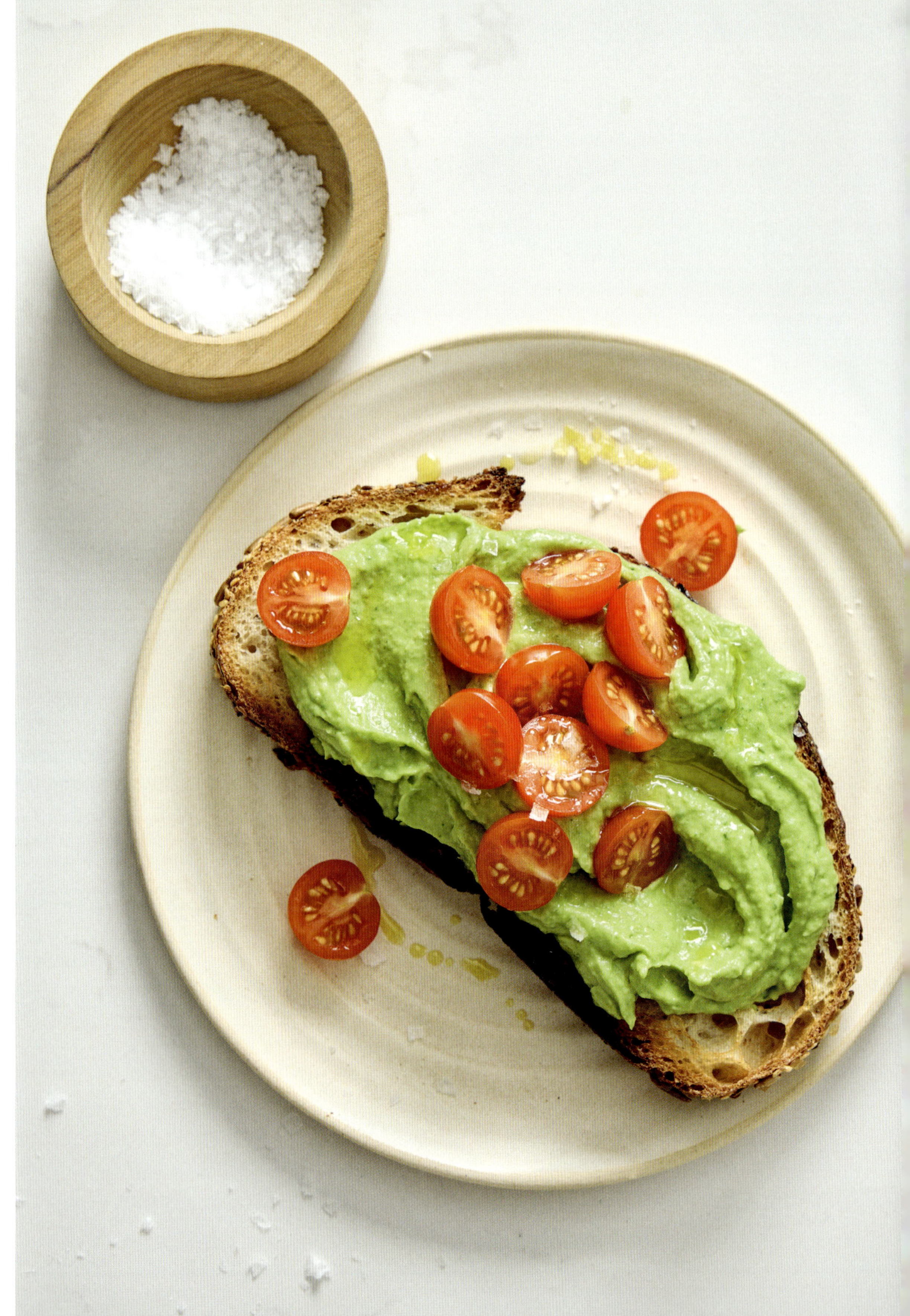

Avocado and Jalapeño Hummus

7 PLANTS

Serves 4

1 × 14 oz can of white beans (I
    use haricot, cannellini or lima
    beans, or chickpeas), drained
    and rinsed
1 avocado, pitted and peeled
2 jalapeños (about ⅕ cup),
    roughly chopped
handful of spinach (about
    2 cups)
2 tablespoons tahini
juice of 2 limes
4 tablespoons olive oil, plus extra
    to serve
sea salt

To serve
crusty sourdough
handful of cherry tomatoes,
    halved

When I first started Deliciously Ella, I used to make avocado cream all the time. Back then it was just avocado, lemon or lime, a splash of apple cider vinegar, and salt and I dipped everything into it! I thought I'd revisit it with a little more flavor and nutrition. This version blends avocado with white beans, spinach, tahini, and jalapeños for a creamy, vibrant, protein-packed twist that's on the table in under 10 minutes.

1. Place all the ingredients in a food processor or high-speed blender with a pinch of salt and blitz until smooth, adding water if necessary to reach your preferred texture. Taste and adjust the seasoning as needed.

2. Pile on to sourdough (toast it if you like) and top with the cherry tomatoes, a drizzle of olive oil, and a sprinkle of salt.

Make it your own: Use this in a sandwich, packed with leaves and cherry tomatoes.

Creamy Miso and Mushroom Broth with Noodles

7 PLANTS

Serves 2

2 tablespoons sesame oil

3 garlic cloves, crushed

small chunk of ginger (about
  1 in), peeled

2 cups mushrooms (any kind you
  like – shiitake will give extra
  flavor but chestnut mushrooms
  are great too), thinly sliced

sea salt

2 servings of noodles (about 6 oz
  for two people; any kind you
  like)

juice of 1 lime

sesame seeds, to serve (optional)

For the sauce

1 × block of silken tofu (about
  9 oz)

2 tablespoons smooth peanut
  butter

2 tablespoons tamari or soy
  sauce

2 tablespoons white miso paste

17 fl oz water

A simple, one-pan lunch that's full of flavor and takes less than 15 minutes from start to finish. Silken tofu blends into a gorgeously creamy sauce with peanut butter, tamari, and miso – all poured over soft mushrooms and tumbled through your favorite noodles. This is delicious served with a spoonful of chili oil.

1. To make the sauce, simply put all the sauce ingredients into a high-speed blender and blend until smooth and creamy.

2. Warm the sesame oil in a large saucepan set over a medium–high heat. Add the garlic and ginger and cook for 1 minute, until fragrant. Add the mushrooms and a pinch of salt and cook for 5 minutes, until the mushrooms are soft and golden.

3. Pour the sauce into the pan, stir and bring to the boil, then reduce the heat to a gentle simmer. Add the noodles to the pan, cover with a lid and cook for as long as the package suggests – usually around 5–10 minutes. Stir occasionally to ensure the noodles don't stick to the bottom of the pan.

4. Once the noodles are cooked, stir in the lime juice and divide between bowls. Scatter over some sesame seeds before serving, if using.

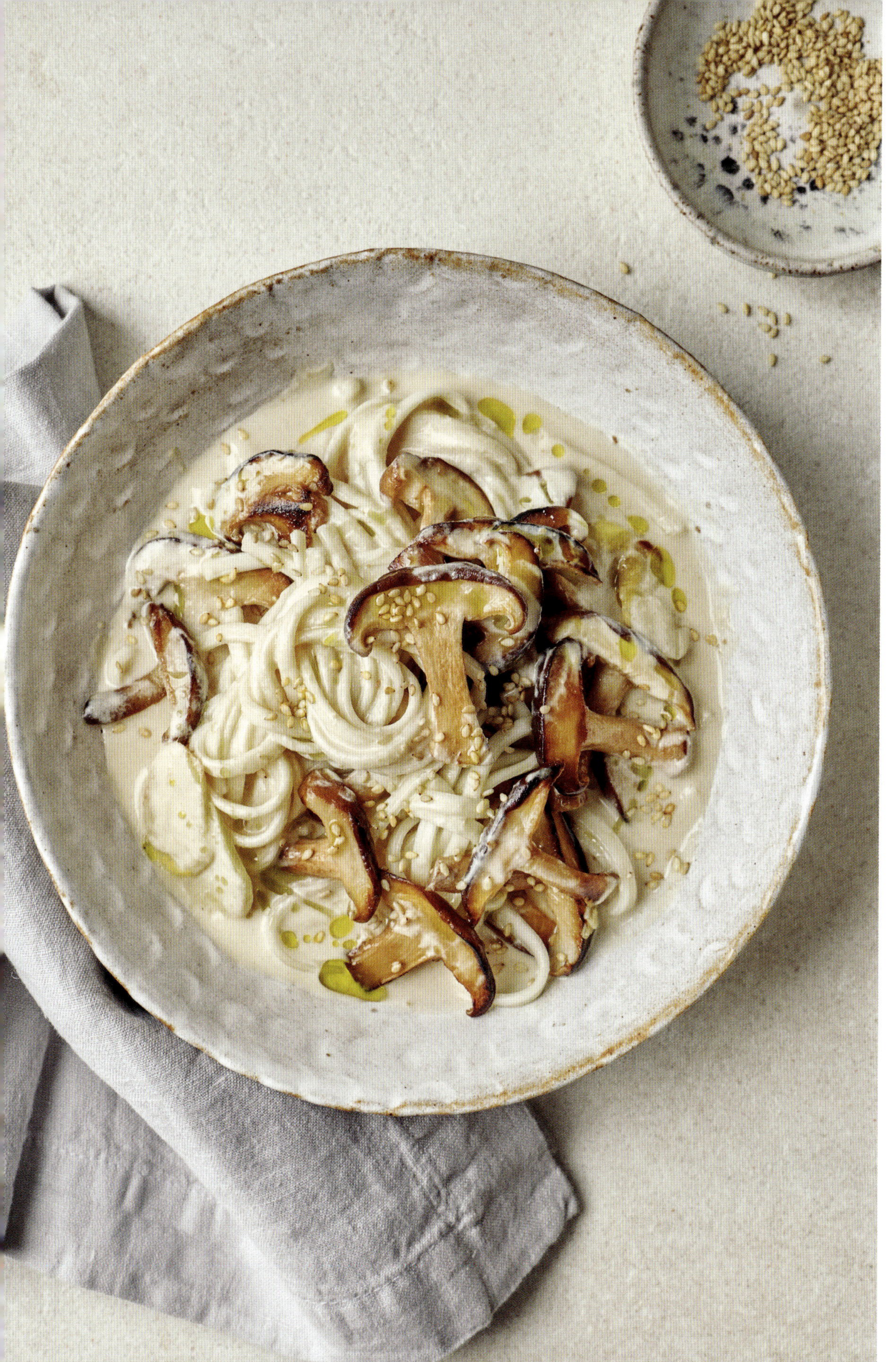

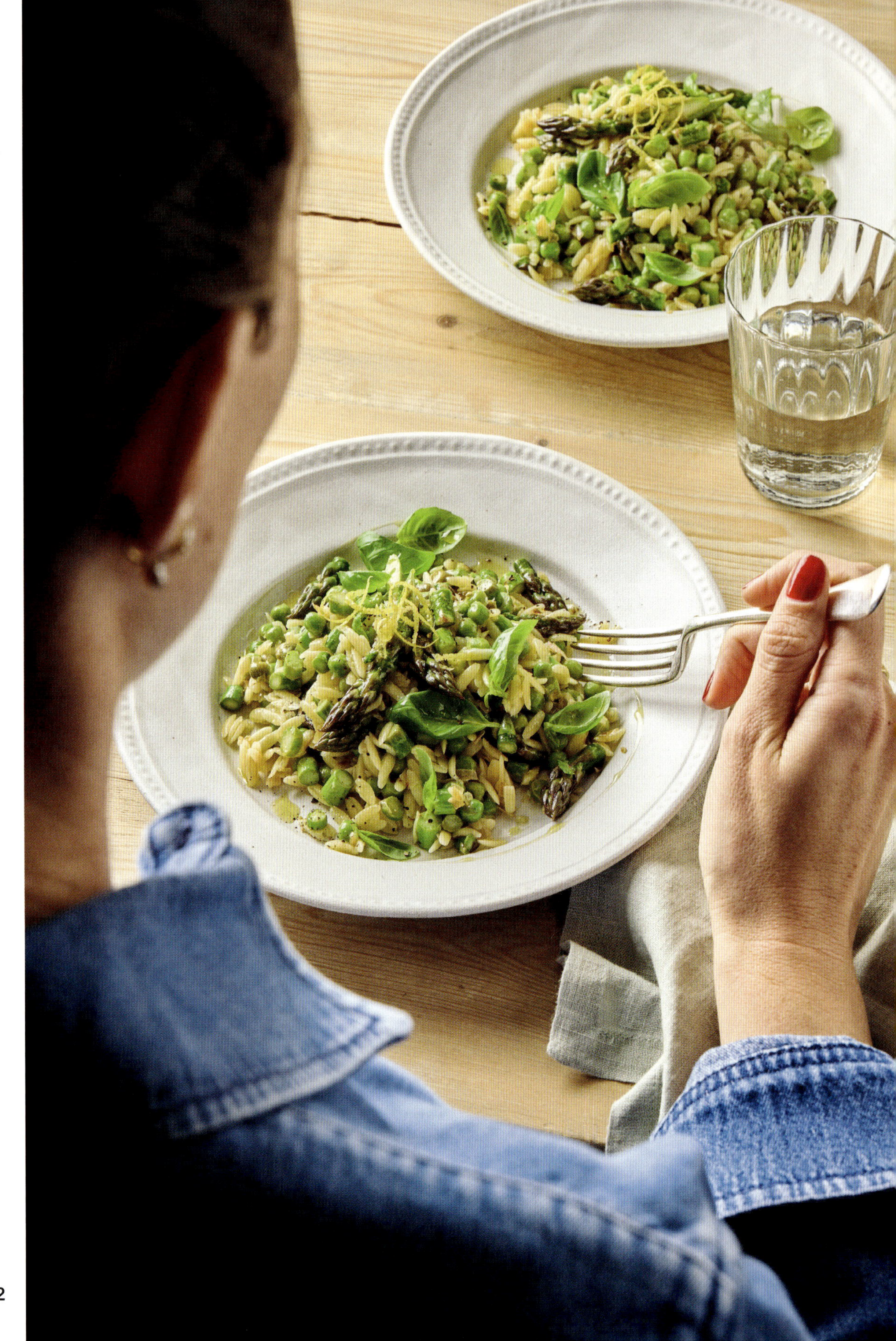

Lemony Pea and Shallot Orzo

6 PLANTS

Serves 2

¾ cup orzo
¾ cup frozen peas, defrosted
olive oil
2 shallots, diced
2 garlic cloves, crushed or finely
  chopped
large handful of asparagus
  (about 1¼ cups), trimmed and
  chopped into bite-sized pieces
grated zest and juice of 1 lemon
handful of basil (about ¾ cup),
  finely chopped, plus extra
  leaves to serve
2 tablespoons plain yogurt
2 tablespoons capers, drained
  and roughly chopped
  (optional)
sea salt and black pepper
extra virgin olive oil, to serve

This light, fresh, and vibrant orzo dish is packed with zingy lemon, sweet peas, and shallots, tender asparagus and fragrant basil. It comes together in just 15 minutes, making it the perfect quick and nourishing meal.

1. Cook the orzo in a saucepan of boiling salted water according to the package instructions, about 6–8 minutes, adding the peas for the last 2 minutes. Drain and set aside.

2. Meanwhile, warm 2 tablespoons of olive oil in a large frying pan set over a medium–low heat. Add the shallots and cook for 8–10 minutes, until softened, adding the garlic for the final 1–2 minutes.

3. Add the asparagus and cook for 2–3 minutes, until al dente.

4. Stir in the orzo, lemon zest (reserving a little for garnish) and juice, basil, yogurt, and capers (if using). Cook for a minute or so then check the seasoning and adjust as needed.

5. Serve in bowls with a drizzle of extra virgin olive oil, the basil leaves, and a little more lemon zest on top.

Make it your own: Swap asparagus for another seasonal green like zucchini, kale, or broccoli.

Chunky Black Bean Soup

Serves 2

olive oil
2 garlic cloves, finely chopped
2 red chilis, finely sliced
1 large red onion, finely chopped
1 tablespoon harissa
1 × 14 fl oz can of coconut milk
1 teaspoon white miso paste
1 × 14 oz can of black beans,
    drained and rinsed
½ vegetable stock cube
juice of 1 lime
small handful of cilantro (about
    ½ cup), stalks finely chopped
    and leaves roughly chopped
sea salt

To serve (optional)
1 avocado, diced
1 large tomato, deseeded and
    diced
plain yogurt
tortilla chips

If you need a quick, comforting, nourishing lunch, this ticks every box. It's thick and luscious, and works brilliantly served simply, just as it is, or piled high with chunks of avocado, cilantro, lots of chili, a dollop of yogurt, and crunchy tortilla chips on the side for dunking.

1. Warm 2 tablespoons of olive oil in a medium saucepan on a medium–high heat. Add the garlic and chili and cook for 1–2 minutes, until fragrant.

2. Set aside a small handful of onion for garnish and add the remainder to the pan, followed by the harissa and a pinch of salt. Cook for 5–7 minutes, stirring frequently, until just softened.

3. Stir in the coconut milk, miso, black beans, vegetable stock cube, and 7 fl oz of water. Bring to a simmer and cook for 10 minutes, stirring occasionally, until thick and creamy.

4. Remove from the heat, then add the lime juice and cilantro stalks. Use a stick blender to blend half the mixture to serve it as a chunky soup (or you can also leave it unblended).

5. Serve with the reserved red onion and the cilantro leaves. If you want to add a bit of texture and extra plant points, top with the avocado, tomato, a dollop of yogurt and serve with some tortilla chips alongside for dipping.

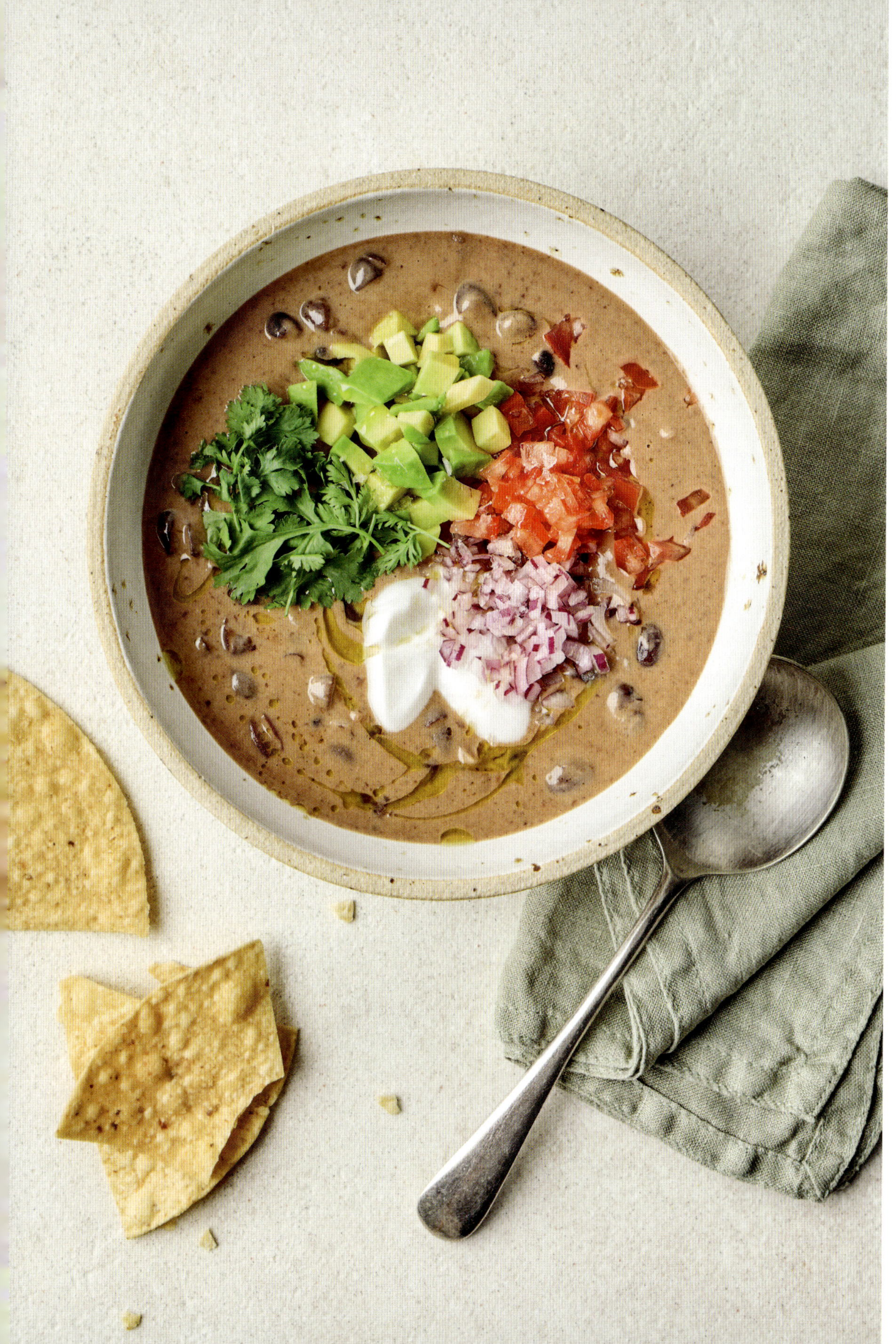

Zesty White Bean, Pea, and Spinach Soup

6 PLANTS

Serves 2

olive oil

3 garlic cloves, finely chopped

1 red chili, finely chopped, plus a
    little extra to serve if wished

6 cups of spinach

¾ cup frozen peas

1 × 14 oz can of lima beans,
    drained and rinsed

juice of ½–1 lemon, to taste, plus
    a little lemon zest, to serve

2 tablespoons plain yogurt, plus
    extra to serve

roughly 3½ fl oz water (or
    enough to blend to your
    desired consistency – I like it
    quite thick)

sea salt and black pepper

A vibrant green soup that takes less than 10 minutes to make. It's creamy, comforting, and packed with plants – white beans and peas bring the protein, spinach adds the greens and lemon gives it a lovely depth. Perfect for a speedy lunch or a light supper served with sourdough on the side.

1. Warm 1 tablespoon of olive oil in a medium–large saucepan over a medium heat. Add the garlic and chili with a pinch of salt and cook for 2 minutes, until soft and fragrant.

2. Add the spinach, peas, and lima beans. Cook for 5 minutes, stirring occasionally, until the spinach has wilted and the peas have defrosted and are tender.

3. Remove the pan from the heat and transfer the contents to a high–speed blender. Add the lemon juice, yogurt, and water. Blend until smooth and creamy, then season to taste. Serve as it is, or topped with a little extra yogurt, olive oil, chili and some lemon zest.

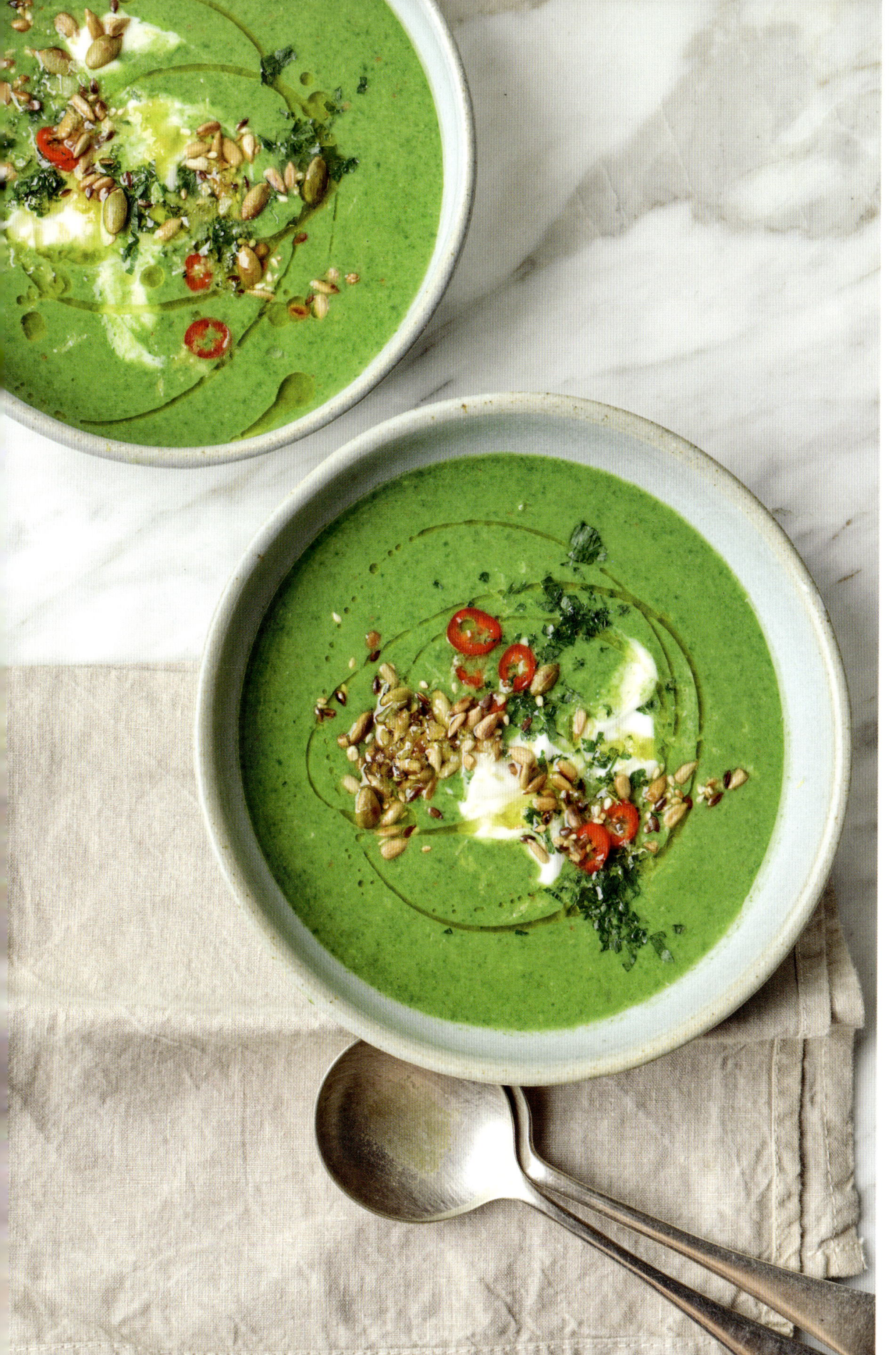

These are the recipes you need when you're tired, hungry, and don't have much energy to shop or inspiration to cook. They all come together in under 20 minutes, and have short ingredient lists built around one hero item you've likely got in your fridge or store cupboard, or can easily grab on your way home. These are all about minimal effort, maximum taste.

FRIDGE-RAID SUPPERS

My Go-To Miso Noodles

7 PLANTS

Serves 2

olive oil or sesame oil
2 garlic cloves, finely chopped
small chunk of ginger (about
   1 in), peeled and finely
   chopped
4 generous cups quick-cook
   veg, roughly chopped (I
   use shredded cabbage,
   Tenderstem broccoli, and
   sliced cavolo nero)
6 oz rice noodles (serving for two
   people)
sea salt and black pepper
crispy chili oil, to serve (optional)
handful of thinly sliced green
   onions, to serve (optional)

For the sauce

2 tablespoons tamari or soy
   sauce
2 tablespoons almond or peanut
   butter
1 tablespoon white miso paste
1 tablespoon maple syrup

These 15-minute bowls of creamy ginger, miso, and veggie-packed goodness are just what you need on rotation. You can use whatever quick-cook veg you have on hand, or try something new to help you up your plant points.

1. Warm 1 tablespoon of oil in a large frying pan set over a high heat, add the garlic and ginger and fry for 1 minute, until fragrant.

2. Add the veg and fry for 4–5 minutes until everything has softened but still has a little bite.

3. Meanwhile, cook the noodles, according to the package instructions.

4. Drain the noodles and add them to the pan with the veg, all the sauce ingredients and $3\frac{1}{2}$ fl oz of water. Stir until you have a smooth glossy sauce and everything is evenly combined.

5. Season to taste and serve with a generous drizzle of crispy chili oil, if using, and a sprinkling of green onions.

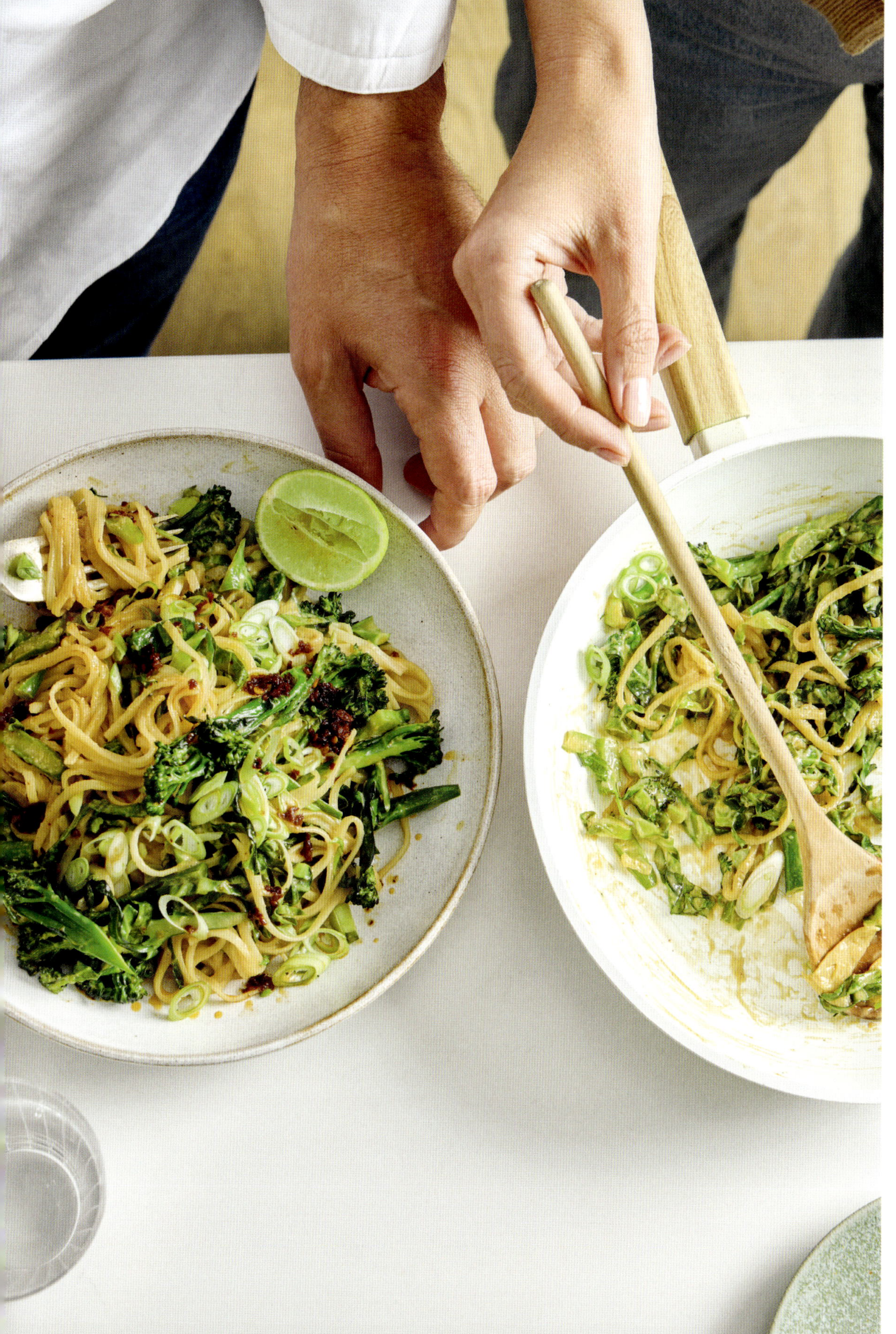

Fancy Lima Beans on Toast

5 PLANTS

Serves 2

olive oil
4 garlic cloves, finely sliced
½ teaspoon dried red chili flakes
  (or to taste)
¾ cup cherry tomatoes, halved
1 × 14 oz can of lima beans,
  drained
6 fl oz passata (you use the rest
  of the jar in the Pulled Miso
  Eggplant Ragu on page 130)
grated zest and juice of ½ lemon
1–2 heaped tablespoons plain
  yogurt (we use unsweetened
  coconut)
sea salt and black pepper
2 slices of crusty bread, to serve

Rich, garlicky lima beans simmered in a spiced tomato sauce – simple, comforting, and packed with goodness. My husband always says, 'not again!' because I make this so much, but it's just the perfect meal when you need something effortless. It's like fancy beans on toast and far more satisfying than anything out of a can. Scoop it up with warm, crusty bread and enjoy.

1. Heat a drizzle of olive oil in a large frying pan over a medium–low heat. Add the garlic, chili flakes and cook for 1–2 minutes until fragrant.

2. Stir in the cherry tomatoes, along with a generous pinch of salt, and cook for 2–3 minutes until they start to soften. Add the lima beans and passata and simmer for 8–10 minutes, stirring occasionally.

3. Stir in the lemon zest and juice and the yogurt, and season to taste.

4. Toast the bread and pile the beans on top with lots of black pepper. For extra flavor, rub a little raw garlic over the toast before adding the beans, along with a big drizzle of olive oil.

Make it your own: Swap lima beans for any white bean. Add Parmesan or tahini for extra richness. Stir in spinach or kale for added greens. Serve with cilantro, chives, a drizzle of tahini, arugula, dukkah, toasted almonds, avocado.

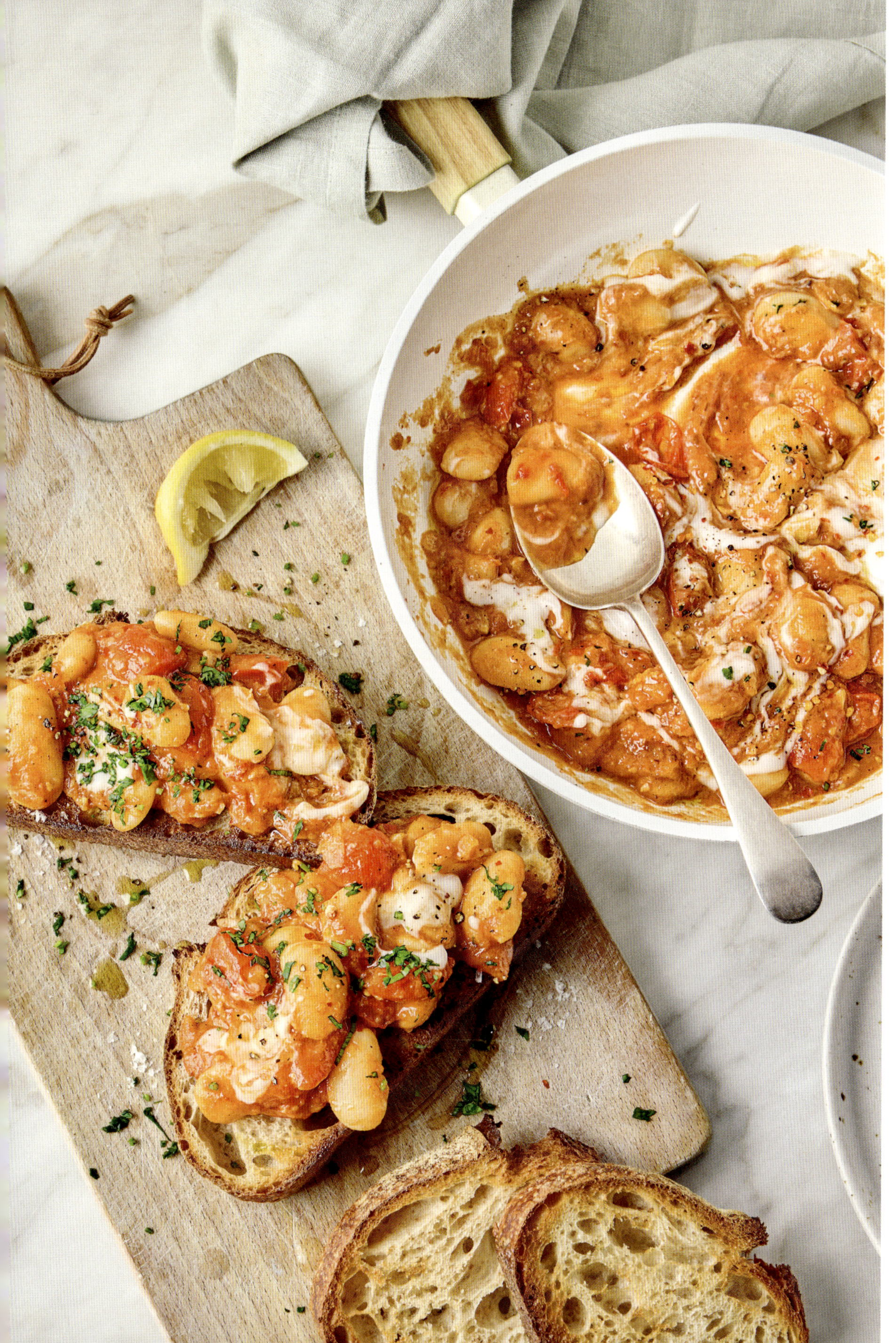

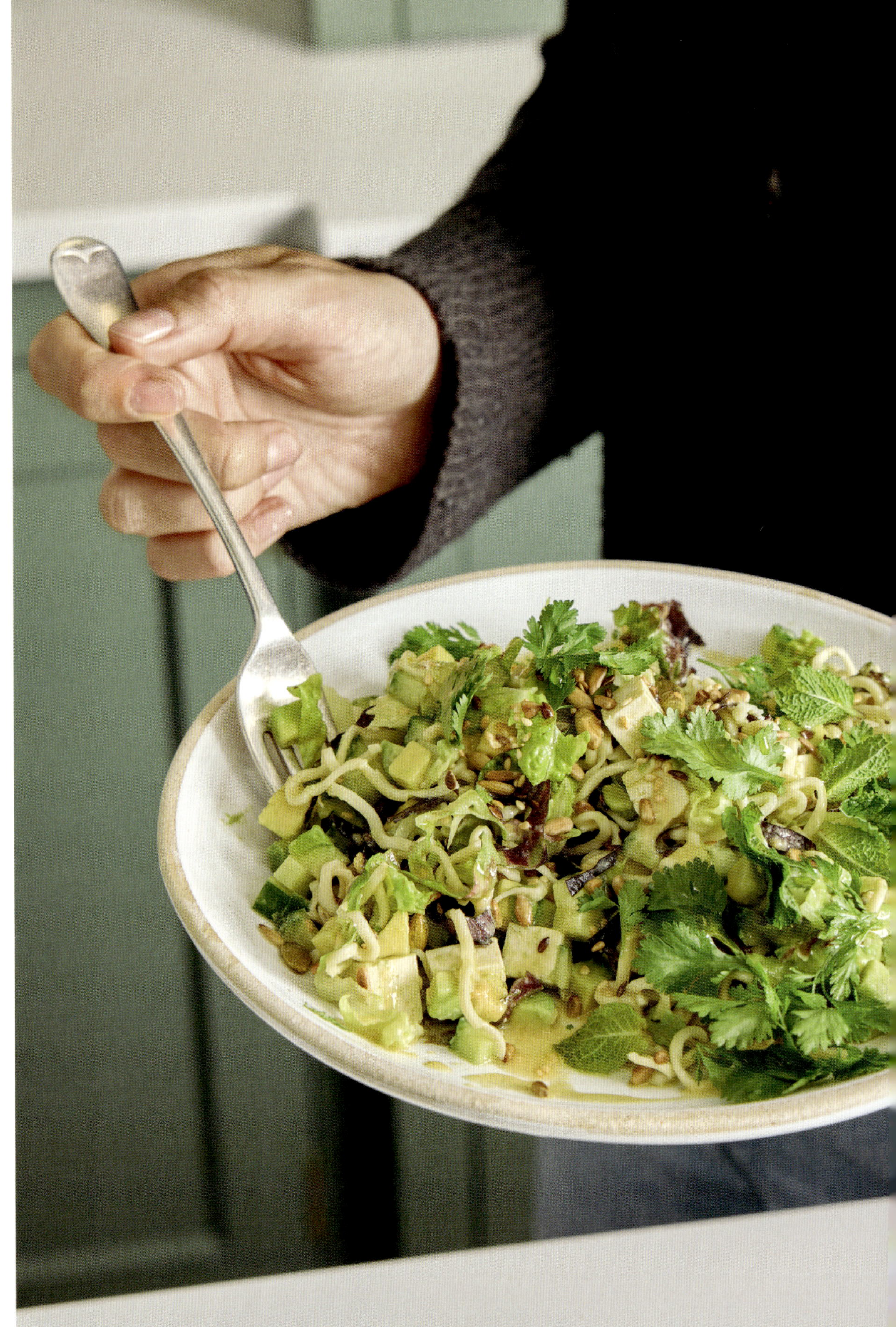

Herby Avocado Noodle Salad with Cucumber

10 PLANTS

Serves 2

2 servings of spelt noodles
   (about 6 oz for two people;
   soba or rice noodles also work
   well)
¼ cucumber, deseeded and
   thinly sliced
1 baby gem lettuce, sliced
1 avocado, diced
2 celery sticks, thinly sliced
½ × block of firm tofu (about
   150g), drained and cut into
   ½ in cubes
handful of mixed seeds (about
   2–3 tablespoons), toasted (see
   page 33), plus extra to serve
2 handfuls of mixed herbs (about
   1½ cups; use what you've
   got but mint and cilantro are
   delicious)
sea salt

For the dressing
1 tablespoon tahini
2 tablespoons extra virgin
   olive oil
1 tablespoon apple cider vinegar
1 tablespoon maple syrup
1 tablespoon white miso paste

Need something healthy and delicious that's on the table in minutes? Here, all you have to do is cook noodles, then toss everything together in the luscious tahini dressing. Getting so many different plants in a single meal has never been easier.

1. Cook the noodles in a saucepan of boiling salted water according to the package instructions. Once ready, drain and refresh under cold water until cool to touch.

2. In a large bowl, toss together the cooked noodles, cucumber, lettuce, avocado, celery, tofu, seeds, and herbs.

3. To make the dressing, simply whisk together all of the ingredients in a bowl. Pour about three-quarters of the dressing over the salad and mix everything together.

4. To serve, divide the noodle salad between bowls, season with a pinch of salt, then scatter over the remaining seeds and herbs. Serve with the remaining dressing on the side.

Creamy Pistachio and Broccoli Pasta

7 PLANTS

Serves 2

2 servings of pasta (about 6 oz
 for two people; short pasta like
 fusilli or rigatoni works well)
1 small head of broccoli (about
 4 cups), chopped into small
 florets
⅓ cup shelled pistachios, plus
 extra to serve
large handful of basil (about
 ¾ cup)
1 garlic clove
1 red chili (optional)
grated zest and juice of ½ lemon
4 tablespoons olive oil
sea salt

This pesto has turned into one of my absolute favorites – it's so creamy and is packed with basil, lemon zest, and loads of pistachios. Blending broccoli into the pesto is such a simple way to sneak more greens into a meal, which has been perfect while one of my kids is firmly in the 'I hate broccoli' phase!

1. Cook the pasta in a saucepan of boiling salted water according to the package instructions, adding the broccoli florets to the pan for the final 3 minutes of cooking. Lift out about half of the broccoli using a slotted spoon and transfer it to a food processor. Drain the remainder of the pan in a colander, reserving a mugful of the cooking water.

2. Add the pistachios, basil, garlic, chili, if using, lemon juice, olive oil, and some salt to the food processor and process until you have a chunky pesto. Add a splash of the reserved pasta water if needed to loosen the sauce.

3. Toss the pesto with the hot pasta and broccoli, adding a little of the reserved pasta water to help it coat the pasta evenly.

4. Serve warm, with extra chopped pistachios sprinkled on top.

Make it your own: Swap pistachios for walnuts or almonds. Stir in tofu or chickpeas for extra protein.

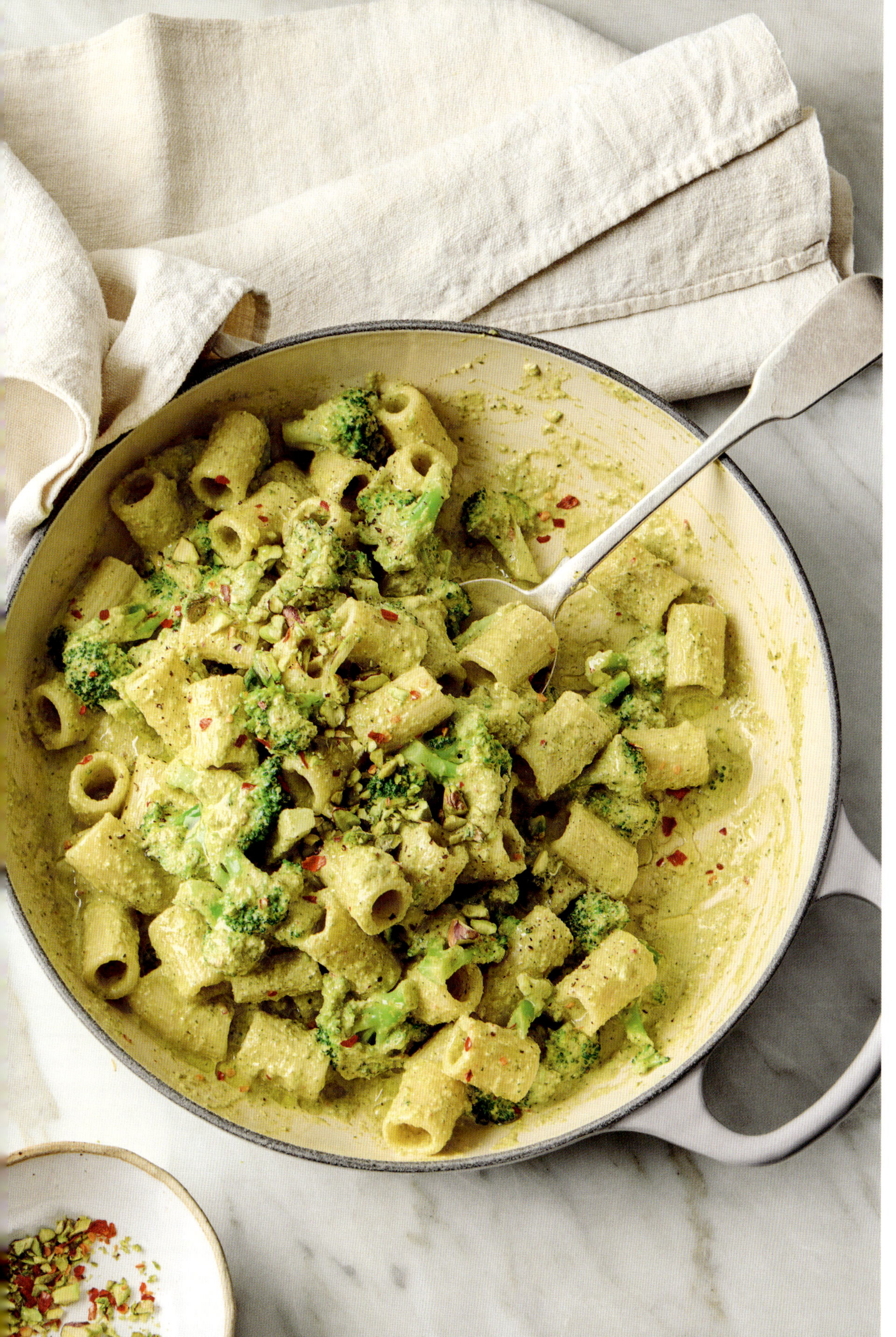

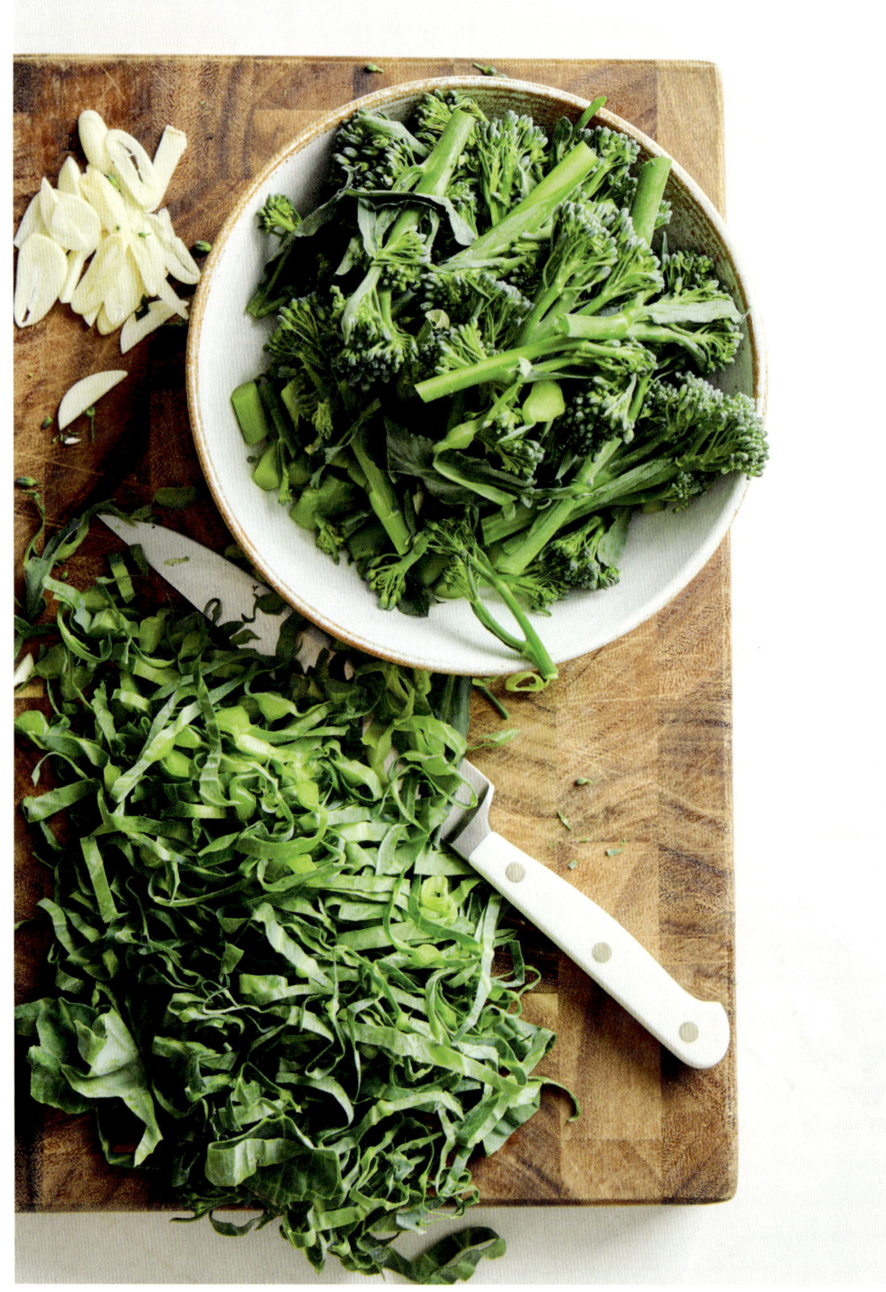

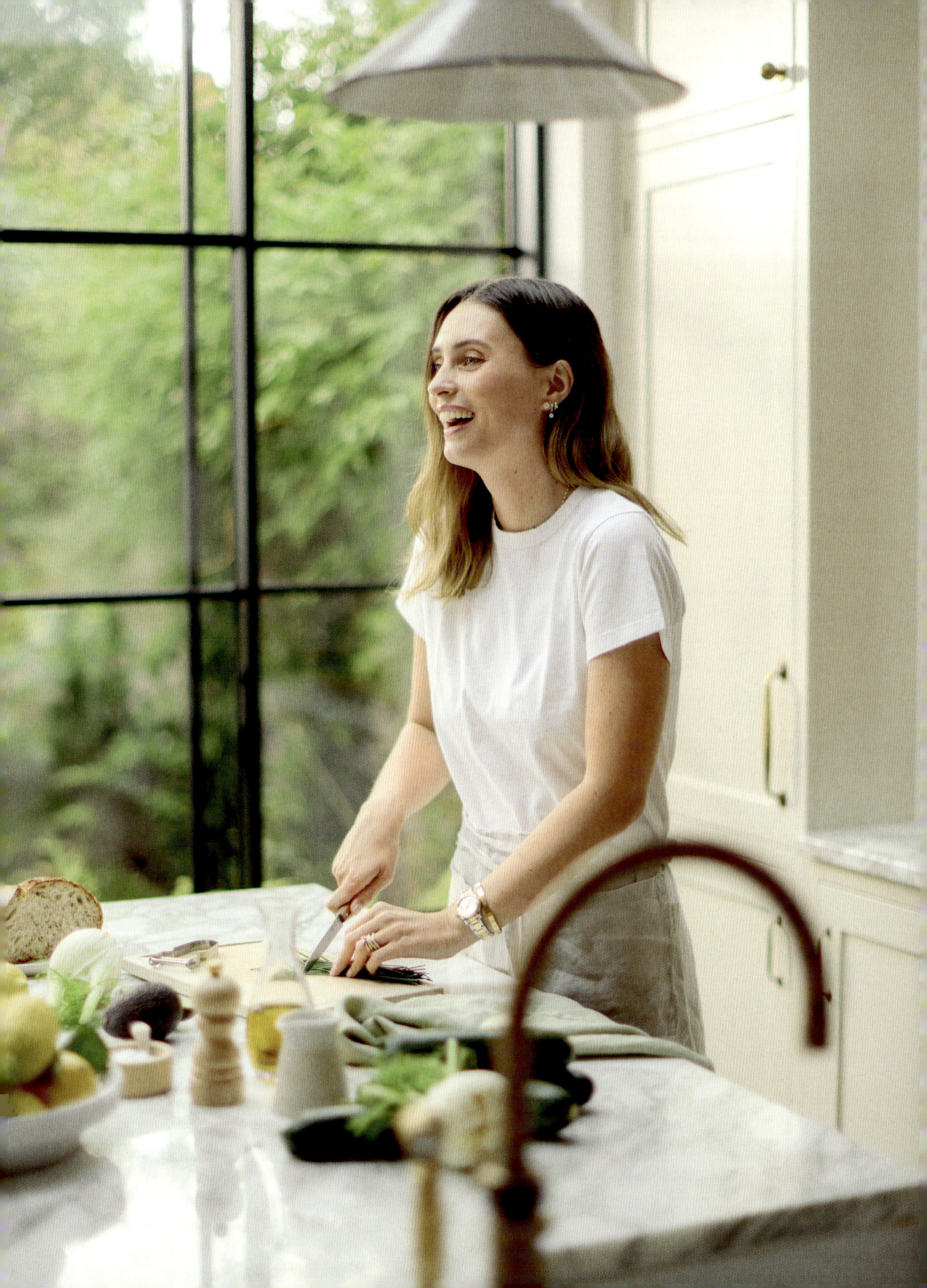

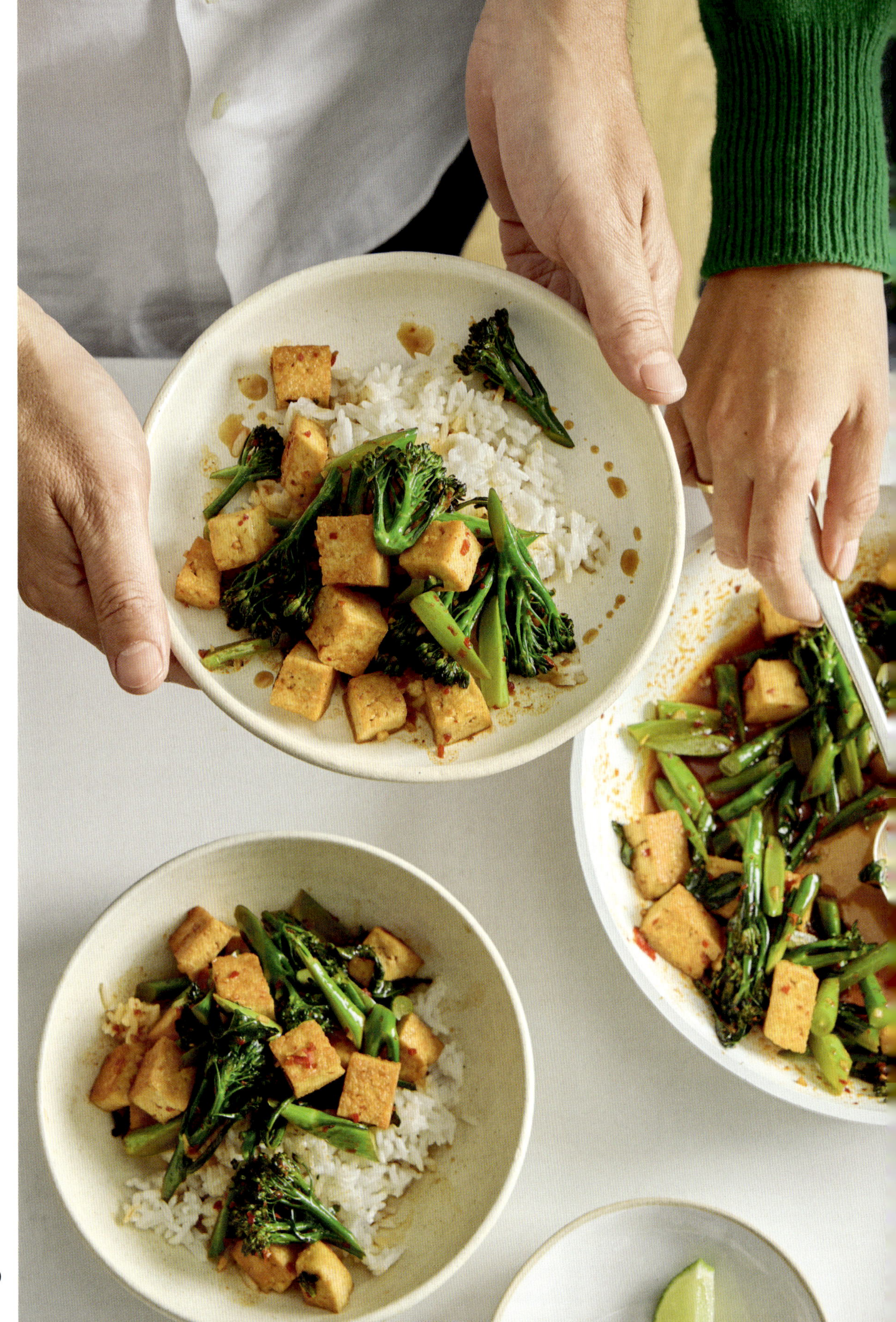

Stir-Fried Harissa Tofu with Broccoli and Rice

6 PLANTS

Serves 2

2 garlic cloves, crushed or finely
   chopped
3 tablespoons tamari or soy
   sauce
1 tablespoon maple syrup
1 tablespoon rice vinegar
1 tablespoon harissa paste
olive oil
1 × block of firm tofu (about
   10 oz), drained and cut into
   bite-sized cubes
3 cups Tenderstem broccoli, cut
   into 1 in pieces

To serve

2 servings of cooked rice (made
   with about ½ cup uncooked
   rice for two people)
juice of 1 lime (optional)
olive or sesame oil

This quick, flavor-packed dish is perfect for those nights when you need something easy but satisfying. The tofu soaks up a rich harissa sauce, while tender broccoli adds freshness and balance. Served over fluffy rice, it's a simple, nourishing meal packed with plant protein, making it as filling as it is delicious.

1. In a small bowl, whisk together the garlic, tamari, maple syrup, rice vinegar, and harissa with $3\frac{1}{2}$ fl oz of water. Set aside.

2. Warm 1 tablespoon of olive oil in a large frying pan set over medium heat. Add the tofu and cook for 8–10 minutes, turning occasionally, until crisp and golden.

3. Pour the sauce into the pan, along with the broccoli and simmer for 4–5 minutes, until the broccoli is just cooked and the sauce is rich and glossy.

4. Serve the tofu and broccoli over warm rice with the lime juice squeezed on top (if using) and a drizzle of olive or sesame oil.

Make it your own: Add dried red chili flakes or fresh chili in step 1 for more heat. Swap the rice for noodles or quinoa. Sprinkle with sesame seeds or toasted cashews for extra crunch. For extra veg, add edamame, peas, or sweetcorn (you can cook them with the rice).

Chunky Chickpea and Lentil Soup with Tahini and Tomatoes

9 PLANTS

Serves 2

olive oil
2 carrots, finely chopped
1 onion, finely chopped
3 celery sticks, finely chopped
1 × 14 oz can of chickpeas,
    drained
1 × 14 oz can of cherry tomatoes
26 fl oz hot vegetable stock
⅓ cup red lentils, rinsed
2 tablespoons tahini
½ bunch of flat-leaf parsley
    (about ½ cup), roughly
    chopped
sea salt and black pepper
extra virgin olive oil, to finish

For the speedy croutons (optional)
2 slices of sourdough
1 garlic clove

This one-pan soup is such a lifesaver – hearty, comforting, and packed with protein from the lentils and chickpeas. You simply throw everything into the pan, and it pretty much cooks itself, making it perfect for those evenings when you're low on energy but still want something nourishing. It also freezes brilliantly, if you want to double the quantities.

1. Warm 1 tablespoon of olive oil in a large saucepan set over a medium heat. Add the carrots, onion, and celery, and cook for 5 minutes until just softened.

2. Tip the chickpeas, cherry tomatoes, stock, and lentils into the pan, add a generous pinch of salt and pepper and bring to the boil.

3. Once the liquid is boiling, turn the heat down to a simmer and cook for 20–25 minutes, stirring occasionally, until the carrots are soft and the lentils are cooked.

4. To make the croutons (if using), toast the bread, then rub the garlic clove on each side and cut into bite-sized pieces.

5. Remove the pan from the heat, then stir in the tahini, parsley, and season to taste. If you've made croutons, stir them through the soup or scatter over the top. To serve, divide into bowls and finish with a drizzle of extra virgin olive oil.

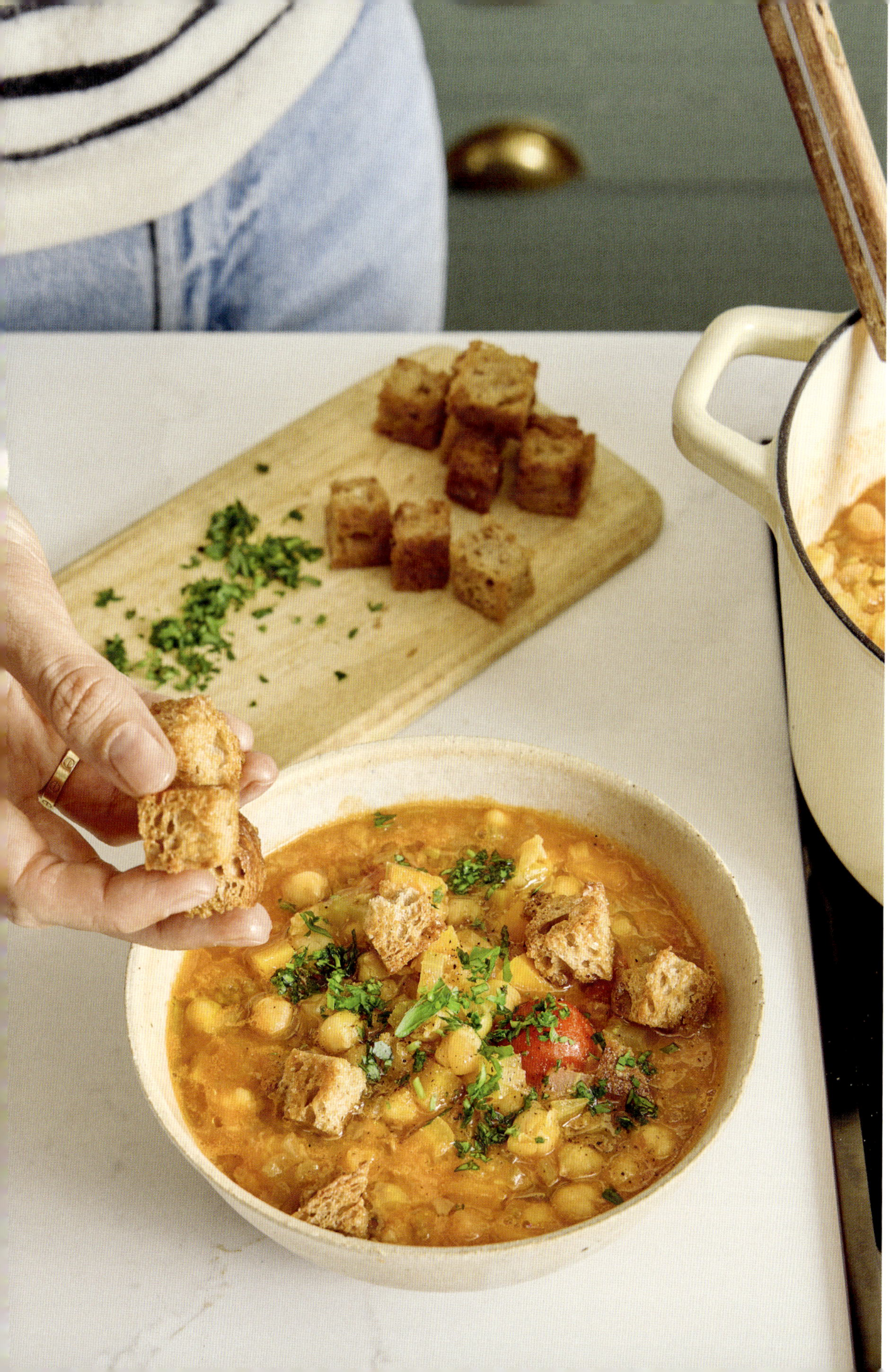

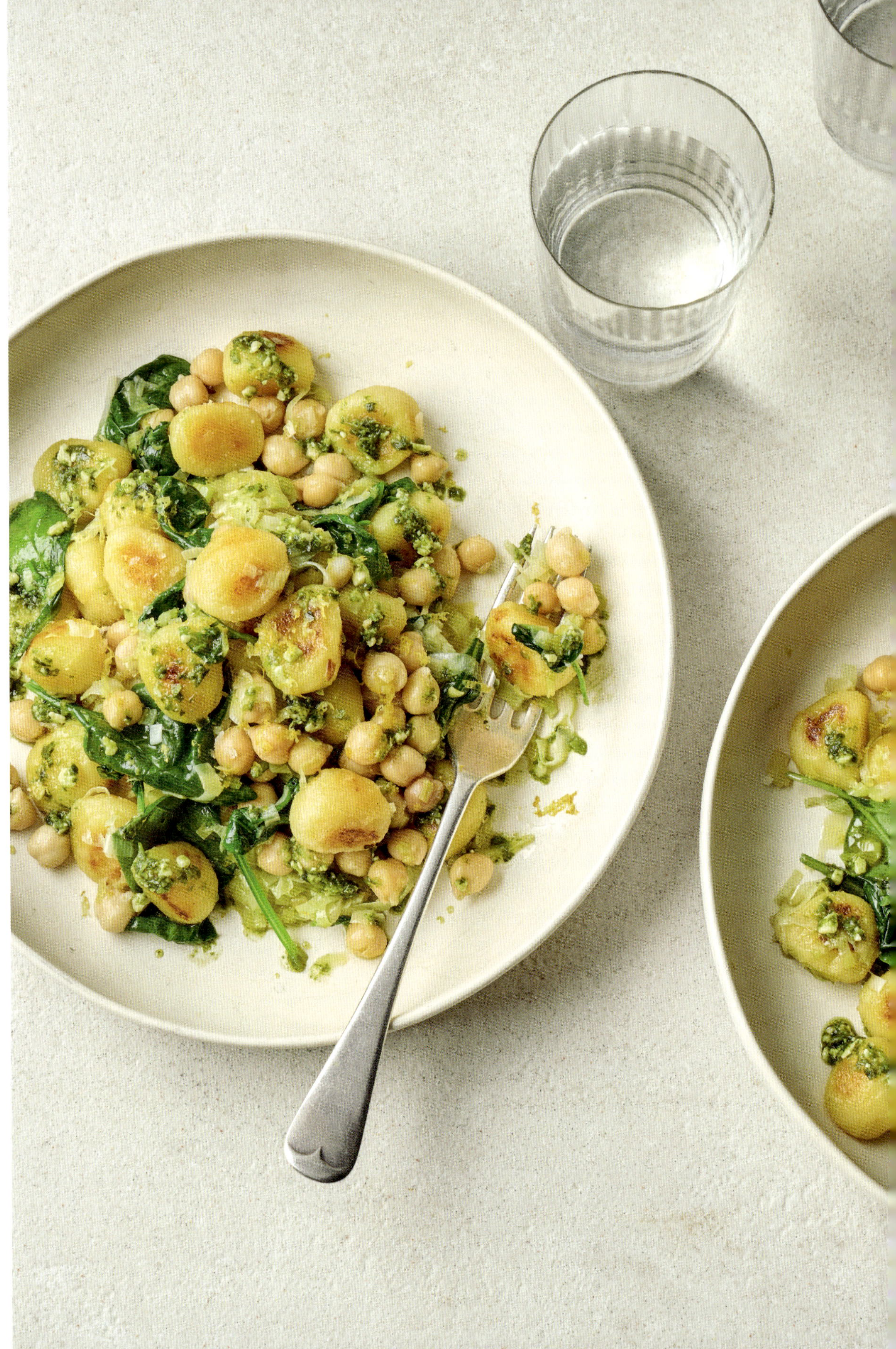

Leek and Chickpea Pesto Gnocchi

5 PLANTS

Serves 2

olive oil
2 leeks, finely sliced
1 garlic clove, crushed or grated
2 servings of gnocchi (about
   18 oz)
1 × 14 oz can of chickpeas,
   drained and rinsed
2 big handfuls of spinach or
   greens (about 3 cups)
3 tablespoons store-bought
   pesto
grated zest and juice of ½ lemon
sea salt and black pepper

Leeks work brilliantly here, adding a little variety to a simple fridge-raid supper that'll be on the table in under 15 minutes. Packed with chickpeas for a creamy, protein-packed bite, jarred pesto for speed, and fresh spinach for extra greens, it's as easy as it is delicious.

1. Warm 1 tablespoon of the olive oil in a large frying pan set over a medium heat. Add the leeks and a sprinkling of salt and cook for 5 minutes until soft. Add the garlic and cook for 1 more minute.

2. Push the leeks to one side of the pan and add the gnocchi with another tablespoon of olive oil. Cook for 5 minutes, stirring occasionally, until golden and slightly crispy.

3. Add the chickpeas and spinach to the pan. Stir everything together and cook for 2 minutes, letting the spinach wilt slightly.

4. Stir in the pesto and lemon juice, tossing everything to combine. Cook for 1 minute to warm through.

5. To serve, season with salt and pepper, then divide into bowls and scatter over the lemon zest.

Make it your own: Swap spinach for kale or arugula for a different green. Add dried red chili flakes for a little heat or a little fresh basil for extra flavor.

Pea and Chickpea Pancakes with Harissa Yogurt

Serves 2

⅓ cup frozen peas
1 × 14 oz can of chickpeas,
   drained and rinsed
½ cup plain flour
¾ tsp baking powder
4 fl oz plant-based milk
⅓ cup fresh herbs (basil, mint,
   and flat-leaf parsley are all
   great), roughly chopped, plus
   extra to serve
olive oil
sea salt

To serve
4 tablespoons plain yogurt
2 tablespoons harissa paste
handful of salad leaves (I like
   arugula)
lemon wedges

These have been a big hit in our house, they're so satisfying, easy, and such a lovely little supper. The harissa yogurt really brings the recipe together, adding a punch of spice to the herby pancakes.

1. Put the peas into a small saucepan of boiling water for 2 minutes, then drain and add to a blender along with the chickpeas, flour, baking powder, milk, herbs, and a big pinch of salt. Pulse until you have a slightly smooth but textured batter.

2. Mix the yogurt with the harissa in a bowl and set aside.

3. Heat 1 tablespoon of olive oil in a large frying pan over a medium heat. Once hot, spoon 2–3 heaped tablespoons of batter into a circle; and repeat until the pan is full. Fry for 5–7 minutes until the outside edges of the pancakes turn golden – a crisp edge will make them easier to flip – then flip and cook for another 5–7 minutes, until golden. Remove the pancakes from the pan and repeat with another tablespoon of oil and the remaining batter. You should have around 4 large pancakes.

4. Serve the pancakes topped with the salad leaves, a spoonful of the harissa yogurt, a sprinkling of extra herbs, and some lemon wedges on the side.

Make it your own: Try using pesto instead of harissa in the yogurt.

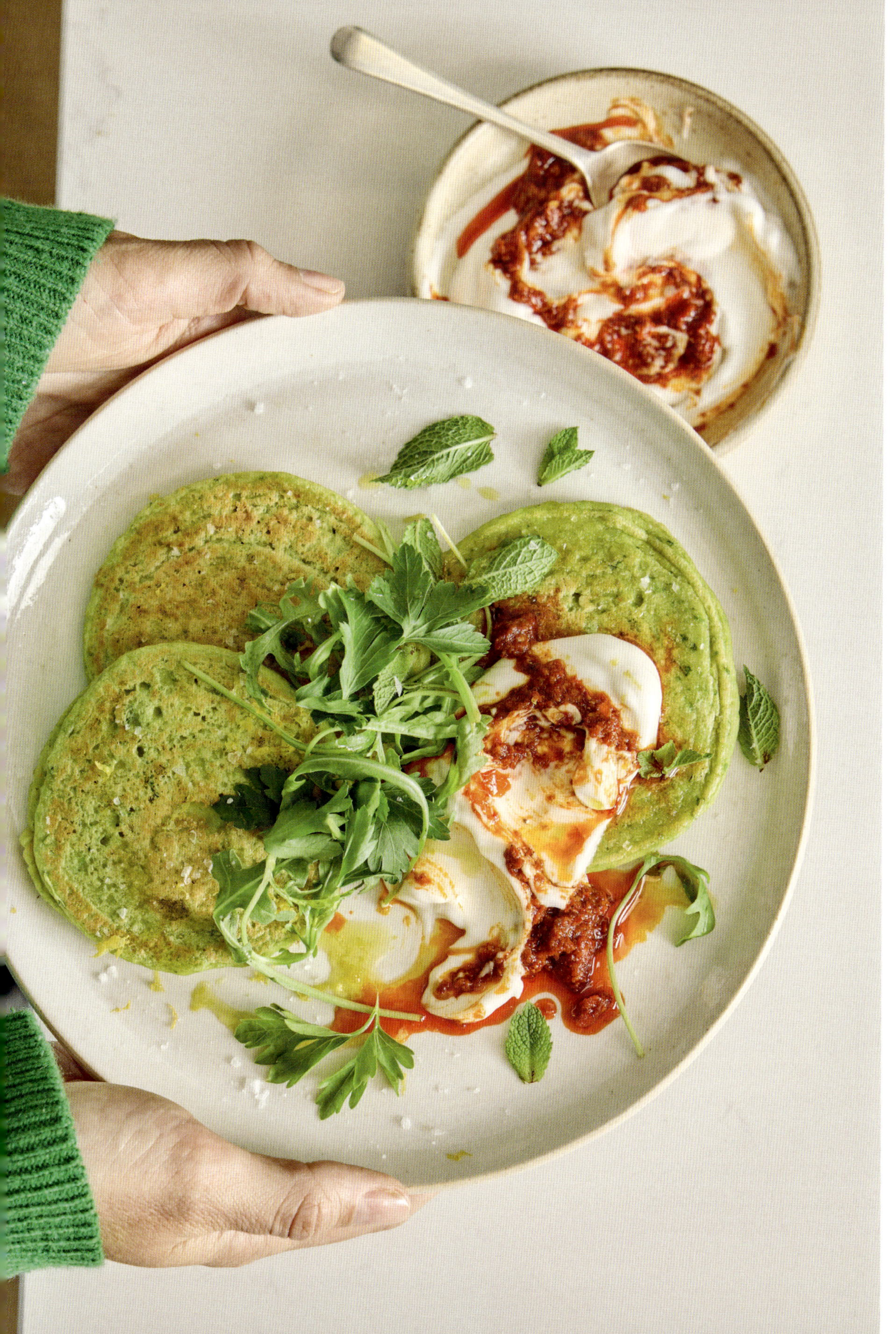

When you've got a bit more time, have friends coming round, or
just fancy making dinner feel a little more special, these recipes are for you.
They look and taste impressive and while they might use an extra
pan or take a little longer to cook, they don't require you to spend hours
in the kitchen and are still simple enough for a midweek meal.

A LITTLE LONGER

Lazy Mushroom Lasagne

—

Zucchini and Black Bean
Tortillas

—

Corn and Zucchini
Orzo

Giant Couscous Salad

—

Pesto Tofu

Squash and Pearl Barley Risotto

—

Chimichurri
Green Beans

—

Mushrooms with Lima Bean
Mash

Lazy Mushroom Lasagne

8 PLANTS

Serves 4

1 lb mushrooms (oyster
   mushrooms work well; you
   can also use shiitake and
   portobello), roughly torn into
   bite-sized pieces
olive oil
4 garlic cloves, grated or crushed
pinch of dried red chili flakes
   (optional)
1 × 14 oz can of cherry tomatoes
   (or use 1 × 14 oz can of
   chopped tomatoes)
1 × 14 oz can of beluga lentils,
   drained and rinsed
1 bay leaf
1 teaspoon dried oregano
1 tablespoon tomato purée
1 teaspoon maple syrup
8 dried lasagne sheets, broken
   in half
sea salt and black pepper

For the creamy sauce
¾ cup cashews
½ × block of silken tofu (about
   5 oz), drained
4 tablespoons nutritional yeast
grated zest and juice of ½ lemon

Make it your own: Swap the
lentils for 1 × 14 oz can of
kidney beans.

Lasagne can feel faffy, but this version makes it so
easy as there's no layering. The mushrooms roast
until golden, then get folded into a rich tomato and
lentil ragu and are then topped with a silky cashew
and tofu sauce.

1. Preheat the oven to 400°F fan. Place the cashews in a
   small bowl and cover with boiling water. Set aside for
   10 minutes to soften.

2. Place the mushrooms in a large shallow baking
   tray, drizzle with 1 tablespoon of olive oil and season
   generously. Cook for 20 minutes in the oven, stirring
   halfway, until crispy and golden.

3. Meanwhile, make the ragu. Warm 1 tablespoon of
   olive oil in a large shallow casserole (about 11 inches
   in diameter) set over a medium heat. Add the garlic
   and chili flakes (if using) and cook for 2–3 minutes
   until fragrant. Stir in the tomatoes, lentils, bay leaf,
   oregano, tomato purée, maple syrup and 17 fl oz
   water, and season generously. Simmer with the lid
   on for 15 minutes until glossy.

4. To make the creamy sauce, transfer the cashews to
   a high-speed blender, along with 3½ fl oz of their
   soaking water, the silken tofu, nutritional yeast,
   lemon zest and juice, and 1 tablespoon of olive oil.
   Blitz until smooth and season to taste.

5. Turn the oven down to 350°F fan. Remove the
   casserole from the heat and stir in the mushrooms.
   Add the lasagne sheets, making sure they're fully
   covered by the sauce and evenly spaced so that they
   don't stick together, then pour over the creamy sauce.
   Bake for 15—20 minutes, until golden and bubbling.

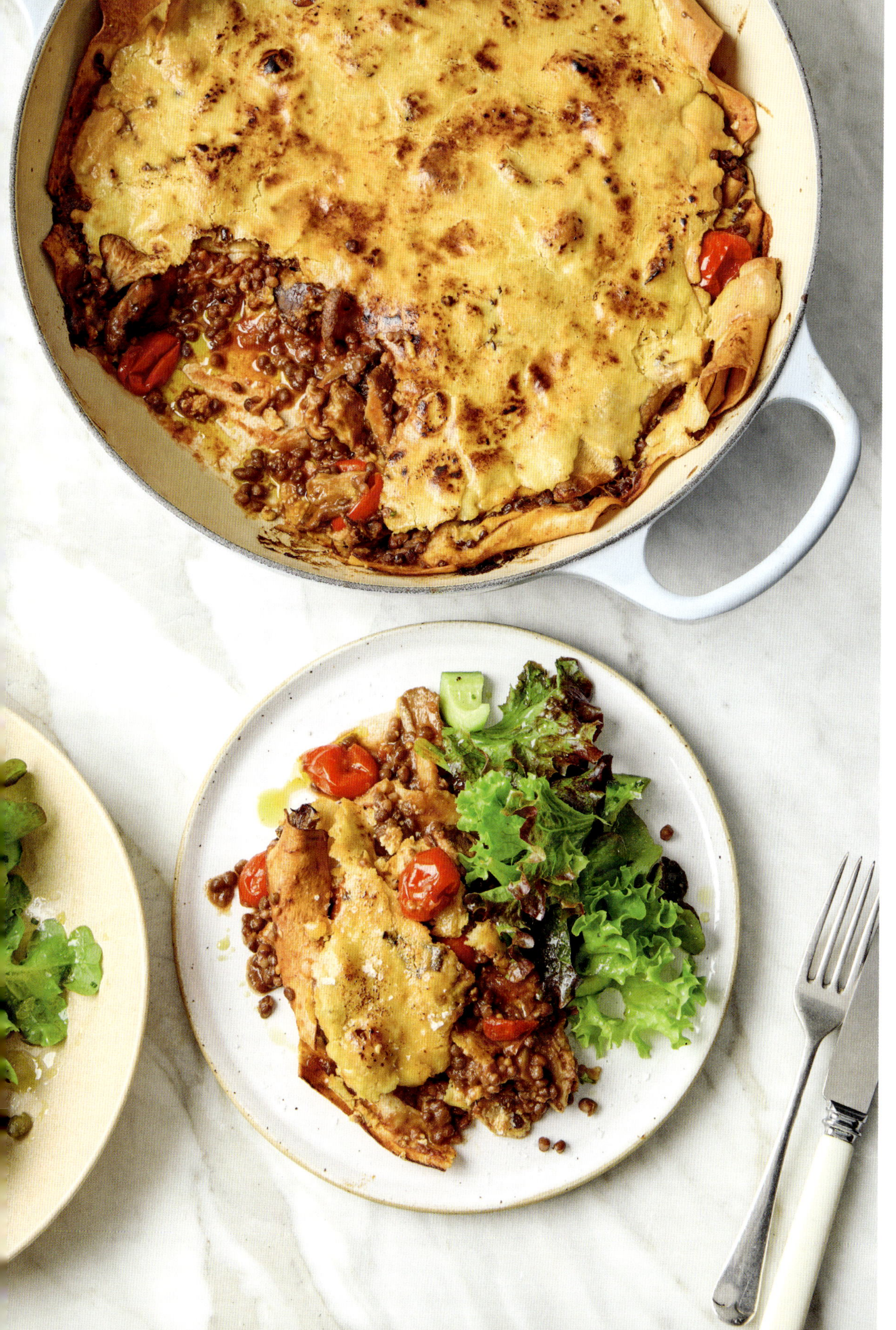

Giant Couscous and Crispy Chickpea Salad with Turmeric Cauliflower

10 PLANTS

Serves 2

1 cauliflower, cut into small
  florets, plus the smaller leaves
1 × 14 oz can of chickpeas,
  drained and rinsed
olive oil
1 teaspoon ground turmeric
1 teaspoon ground cumin (or use
  cumin seeds)
1 teaspoon smoked paprika
⅓ cup giant couscous
2 tablespoons tahini
grated zest and juice of ½ lemon
2 teaspoons maple syrup
about ¾ cup of pomegranate
  seeds
large handful of salad leaves
  (about ⅔ cup)
sea salt and black pepper

Make it your own: Swap the
couscous for orzo or pearl barley
for a different base. Add toasted
almonds or sunflower seeds
for crunch, some cilantro, basil,
or flat-leaf parsley for a fresh,
herby flavor or roast some cubes
of tofu with the chickpeas and
cauliflower for additional protein.

This hearty, flavor-packed bowl is packed with protein and fiber. It's delicious to enjoy on repeat too, with crispy roasted cauliflower, cumin-spiced chickpeas, sweet pomegranates and chewy giant couscous all tossed with a creamy tahini dressing.

1. Preheat the oven to 400°F fan. In a large, shallow baking tray toss the cauliflower florets and chickpeas with 1 tablespoon of olive oil, the turmeric, cumin, smoked paprika, salt, and a pinch of black pepper. Spread into an even layer and roast for 25 minutes, stirring halfway through, until golden and crispy.

2. Meanwhile, cook the giant couscous in a saucepan of salted boiling water according to the package instructions. Drain, then return to the pan to steam dry.

3. To make the dressing, in a small bowl, simply mix the tahini, lemon zest and juice, maple syrup, a pinch of salt and pepper, and 3 generous tablespoons of olive oil until smooth and pourable – adding a splash of water to loosen if needed (depending on the consistency of your tahini).

4. Toss the crispy cauliflower, chickpeas, couscous, and pomegranate together in a large bowl, then transfer to serving bowls, drizzle the tahini dressing over the top, top with the salad leaves, and season as needed.

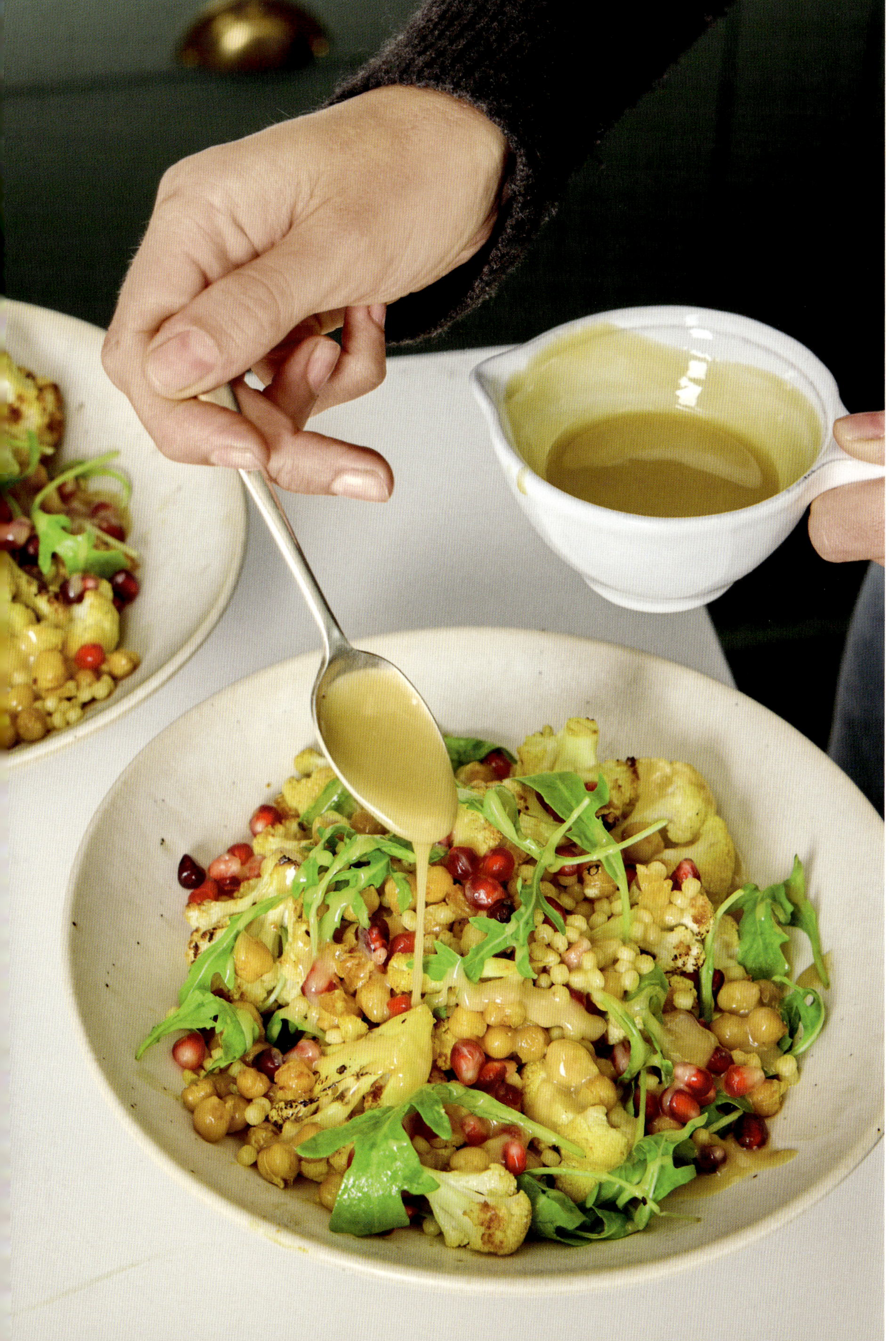

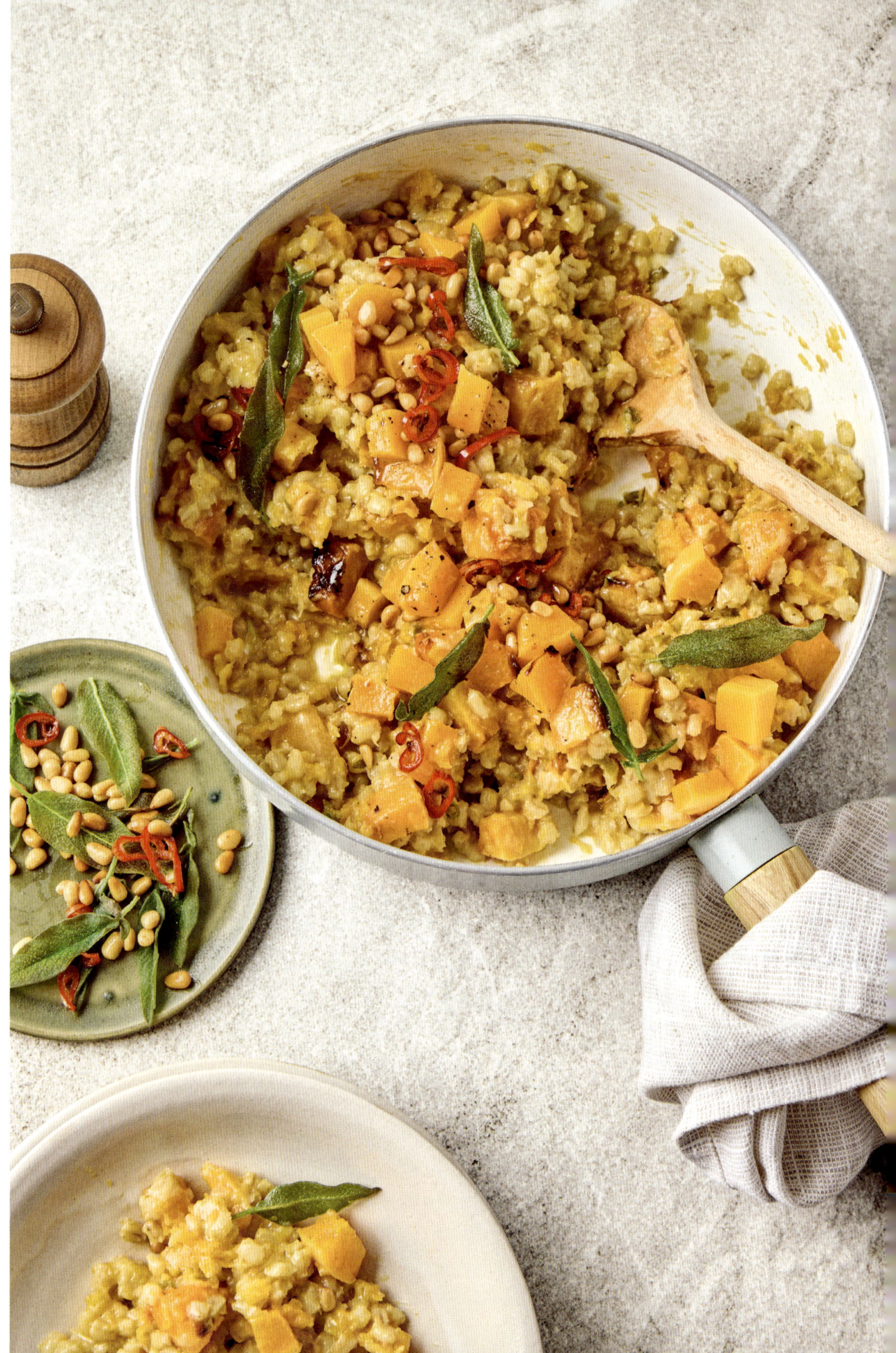

Roasted Squash and Pearl Barley Risotto with Crispy Sage

7 PLANTS

Serves 2

1 small butternut squash or
   pumpkin (about 1½ lb), cut into
   ½ in cubes
olive oil
1 garlic bulb
1 onion or shallot, finely chopped
handful of sage leaves (about
   2–3 tablespoons), half thinly
   sliced, half left whole
⅔ cup pearl barley, rinsed
26 fl oz hot vegetable stock
3½ fl oz almond milk
sea salt and black pepper

For the chili and pine nuts
handful of pine nuts (about
2–3 tablespoons)
1–2 red chilis, thinly sliced/finely
   chopped

Make it your own: Stir in half a
can or pouch of lentils for extra
plant protein. Add a squeeze of
lemon zest for more zing.

This nutty risotto is one of my favorite cosy meals —
half the roasted squash is stirred into the risotto, the
rest is blended into a rich velvety sauce. I love that
pearl barley has more bite than risotto rice, plus it's
much higher in fiber.

1. Preheat the oven to 350°F fan. Toss the squash with
   2 tablespoons of olive oil, salt and pepper and spread
   over a large baking tray. Slice off the top of the garlic
   bulb, wrap it in foil and place it in the corner of the
   tray. Roast for 30 minutes until tender and golden.

2. Warm a generous glug of oil in a medium saucepan
   set over a medium heat. Add the onion, sliced
   sage, and a pinch of salt. Cook for 8–10 minutes,
   stirring frequently, until softened. Stir through the
   pearl barley and cook for 2 minutes, then add the
   vegetable stock. Simmer on a medium–low heat for
   30 minutes, stirring frequently, until all of the stock
   has been absorbed and the barley is tender.

3. Meanwhile, warm 2 tablespoons of olive oil in a
   small frying pan set over a medium–low heat. Gently
   fry the whole sage leaves, pine nuts, and chili, for
   4–5 minutes, until crisp and golden. Remove from
   the heat and set aside.

4. Once the squash is cooked, remove from the oven
   and roughly mash half of it with a potato masher.
   Transfer all of the squash to the risotto, squeeze the
   garlic cloves out of their skins and add them to the
   pan along with the almond milk, stirring until rich
   and creamy. Season to taste.

5. Spoon the risotto into bowls, then top with the crispy
   sage, chili, and pine nuts and lots of black pepper.

Spicy Zucchini and Black Bean Tortillas with Aïoli

8 PLANTS

Serves 2

1 zucchini, peeled into thick
   ribbons (easiest with a potato
   peeler)
olive oil
3 garlic cloves
1 red onion, finely diced
1 × 14 oz can of black beans,
   drained and rinsed
2 teaspoons smoked paprika
2 teaspoons maple syrup
juice of ½ lime (serve the other
   half as quarters on the plates)
4 tortillas
sea salt

For the cashew aïoli
¾ cup cashews, soaked in
   3½ fl oz hot water for 5–10
   minutes
1 garlic clove, crushed
juice of 1 lime
1 teaspoon maple syrup
1 red chili

Note: If you want to make some
quick pickled onions – a simple
addition that cuts through the
richness – finely slice ½ small red
onion and toss with 1 tablespoon
of apple cider vinegar and a
pinch of salt in a small bowl. Let
sit while you prepare the tortillas,
stirring occasionally, until
softened and lightly pickled.

This is one of my favorite meals to make for friends, because who doesn't love lightly charred zucchini with smoky black beans and creamy, spicy cashew aïoli, all wrapped in warm tortillas? Packed with protein and fiber, they're not only deeply satisfying but loaded with goodness.

1. Toss the zucchini ribbons with 1 tablespoon of olive oil and a pinch of salt. Heat a frying pan over a high heat. Add the zucchini and cook for 3–5 minutes, turning occasionally. In the last minute of cooking, stir in 1 clove of crushed garlic for extra flavor. Remove from the pan and set aside.

2. Next, put the pan back on a medium heat, add a drizzle of olive oil, along with the red onion. Cook for 5 minutes, then add the other two cloves of crushed garlic, along with the black beans, smoked paprika, and maple syrup. Cook for a further 5–10 minutes, stirring occasionally, adding a splash of water if needed, until tender. Then stir in the lime juice.

3. While the beans cook, add the soaked cashews, along with their water, and all the aïoli ingredients, plus 2 tablespoons of olive oil and a pinch of salt to a high-speed blender, and blend until smooth and creamy. Add more water or olive oil if needed to reach a consistency for drizzling.

4. Warm the tortillas in a dry frying pan for 30 seconds per side.

5. Fill each tortilla with the black beans and softened zucchini, then drizzle with the cashew aïoli.

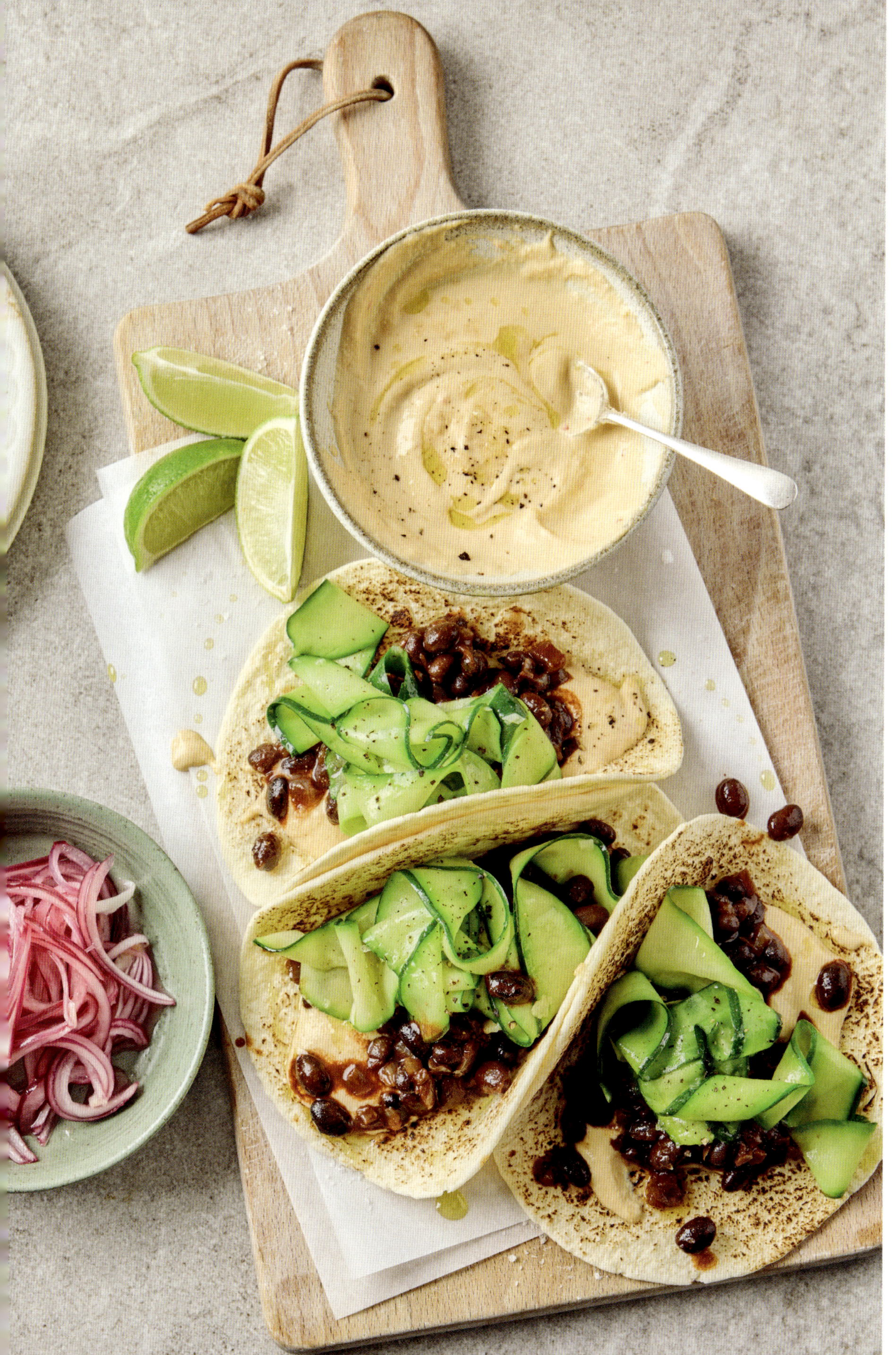

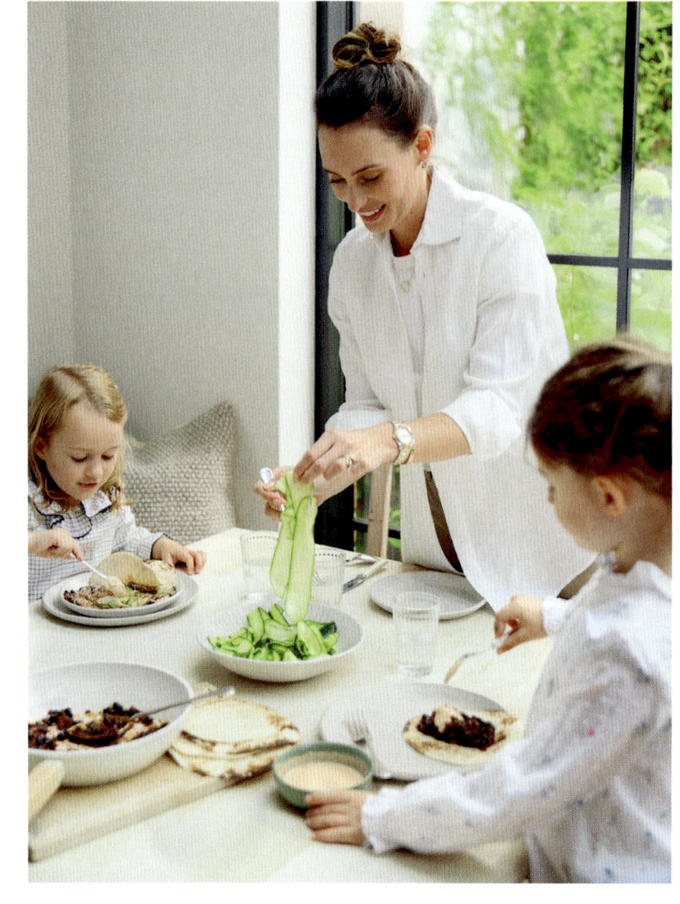

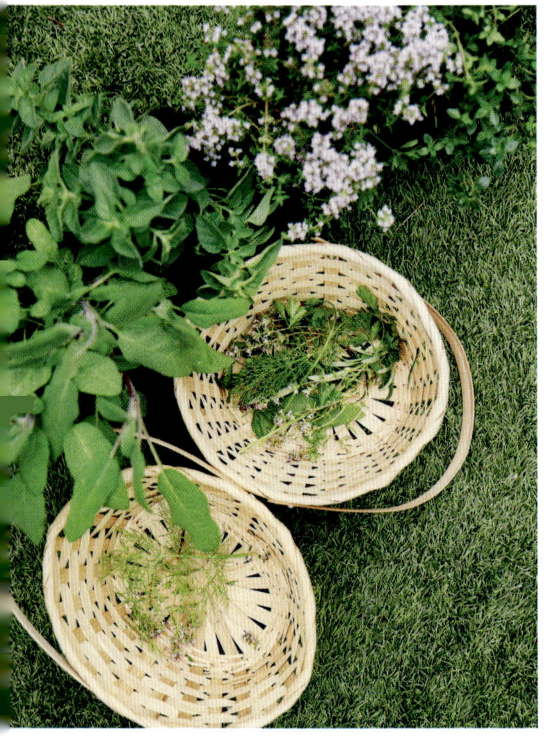

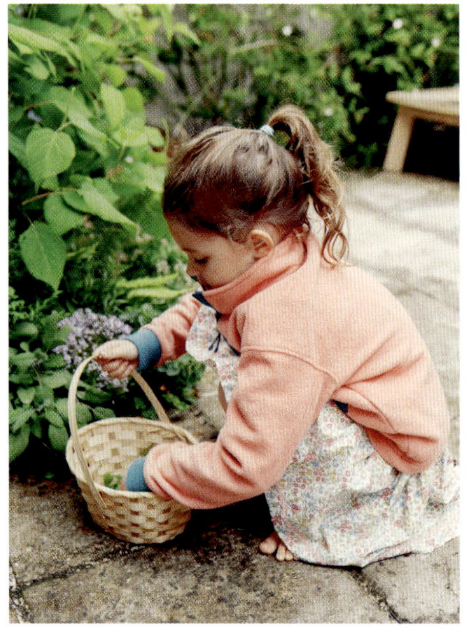

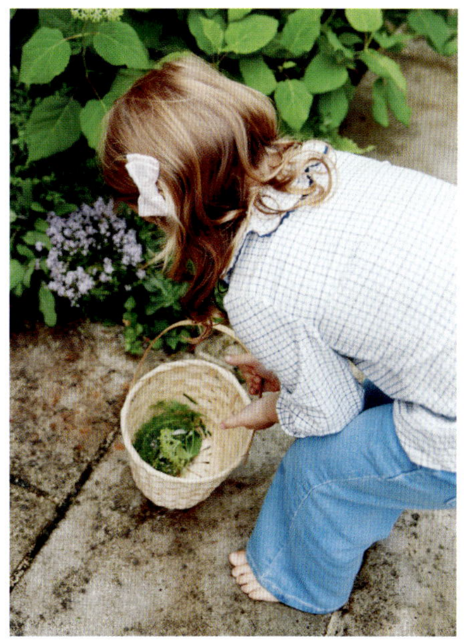

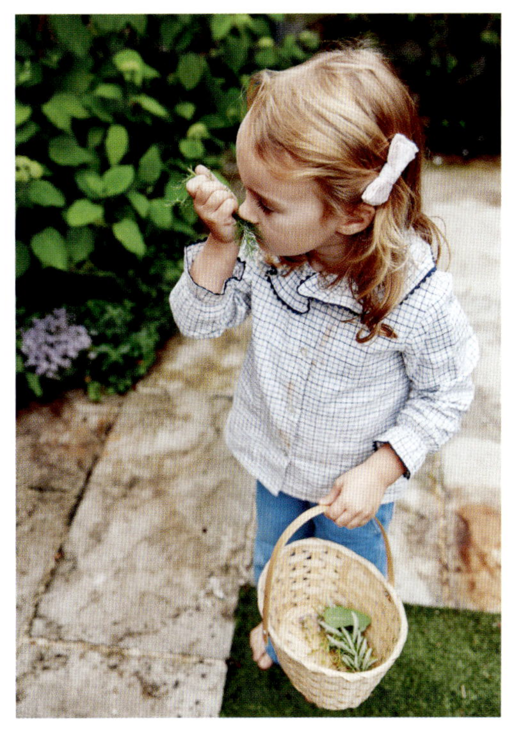

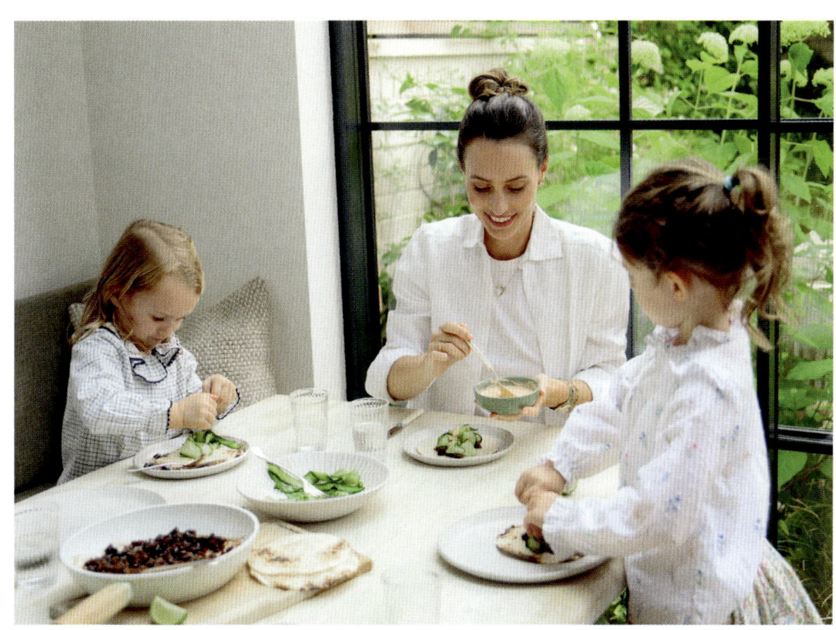

Pesto Tofu with Chili Almond Crunch and Quinoa

9 PLANTS

Serves 2

½ cup quinoa
olive oil
large handful of soft herbs (about
   ¾ cup cilantro, flat-leaf parsley,
   or mint work well; see Note),
   roughly chopped
grated zest and juice of ½ lemon
sea salt

For the chili almond crunch

1 cup almonds, roughly chopped
2 garlic cloves, thinly sliced
1 red chili, thinly sliced

For the tofu

1 × block of firm tofu (about
   10 oz), drained and halved
   lengthways and cut into 1cm
   slices
2 heaped tablespoons store-
   bought pesto, plus extra to
   serve

Note: If you're doing the meal plan, use the rest of the herbs in the Pea and Chickpea Pancake batter (see page 106).

Make it your own: Serve the bowls with a handful of arugula or spinach tossed through the quinoa. Add sliced avocado.

The best thing about this recipe is the crunchy almonds with fresh chili and golden slices of pan-fried garlic. Once you start making these, you'll be sprinkling them on everything! Here they're brilliant with herby quinoa, pesto tofu, and lots of olive oil and black pepper. It's a really fresh, vibrant recipe that's equal parts nourishing and delicious.

1. Pour the quinoa into a small saucepan and cook according to the package instructions, about 8–10 minutes. When it's cooked the liquid should have been fully absorbed – if not, drain off any excess. Remove from the heat and leave to stand.

2. While the quinoa cooks, make the chili almond crunch. Warm 2 tablespoons of olive oil in a large frying pan set over a medium–low heat. Add the almonds, garlic, and chili and cook for 5–7 minutes until crisp and golden, stirring occasionally. Remove from the pan and set aside.

3. Set the pan back over a medium heat and warm another tablespoon of olive oil. Add the tofu and cook for 4–5 minutes on each side until crisp and golden. Remove the pan from the heat and gently stir through the pesto.

4. Fluff up the quinoa with a fork and stir through the herbs, lemon zest and juice, a tablespoon of olive oil, and a good pinch of salt.

5. Spoon the herby grains into bowls, top with the pesto tofu and scatter over the chili almond crunch. You can add an extra drizzle of pesto over the top of each bowl to serve, if you like.

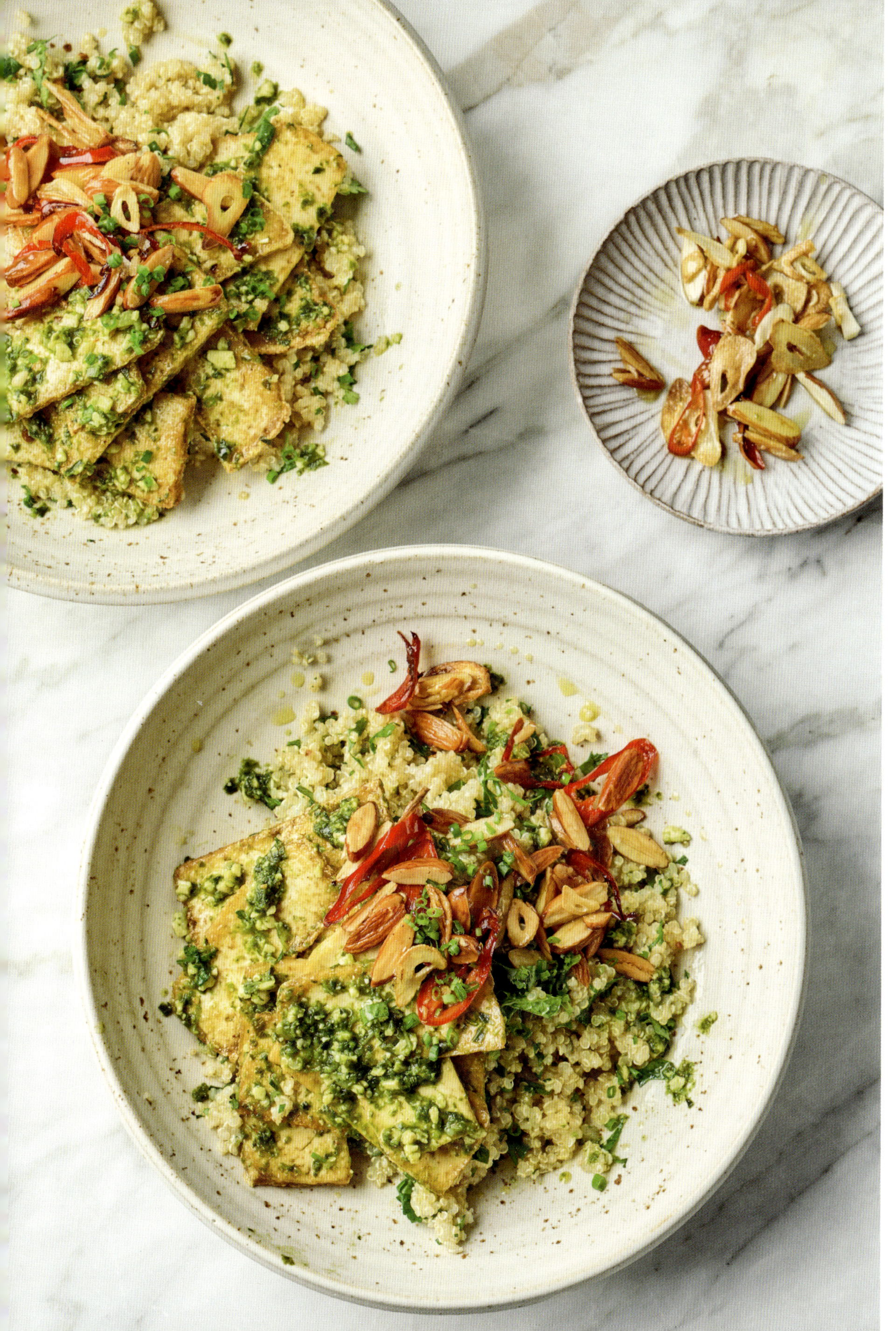

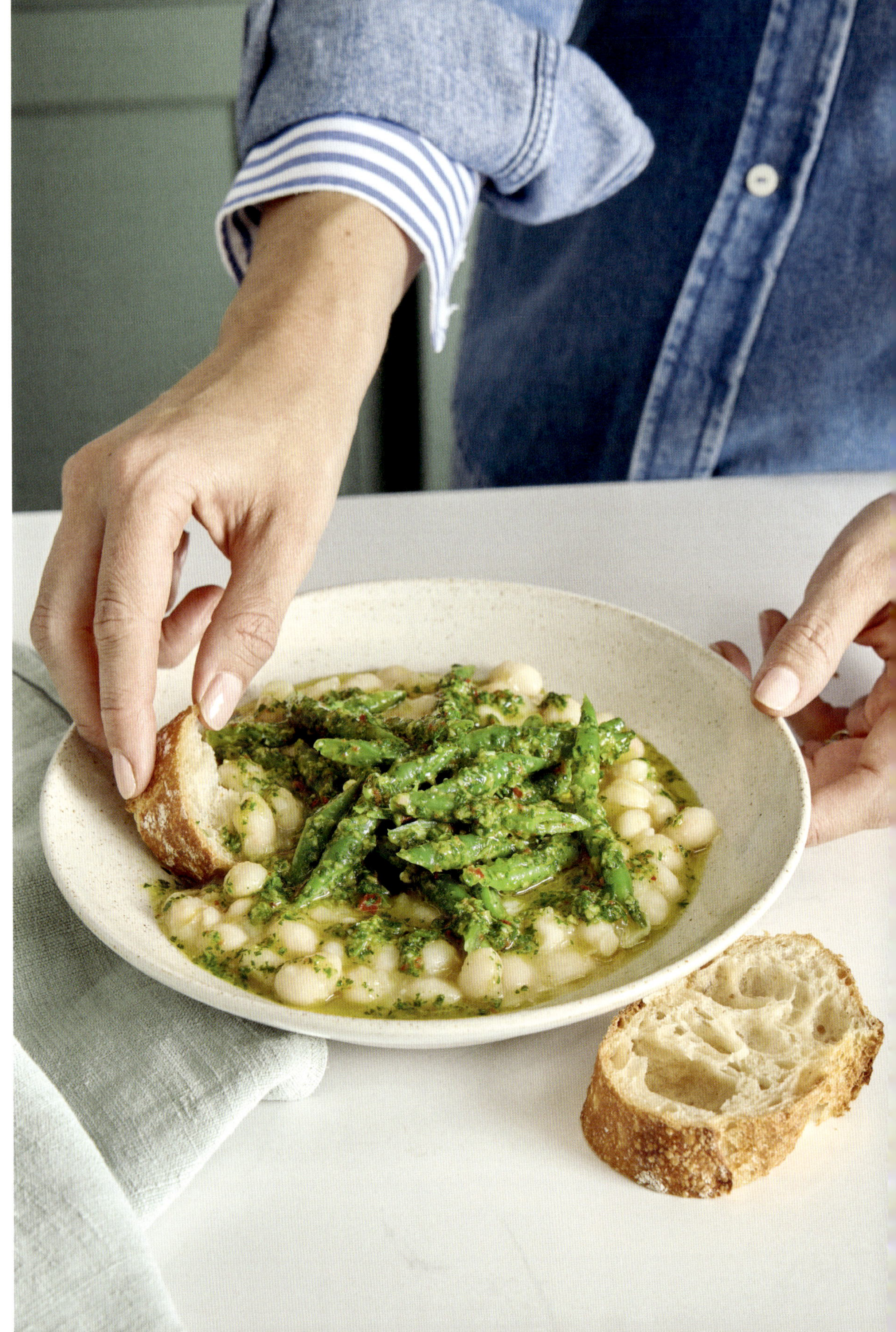

Chimichurri Green Beans with Brothy Beans

Serves 2

For the brothy beans
olive oil
3 garlic cloves, thinly sliced
1½ shallots, finely chopped
1 × 20 oz jar of white beans
  (you can use lima beans or
  cannellini beans), plus the
  stock from the jar
1–2 tablespoons plain yogurt
sea salt and black pepper

**For the chimichurri
green beans**
½ shallot, finely chopped
1 garlic clove
large handful of parsley (about
  ¾ cup)
small handful of cilantro (about
  ½ cup)
1–2 red chilis
2 tablespoons apple cider
  vinegar
olive oil
1⅓ cups green beans, trimmed

To serve
crusty sourdough, flatbread, or
  toasted pitta bread

Possibly my favorite recipe in this book, this bright, comforting stew has a deliciously zesty lemon kick and wonderful creamy finish from the yogurt. But it's the chimichurri that makes it sing – a punchy blend of parsley, cilantro, garlic, apple cider vinegar, and a little chili.

1. For the brothy beans, warm 1 tablespoon of olive oil in a large frying pan (with a lid) set over a medium heat, then add the garlic and shallots. Cook for 5 minutes until softened.

2. Stir in the white beans, along with the stock from the jar, cover with a lid, and simmer for 10 minutes until thickened slightly. Remove the pan from the heat, stir in the yogurt and season to taste.

3. To make the chimichurri, place the shallot, garlic, herbs, chili, cider vinegar, 5 tablespoons of olive oil, and a generous pinch of salt in a mini-chopper or food processor and blitz until combined. Taste and adjust the seasoning as needed.

4. While the beans are cooking, place the green beans in a steamer and steam for 4–5 minutes until just tender, then toss through the chimichurri.

5. Spoon the brothy beans into bowls and top with the chimichurri green beans. Serve with bread on the side for dipping.

Charred Corn Orzo with Almond Pesto

8 PLANTS

Serves 2

olive oil
2 corn on the cob (about 1 lb)
2 garlic cloves, grated
1 onion, finely chopped
1 zucchini, grated
¾ cup orzo
20 fl oz hot vegetable stock
grated zest and juice of ½ lemon
sea salt and black pepper

For the chunky almond pesto
large handful of basil (about
   ¾ cup basil)
about 2–3 tablespoons chives
¾ cup almonds
½ garlic clove
3 tablespoons olive oil

When I want something comforting and easy that I know will be a huge hit, this is my go-to. The charred corn adds a delicious sweetness, while the chunky chive and almond pesto freshens up the creamy orzo. I often double up the pesto and use the leftovers later in the week.

1. Warm a heavy-based frying pan set over a high heat. Add 1 tablespoon of olive oil and the corn cobs and cook for 13–15 minutes, turning frequently, until evenly charred. Transfer to a plate and slice vertically down each side to remove the corn kernels in chunks.

2. Meanwhile, warm 1 tablespoon of olive oil in a large frying pan set over a medium heat, then add the garlic and cook for 1 minute, until fragrant. Next, add the onion along with a pinch of salt and cook for 10 minutes until softened. Stir in the zucchini and cook for 5 minutes until most of the water has evaporated.

3. Stir in the orzo and vegetable stock. Simmer for 8–10 minutes until al dente, stirring occasionally so it doesn't stick to the pan.

4. Meanwhile, make the pesto. Simply add all of the ingredients to a food processor or mini-chopper and pulse until you have a chunky pesto, adding a splash of water to loosen as needed.

5. Once the orzo is cooked, stir in the corn, along with the lemon zest and juice and season to taste with salt and lots of pepper. Serve with a swirl of the chunky almond pesto on top.

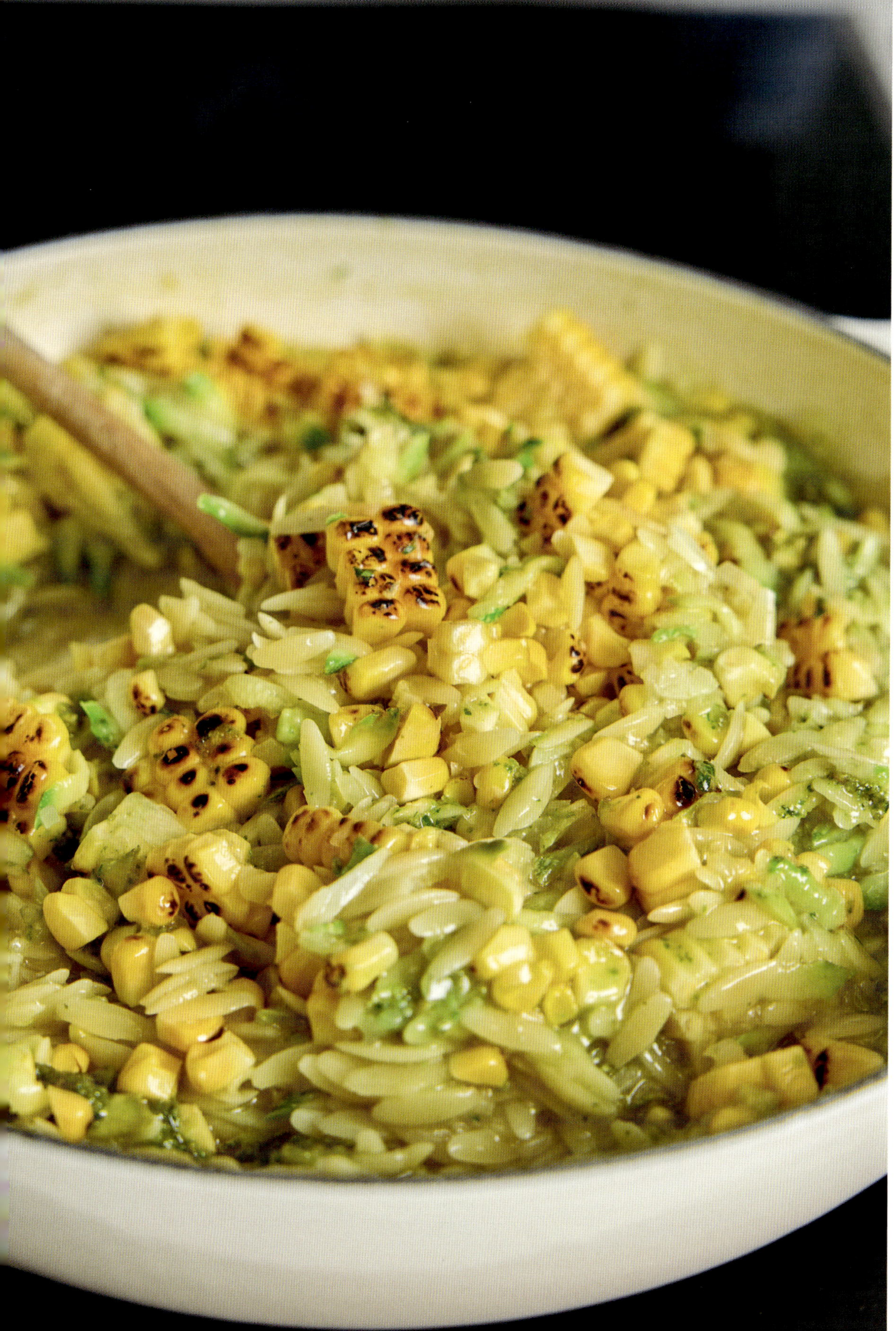

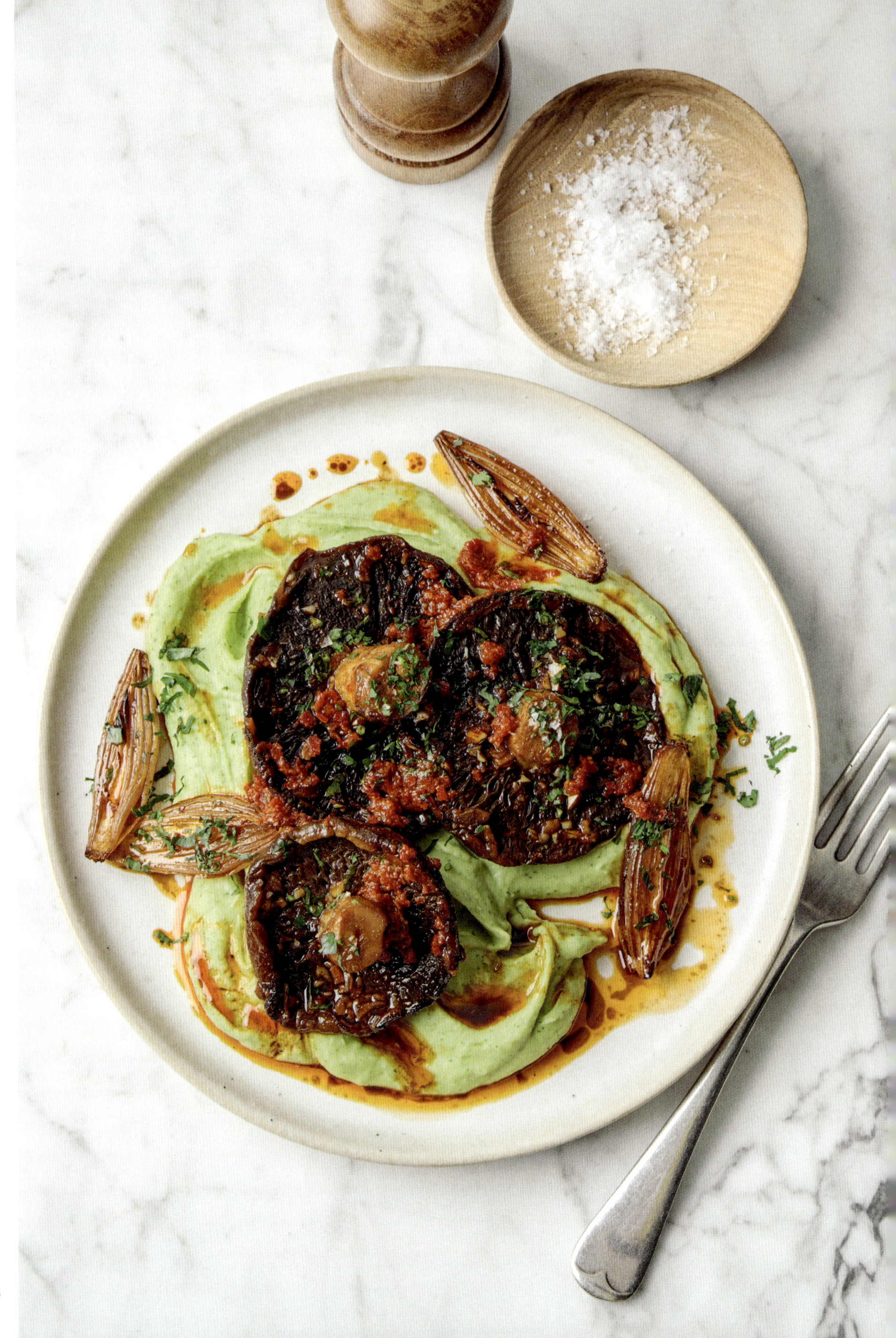

Balsamic-Roasted Portobello Mushrooms with Lima Bean Mash

8 PLANTS

Serves 2

olive oil
2 tablespoons balsamic vinegar
1 tablespoon maple syrup
4 garlic cloves, crushed
1 tablespoon harissa paste
6 large portobello mushroom
   caps
2 shallots, quartered
sea salt

For the lima bean mash
1 shallot, finely chopped
1 garlic clove, crushed
1 × 20 oz jar of lima beans,
   drained
large handful of basil (about
   ¾ cup), half in the mash, half
   finely chopped to serve
large handful of cilantro, (about
   ¾ cup), half in the mash, half
   finely chopped to serve

This recipe is all about simple, comforting flavors with a little smoky punch. Tender roasted portobello mushrooms are coated in a garlicky, balsamic vinegar and harissa marinade – the perfect partner to a creamy, herby white bean mash. I've specified using a jar of beans in this recipe as I really think it helps give the mash the best flavor but you can use a can of beans if you'd prefer.

1. Preheat the oven to 350°F fan. To make the marinade, mix 3 tablespoons of olive oil with the balsamic vinegar, maple syrup, garlic, harissa, and a pinch of salt in a bowl.

2. Place the mushroom caps and shallots in a deep baking tray and coat with the marinade. Roast for 25 minutes until tender and glossy.

3. Meanwhile, make the mash. Heat 1 tablespoon of olive oil in a frying pan set over a medium heat. Add the shallot, garlic, and a pinch of salt and cook for about 2 minutes, until fragrant. Then add the lima beans and cook for 5–10 minutes, stirring occasionally, until soft and warmed through.

4. Tip the lima beans into a food processor with 2 more tablespoons of olive oil, and the basil and cilantro and blitz until smooth and creamy.

5. Spread the mash on to two plates, then pile the mushrooms, shallots, and all the roasting juices on top. Garnish with the finely chopped basil and cilantro to serve.

This is a chapter of hearty dishes designed to help you get ahead. Eight core recipes will give you two batches of a meal that can be enjoyed twice in the week – in two different ways. You cook the main recipe, then a second recipe on the following page shows you how to give the second batch a different twist, guaranteeing that your leftovers will never feel boring.

BATCH COOK

Miso Eggplant Ragu

Coconut Lentils with Flatbreads

Sweet Potato Thai Curry

Loaded Chili Bowls

Lima Bean and Carrot Soup

Eggplant Tortillas

Romano Pepper Stew

Speedy Thai Noodles

Smoky White Bean Chili

Lima Bean Soup with Cavolo

Curry with Chickpea Salad

Creamy Coconut Lentils

Pepper and Orzo Soup

Quinoa Bean Chili

Chili with Baked Potato

Cauliflower and Coconut Curry

Pulled Miso Eggplant Ragu

8 PLANTS

Serves 4

4 eggplant
olive oil
3 garlic cloves, crushed or
    minced
1 teaspoon ground cumin
2 onions, finely chopped
1 × 14 oz can of beluga (or green)
    lentils, drained and rinsed
1 tablespoon tomato purée
1 tablespoon almond butter
18 oz passata (from a 24 oz jar;
    you use the rest in the Fancy
    Lima Beans on Toast on
    page 92)
juice of ½ lemon
2 teaspoons white miso paste
    (optional)
2 teaspoons maple syrup
sea salt and black pepper
pasta or grains, to serve

To store: Store in a sealed
container in the fridge for up to
5 days or store in the freezer
for up to 3 months.

Make it your own: Stir in a
spoonful of tahini for extra
richness or add a sprinkling of
dried red chili flakes for a little
heat. If you're serving it with
rice, a dollop of yogurt makes a
delicious addition, as does basil.

A hearty and flavorful pulled eggplant ragu with lentils, perfect as a main dish on its own or served over pasta or grains. The eggplant is roasted until tender, shredded, then combined with lentils and a spiced tomato sauce to create a rich, satisfying sauce.

1. Preheat the oven to 400°F fan. Pierce the eggplants all over with a knife to stop them from bursting and place in a deep baking tray. Roast for 40–45 minutes, turning halfway, until softened and collapsed.

2. Meanwhile, warm 2 tablespoons of olive oil in a large frying pan set over a medium–low heat. Add the garlic and cumin and cook for 2–3 minutes, until fragrant. Add the onion, along with a pinch of salt and cook for 10–15 minutes, until golden.

3. Stir in the lentils, tomato purée, almond butter, passata, lemon juice, miso, and maple syrup. Half-fill the empty passata jar with water and add this too. Simmer for 10–15 minutes, stirring occasionally, until glossy and thickened. Turn the heat right down, cover with a lid and leave to simmer very gently until the eggplants are ready.

4. Let the eggplants cool slightly then carefully cut in half and use a fork to scrape out the soft, silky flesh — it should melt away from the skin. Stir into the sauce and season to taste.

5. Serve half the ragu with your favorite pasta or grain and keep the other half for later in the week (see the next page for my suggestion of how to serve it).

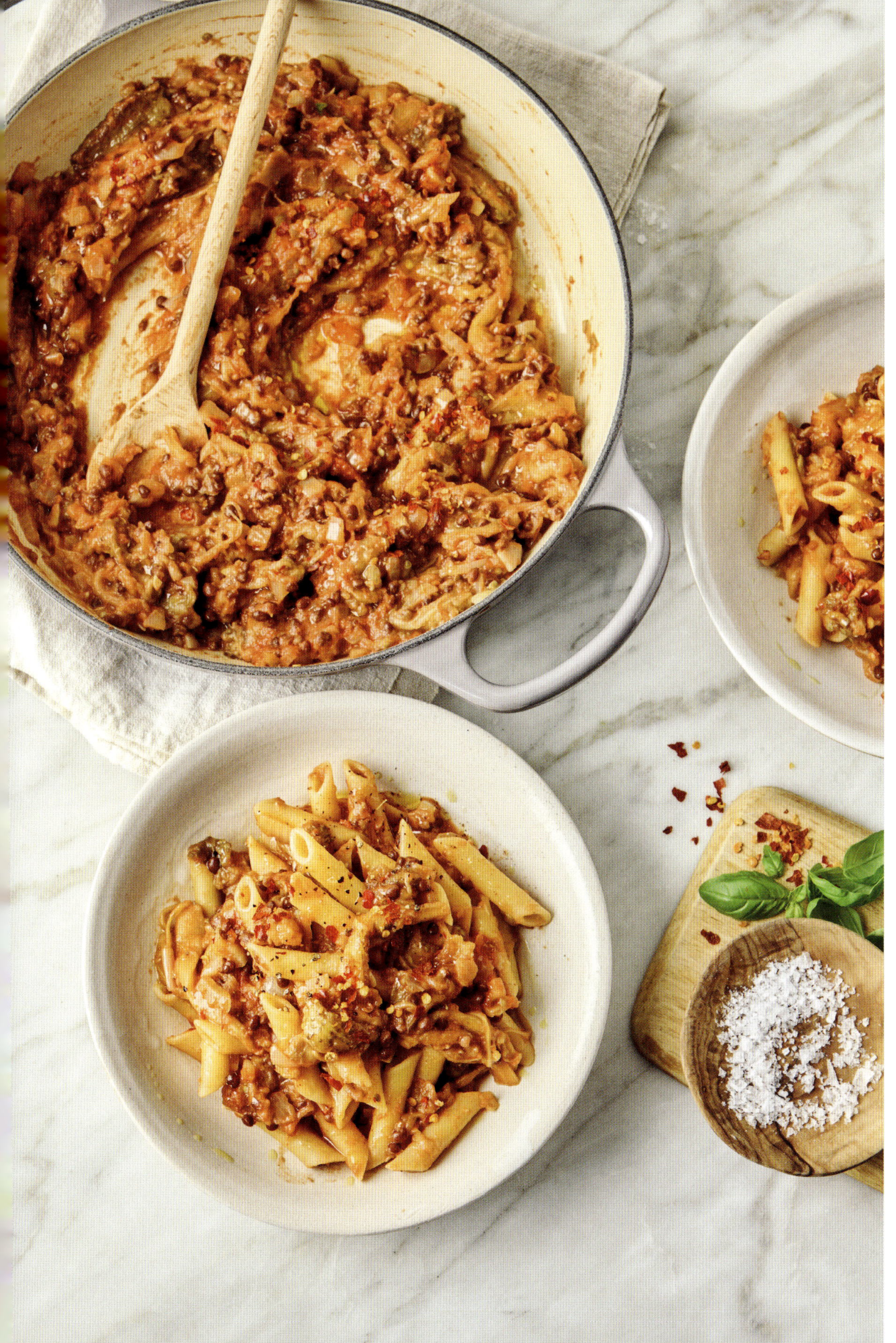

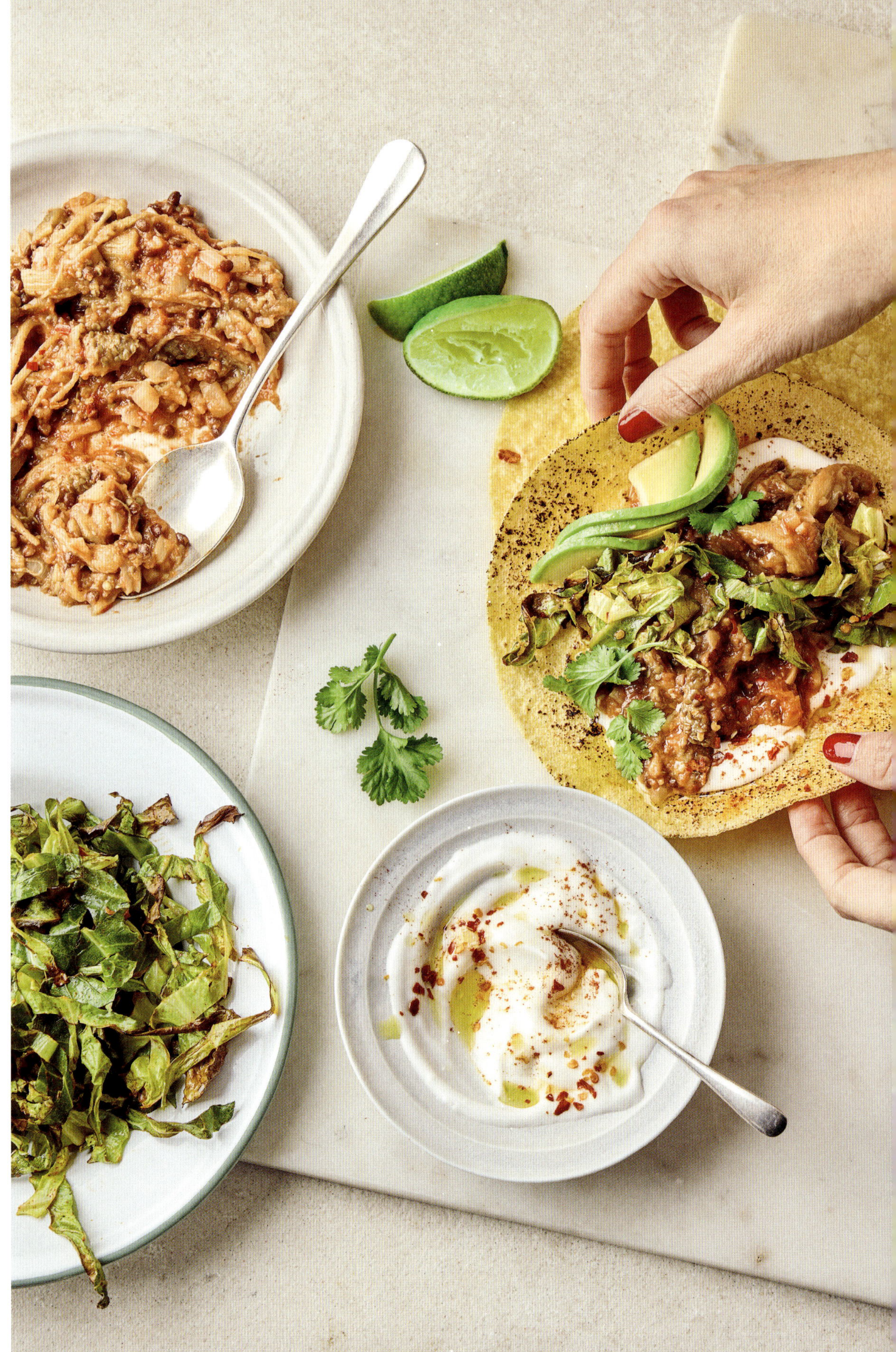

Pulled Eggplant Tortillas with Crispy Roasted Cabbage

Serves 2

⅔ cabbage (use the rest of the cabbage from the Crunchy Cabbage, Sesame and Mango Salad on page 73), thinly sliced
½ teaspoon smoked paprika
pinch of dried red chili flakes
olive oil
4 small whole-wheat tortillas (or use 2 large ones)
1 lime, halved
1–2 avocados, thinly sliced
2 servings of Pulled Miso Eggplant Ragu (see page 130)
handful of cilantro (about ¾ cup) roughly chopped
sea salt
plain yogurt, to serve (optional)

Pile your leftovers of the Pulled Miso Eggplant Ragu into lightly toasted tortillas with thin slices of roast cabbage and a dollop of yogurt. The cabbage adds texture and a smoky flavor that works brilliantly with the rich ragu.

1. Preheat the oven to 400°F fan. On a large baking tray, toss together the cabbage, paprika, chili flakes, a tablespoon of olive oil, and a generous pinch of salt and spread out in a single layer.

2. Roast for 20 minutes, stirring halfway, until crisp and lightly charred.

3. Meanwhile, warm the tortillas in a dry pan or in the oven for 2–3 minutes. Squeeze the juice from half of the lime over the avocado.

4. To assemble the tortillas, spoon a generous amount of ragu on to each tortilla, then pile on some crispy cabbage, avocado, cilantro, and a spoonful of yogurt (if using). Squeeze over a little lime juice and serve immediately.

My Go-To Creamy Coconut Lentils

Serves 4

1 cup red split lentils, rinsed
1 × 14 fl oz can of coconut milk
1 × 14 oz can of chopped
  tomatoes
2 large handfuls of baby spinach
  (about 3 cups), roughly
  chopped
juice of 1 lime or lemon
steamed rice, to serve (optional)
plain yogurt, to serve (optional)

For the curry paste

1 red onion, peeled and roughly
  chopped
3 garlic cloves, peeled
small chunk of ginger root (about
  1 in), peeled
2 teaspoons medium curry
  powder
1–2 red chilis, stalks removed
olive oil
sea salt and black pepper

This is one of those recipes that I make again and again, ready for a busy week. It's comforting, creamy, and easy to throw together. The mix of onion, chili, and fresh ginger brings so much warmth, while the red lentils turn soft and rich in the coconut-tomato sauce. The flavors only get better with time, so your leftovers will be fantastic later in the week. For a super-nourishing bowl, I love serving it with fluffy rice and a dollop of coconut yogurt.

1. To make the curry paste, simply place the onion, garlic, ginger, curry powder, chili, 3–4 tablespoons of olive oil, a large pinch of salt, and lots of black pepper in a small food processor or high-speed blender. Blitz to form a coarse paste.

2. Warm 1 tablespoon of olive oil in a shallow casserole dish or large frying pan set over a low–medium heat. Add the curry paste and cook for 10 minutes, stirring often, until fragrant and the color deepens.

3. Pour in the lentils and 14 fl oz of water. Bring to a simmer and cook for 5–7 minutes, until all of the water has been absorbed.

4. Add the coconut milk and canned tomatoes. Simmer gently for 20 minutes, stirring occasionally to prevent it sticking, until the lentils are completely tender.

5. Season generously with salt, then stir in the spinach and lime juice. Serve warm with steamed rice and a dollop of yogurt.

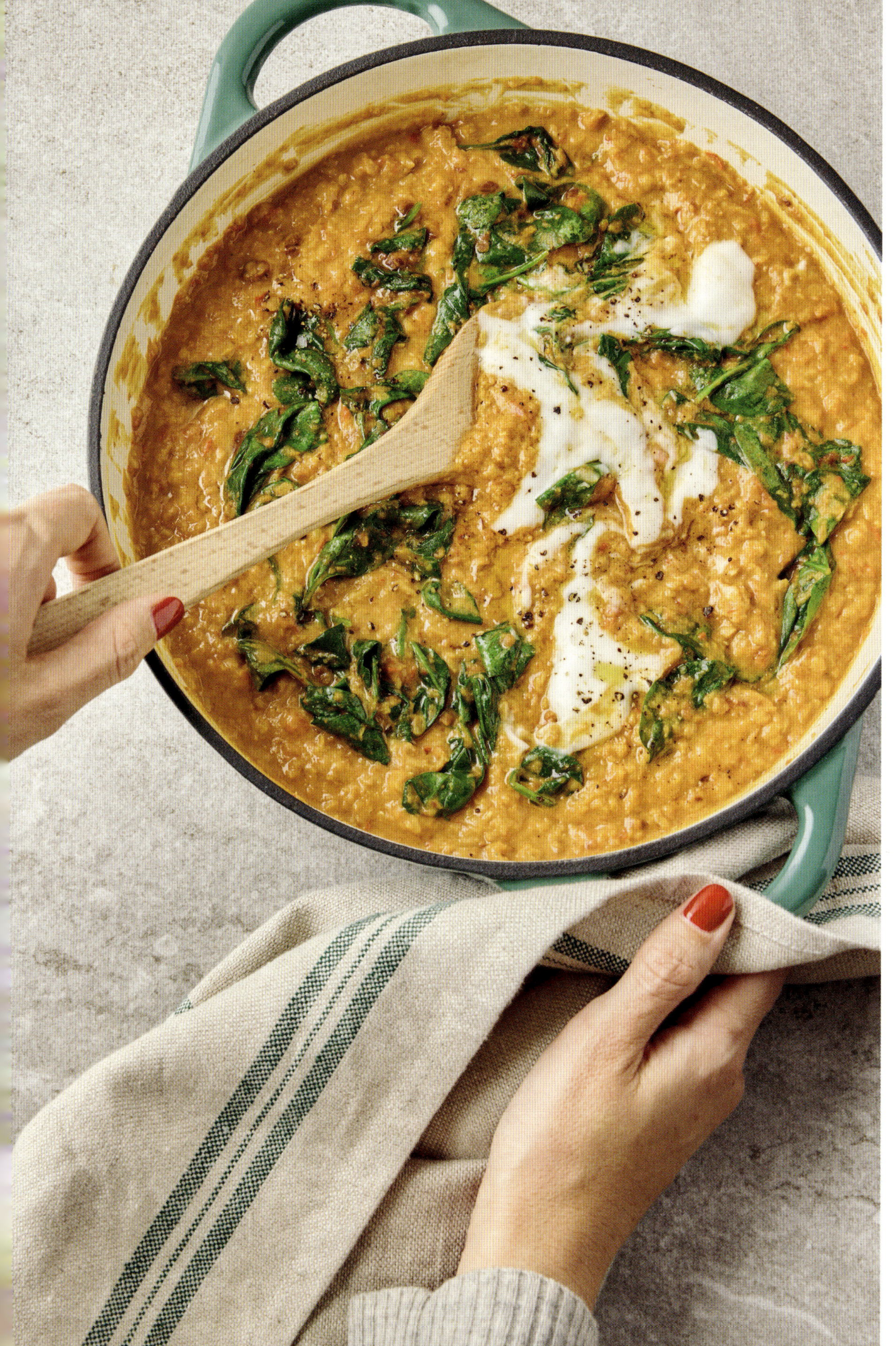

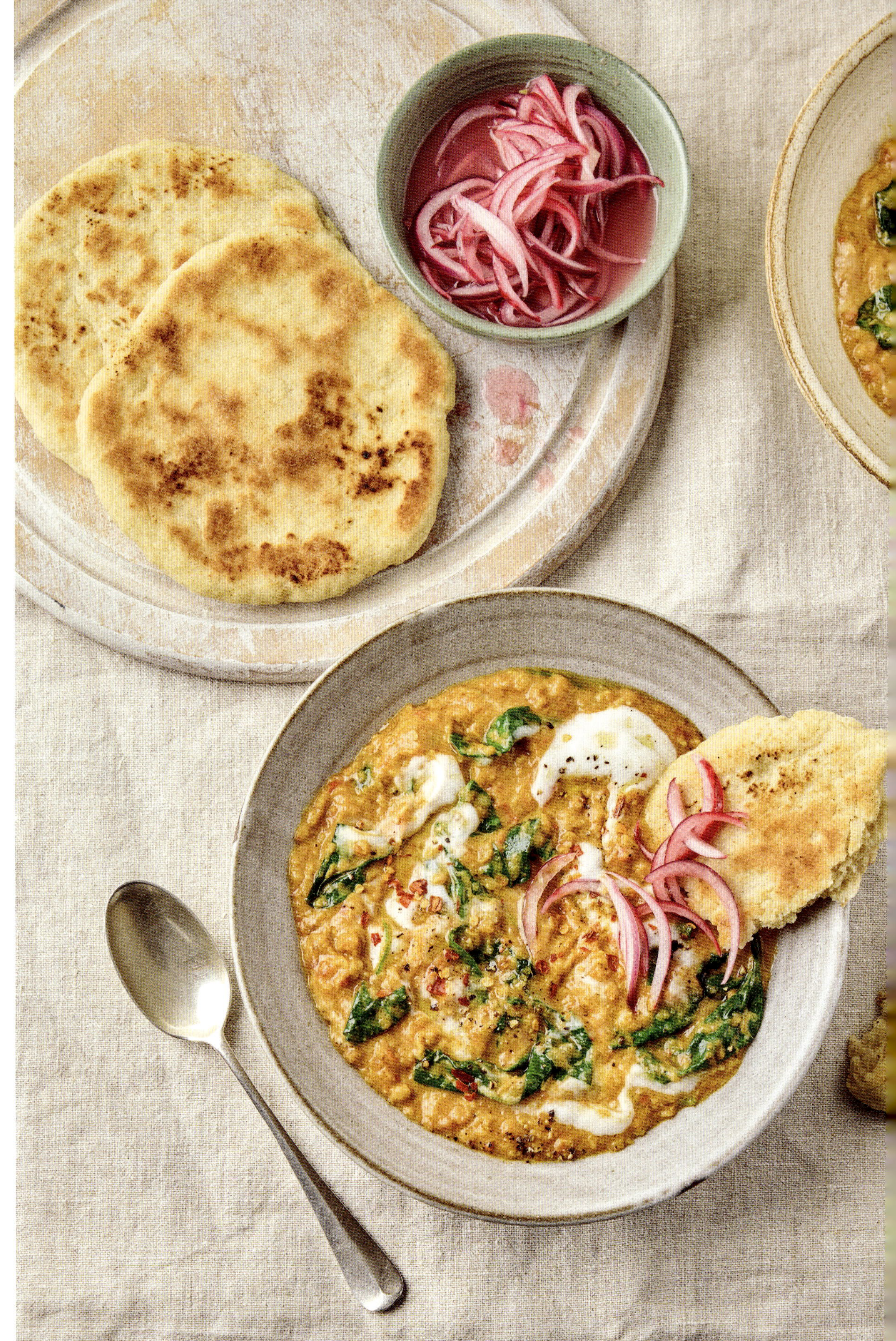

Creamy Coconut Lentils with Flatbreads and Quick Pickled Onions

10 PLANTS

Serves 2

2 servings of My Go-To Creamy
  Coconut Lentils (see page 134)

For the quick pickled onions
1 red onion, thinly sliced (use a
  mandoline if you have one)
juice of 2 limes
drizzle of maple syrup (optional)
pinch of salt

For the flatbreads
1¼ cups plain flour, sifted, plus
  extra for dusting
1 tsp baking powder
7 oz plain yogurt
2 tablespoons olive oil
1 teaspoon fine sea salt

Instead of simply reheating the lentils and having them with a grain again, try scooping them up with hot flatbreads topped with pickled red onions. The combination of creamy, crunchy, tangy, sweet, and spice is just heaven. You can, of course, buy the flatbreads, or they're super easy to make yourself! You can also add a little herby salad on the side, if you have cilantro, mint, and other fresh herbs in the house.

1. To make the quick pickled onions, simply combine all the ingredients in a small bowl, and set aside to marinate while you make the flatbreads.

2. To make the flatbreads, sift the flour and baking powder into a large bowl, then add the yogurt, olive oil, and salt, and gently mix together to form a dough.

3. Lightly dust a work surface with flour and tip out the dough. Knead briefly until smooth. Divide the dough into two balls and using a rolling pin, roll each one out into a large circle, roughly the same size as your frying pan.

4. Warm a large frying pan set over a medium heat, add one circle of dough and cook for 2–3 minutes on each side until puffy and golden. Repeat with the second one.

5. Serve right away with the lentils and pickled onions.

Spicy Carrot and Romano Pepper Stew

10 PLANTS

Serves 4

olive oil
4 garlic cloves, thinly sliced or
    finely chopped
small chunk of fresh ginger root,
    (about 1 in), peeled and finely
    chopped
2 shallots, finely diced
3 carrots, diced
2 Romano peppers, thinly sliced
1 tablespoon harissa
1 × 14 oz can of haricot or
    cannellini beans, drained and
    rinsed
1 × 14 oz can of chopped
    tomatoes
1 teaspoon maple syrup
large handful of cilantro (about
    ¾ cup), stalks finely chopped,
    leaves roughly chopped
sea salt and black pepper

To serve

2 servings of pasta, brown rice,
    or baked potatoes
plain yogurt, cilantro, and tahini
    (optional)

Make it your own: Top with
flaked or toasted almonds for
crunch. Stir through a handful of
baby spinach at the end for extra
greens, or add a pinch of dried
red chili flakes for more heat.

There's so much to love about this stew – the smoky harissa, the sweetness of the carrots and peppers, the way it thickens into something rich and comforting without needing much effort at all. It's the kind of easy, throw–it–all–in meal I rely on when I want something packed with goodness but don't feel like spending ages in the kitchen.

1. Warm 2 tablespoons of olive oil in a large saucepan or casserole set over a medium–low heat. Add the garlic, ginger, shallot, carrot, and a generous pinch of salt. Cook for 5 minutes until glossy.

2. Add the pepper and cook for 5 minutes until just softened.

3. Stir in the harissa, beans, chopped tomatoes, and maple syrup, along with 7 fl oz water. Bring to the boil, then reduce the heat and simmer with the lid off for 15 minutes, until thickened.

4. Remove the pan from the heat and stir in the cilantro stalks. Season generously.

5. Divide half the stew between two bowls, top with the remaining cilantro and a drizzle of tahini and yogurt (if using).

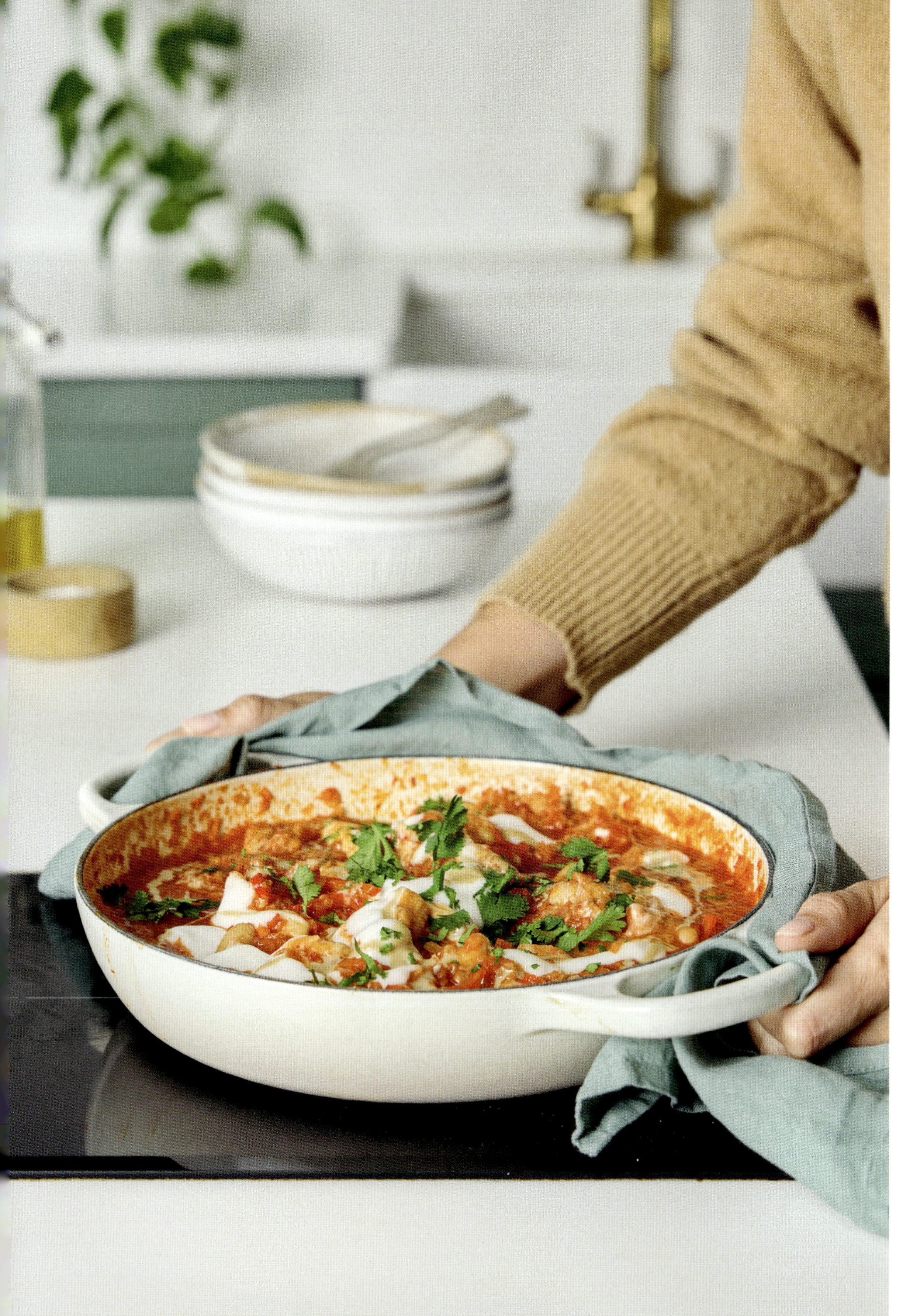

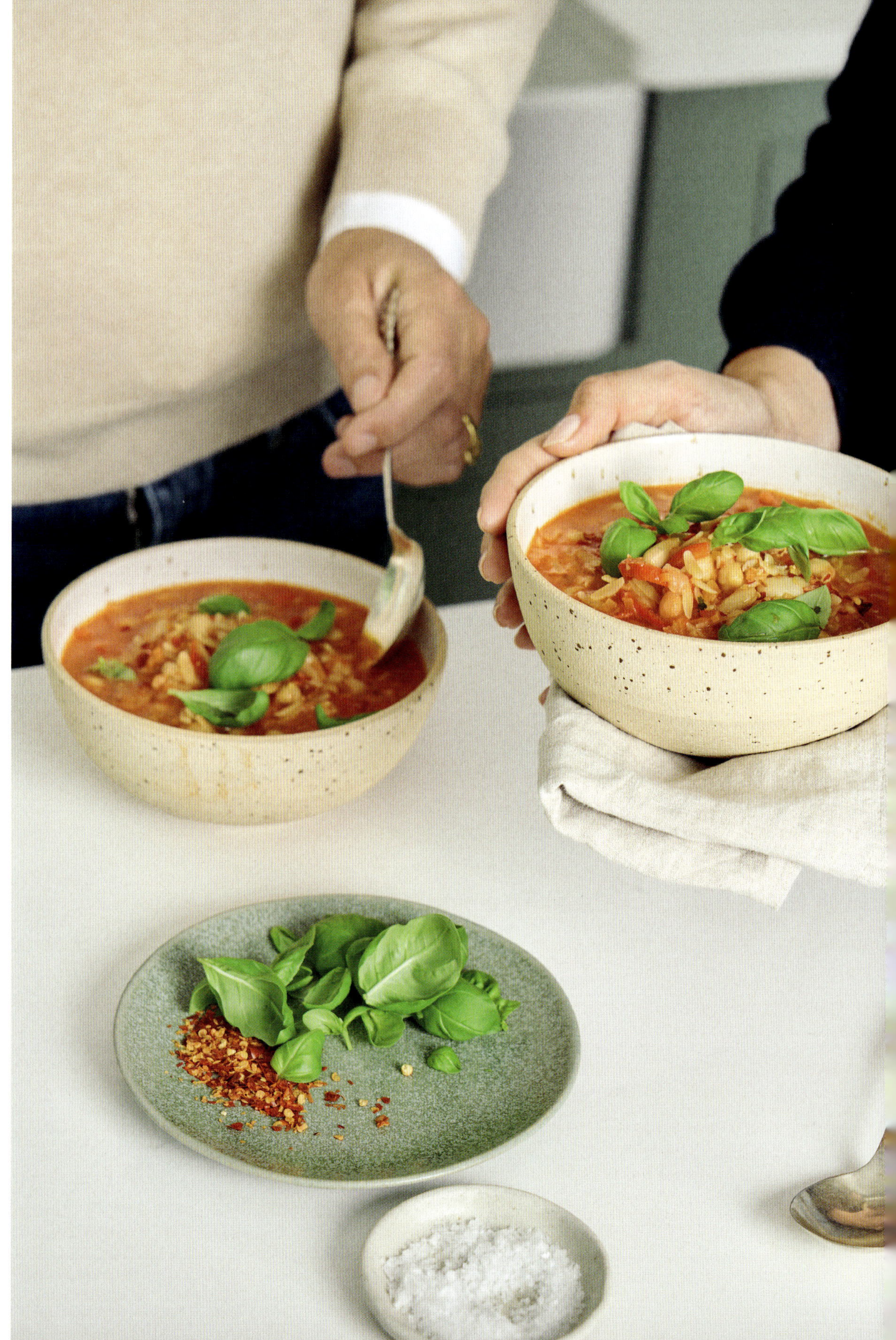

Chunky Romano Pepper Soup with Orzo and Chickpeas

12 PLANTS

Serves 2

2 servings of Spicy Carrot and Romano Pepper stew (see page 138)

26 fl oz hot vegetable stock (or use water)

1 × 14 oz can of chickpeas, drained and rinsed

¾ cup orzo

large handful of basil (about ¾ cup), roughly chopped, plus extra to garnish

sea salt and black pepper

extra virgin olive oil, to finish

dried red chili flakes, to serve (optional)

Turn your leftover stew into delicious minestrone-inspired bowls in minutes. This is the ultimate quick win on a busy week! With orzo, extra chickpeas, and lots of fresh basil, it's brilliantly nourishing and satisfying.

1. Pour the leftover stew portions into a saucepan set over a medium–high heat, then stir in the vegetable stock and chickpeas.

2. Bring to a gentle boil, then add the orzo and cook for 6–8 minutes until al dente.

3. Remove the pan from the heat, stir in the basil and season to taste.

4. To serve, spoon the soup into bowls, drizzle over some extra virgin olive oil, add a pinch of chili flakes, if using, and garnish with the remaining basil.

Make it your own: Garnish with lemon zest; stir in a spoonful of plain yogurt; add diced tofu for extra protein; use pesto instead of basil; swap the chickpeas for lima beans or borlotti beans.

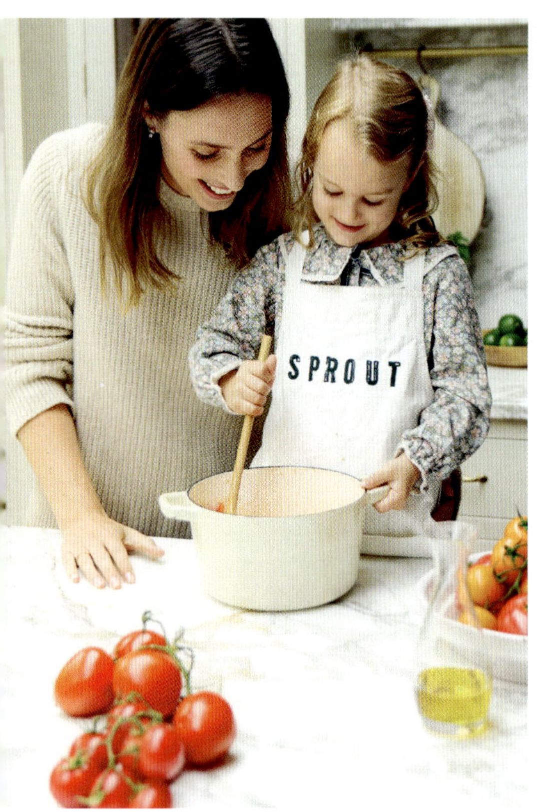

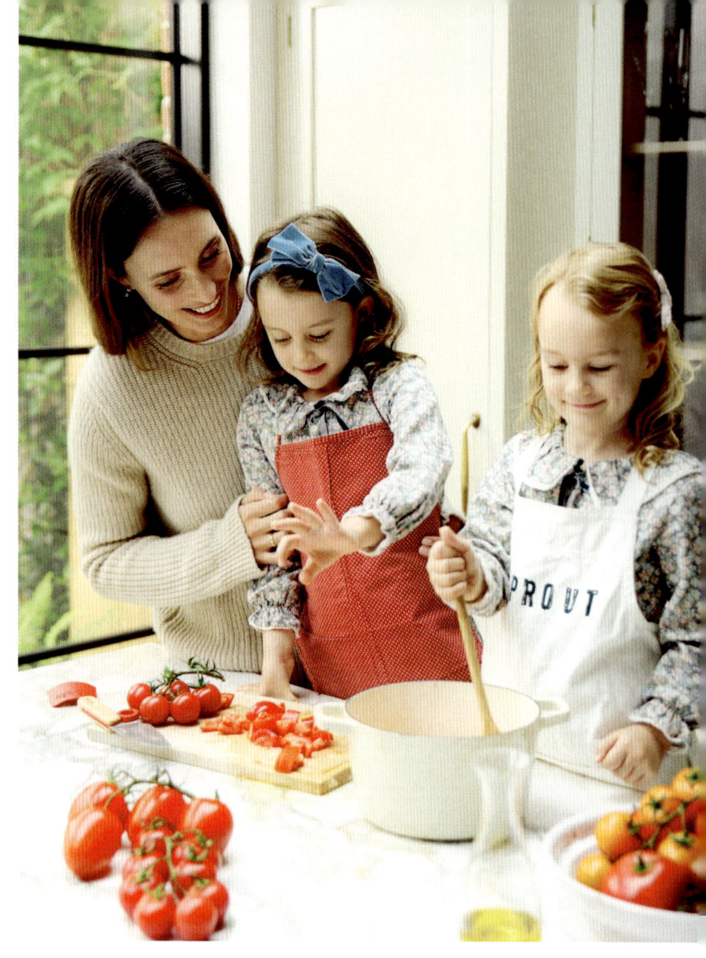

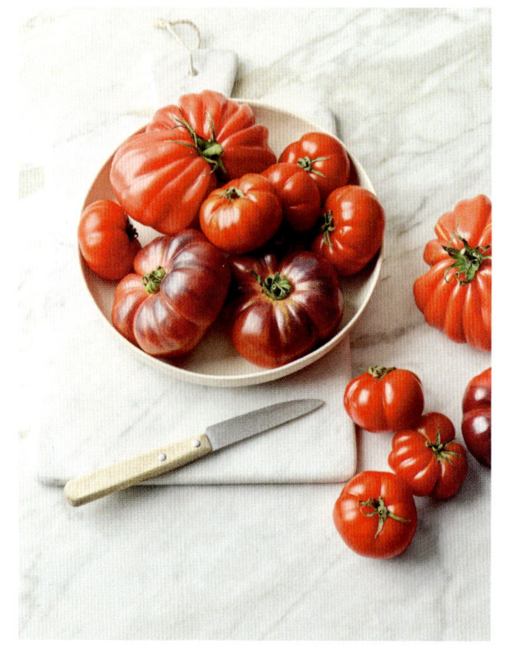

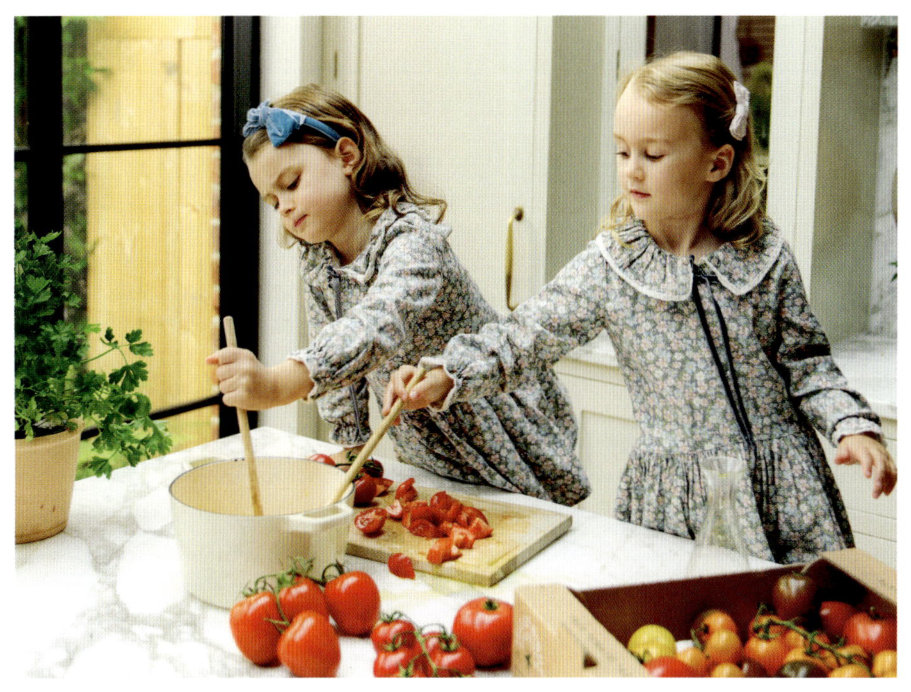

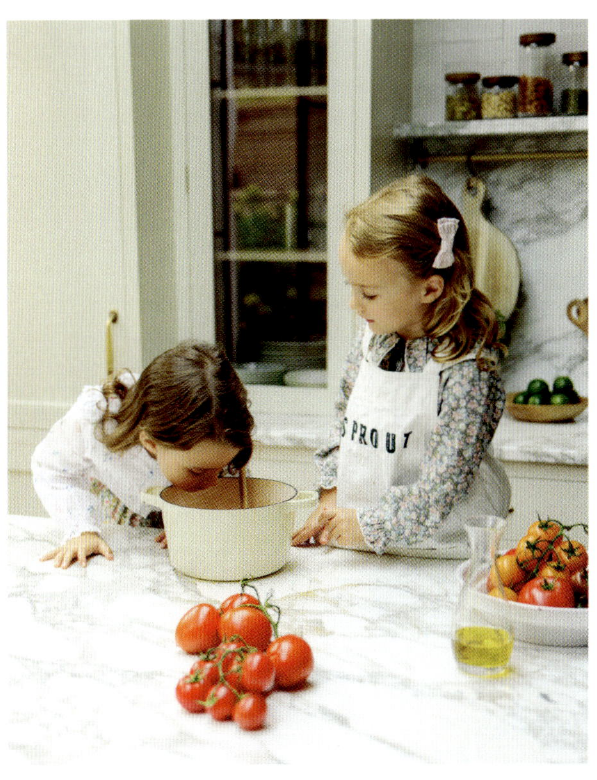

Sweet Potato Red Thai Curry

10 PLANTS

Serves 4

olive oil

3 garlic cloves, finely chopped

small chunk of fresh ginger root
(about 1 in), finely chopped

2 bird's eye chilis, finely chopped

3 tablespoons red Thai curry
paste

2 sweet potatoes (about
2¼ cups), cut into 1 in chunks

2 Romano peppers, cut into ½ in
slices

1 cup red lentils, rinsed

1 × 400ml tin of coconut milk

splash of tamari or soy sauce (or
use a pinch of salt)

4 cups spinach

juice of 1 lime

1 tablespoon maple syrup

handful of Thai basil (about
¾ cup), plus extra to garnish

sea salt

steamed rice or cooked quinoa,
to serve

Packed with flavor, this spicy sweet potato curry with Romano peppers, red lentils, ginger, and chili is just what you need on a cold day. Packing in 10 different plants in one meal, it's an easy way to hit your 30-plants-a-week goal in a super-warming, creamy way. If you're following the meal plan, I'd recommend serving around 60 percent of the recipe for this meal, as you'll be turning the leftovers into brothy noodle bowls (see page 147), so won't need as much of the curry the second time around.

1. Warm 1 tablespoon of olive oil in a large saucepan or casserole set over a medium–low heat. Add the garlic, ginger, chili, and curry paste and cook for 5–7 minutes, stirring frequently, until fragrant.

2. Add the sweet potatoes, peppers, lentils, coconut milk, tamari, and 17 fl oz water. Bring to the boil, then reduce the heat and allow to simmer with the lid off for 20–25 minutes, until thickened.

3. Stir in the spinach, lime juice, maple syrup, and about three quarters of the Thai basil. Taste and adjust the seasoning as needed.

4. To serve, divide into bowls and scatter over the remaining Thai basil. This is delicious served with steamed rice or quinoa.

Make it your own: Serve with juicy lime wedges. Swap the sweet potatoes for carrots.

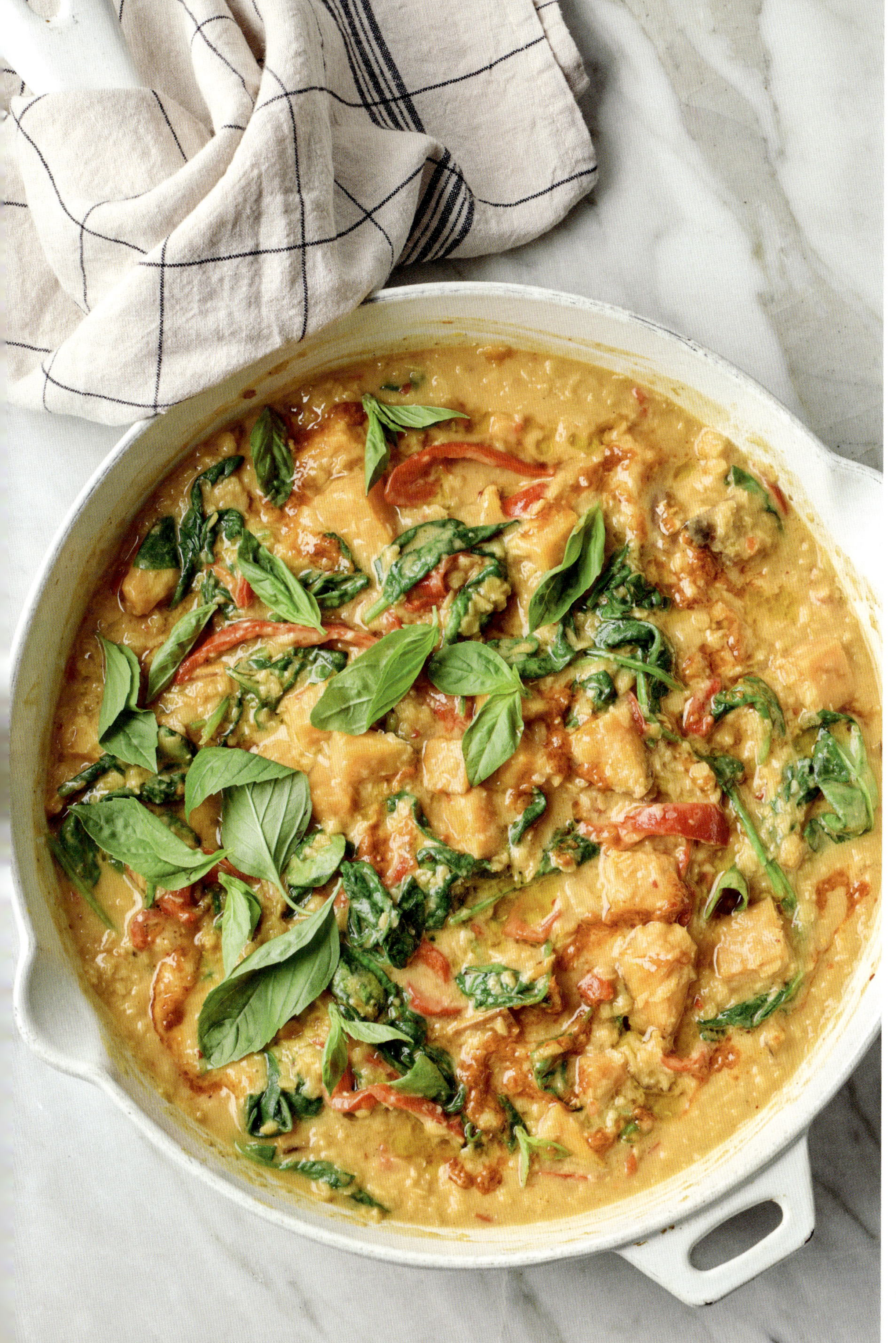

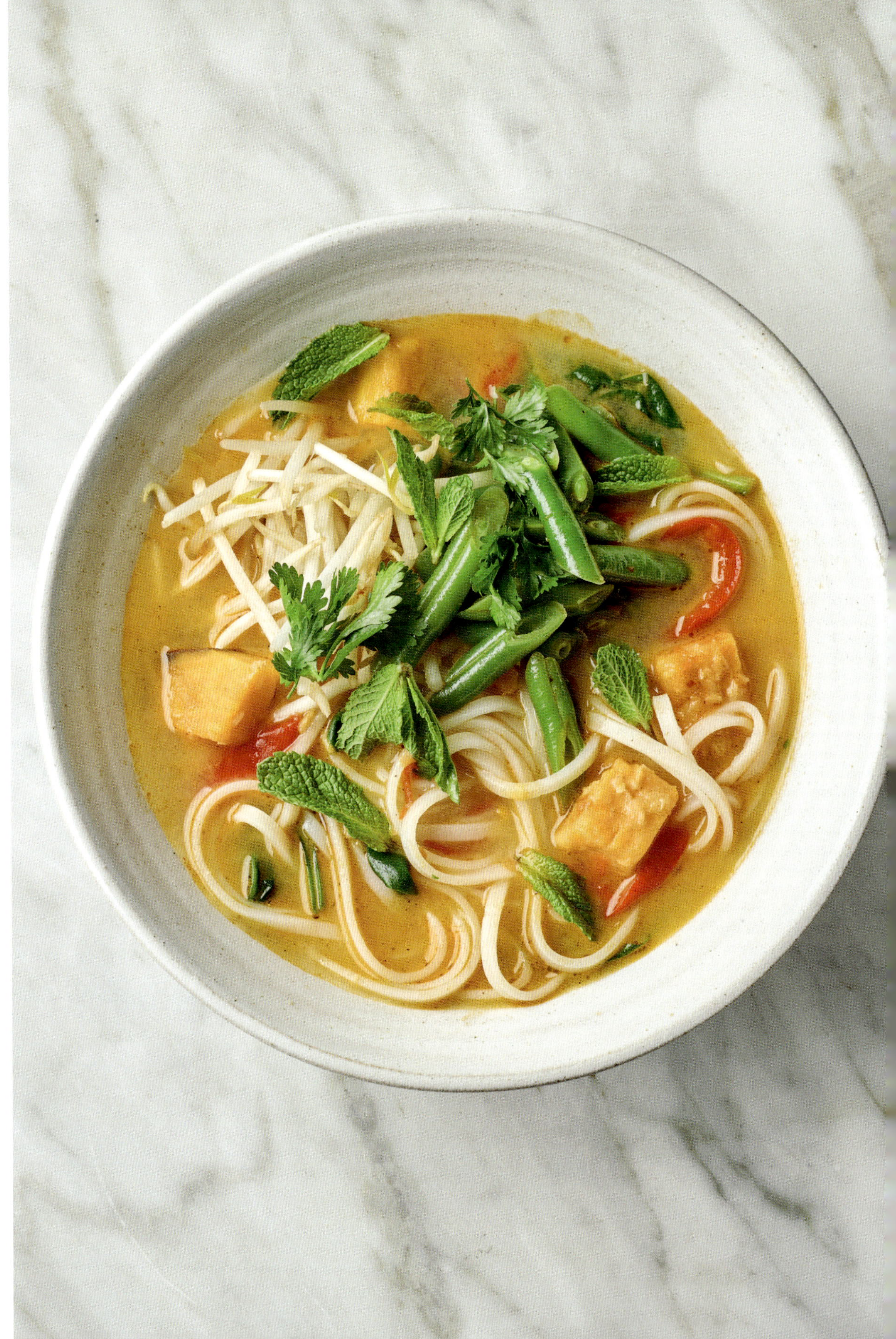

Speedy Red Thai Curry Noodles

Serves 2

2 servings of Sweet Potato Red
  Thai Curry (see page 144)
17 fl oz hot vegetable stock or
  water
⅔ cup green beans, trimmed
1 cup beansprouts
2 servings of spelt noodles (or
  use rice noodles)
handful of mint (about ⅓ cup),
  roughly chopped
handful of cilantro (about ⅓ cup),
  roughly chopped

There's nothing more satisfying than coming home from a busy day and having a delicious dinner ready to go. All you do to prepare these noodles is warm up your leftovers and stir green beans, beansprouts, and noodles into the pan for a few minutes before ladling into bowls. It's a very comforting quick win!

1. Put the leftover curry into a large saucepan, pour in the vegetable stock, and bring to a vigorous simmer.

2. Add the green beans, beansprouts, and noodles. Cook for 4–5 minutes, stirring every so often to disperse the noodles, until both the beans and noodles are just cooked.

3. To serve, divide the broth between bowls and garnish with the mint and cilantro.

Five-Bean and Quinoa Chili

13 PLANTS

Serves 4

olive oil
1 red onion, finely chopped
1–2 red chilis, finely chopped (use
    as many as is to your taste)
1 teaspoon ground cumin
2 × 14 oz cans of mixed beans (or
    1 × can of beans and 1 × can of
    lentils), drained and rinsed
½ cup quinoa
1 × 14 oz can of chopped
    tomatoes
1 teaspoon maple syrup
9 fl oz hot vegetable stock
1 × 14 fl oz can of coconut milk
2 limes (1 juiced, 1 cut into
    wedges)
handful of cilantro (about ½ cup),
    roughly chopped
2 green onions, thinly sliced
sea salt and black pepper

Note: If you're making this as
part of the meal plan, you'll have
half a block of tofu left over from
the Ginger and Tahini Noodles
(see page 22). Crumble or cube
it and stir it into the pan with the
coconut milk. It melts into the
sauce for a creamy texture.

Make it your own: Stir through a
handful of spinach or kale at the
end to add some extra greens.

This is one of those recipes I come back to again
and again as it's easy, nourishing, and endlessly
adaptable. Everything cooks in one pan, which
means minimal dish washing, and it's packed with
plant-based protein. The quinoa soaks up all the
flavor from the spices, beans, and tomatoes, while
the coconut milk adds a creamy richness that makes
it feel a little indulgent, without being heavy. The
leftovers are even better the next day in the Loaded
Chili Bowls with Sweet Potato Wedges (see page 151).

1. Warm 2 tablespoons of olive oil in a large saucepan
   set over a medium–low heat. Add the onion, chili,
   and cumin, along with a pinch of salt. Cook the onion
   for 8–10 minutes, until softened and fragrant.

2. Stir in the beans, quinoa, chopped tomatoes, maple
   syrup, and stock. Bring to a gentle simmer and cook
   for 10 minutes.

3. Pour in the coconut milk and continue simmering for
   another 10–15 minutes, until the quinoa is tender and
   the chili is thick and creamy.

4. Add the lime juice, season to taste, and stir through
   half the cilantro.

5. Ladle into bowls and top with the remaining cilantro,
   green onions, and a wedge of lime. This is delicious
   on its own or served with avocado slices, warm
   tortillas and/or a scoop of plain yogurt.

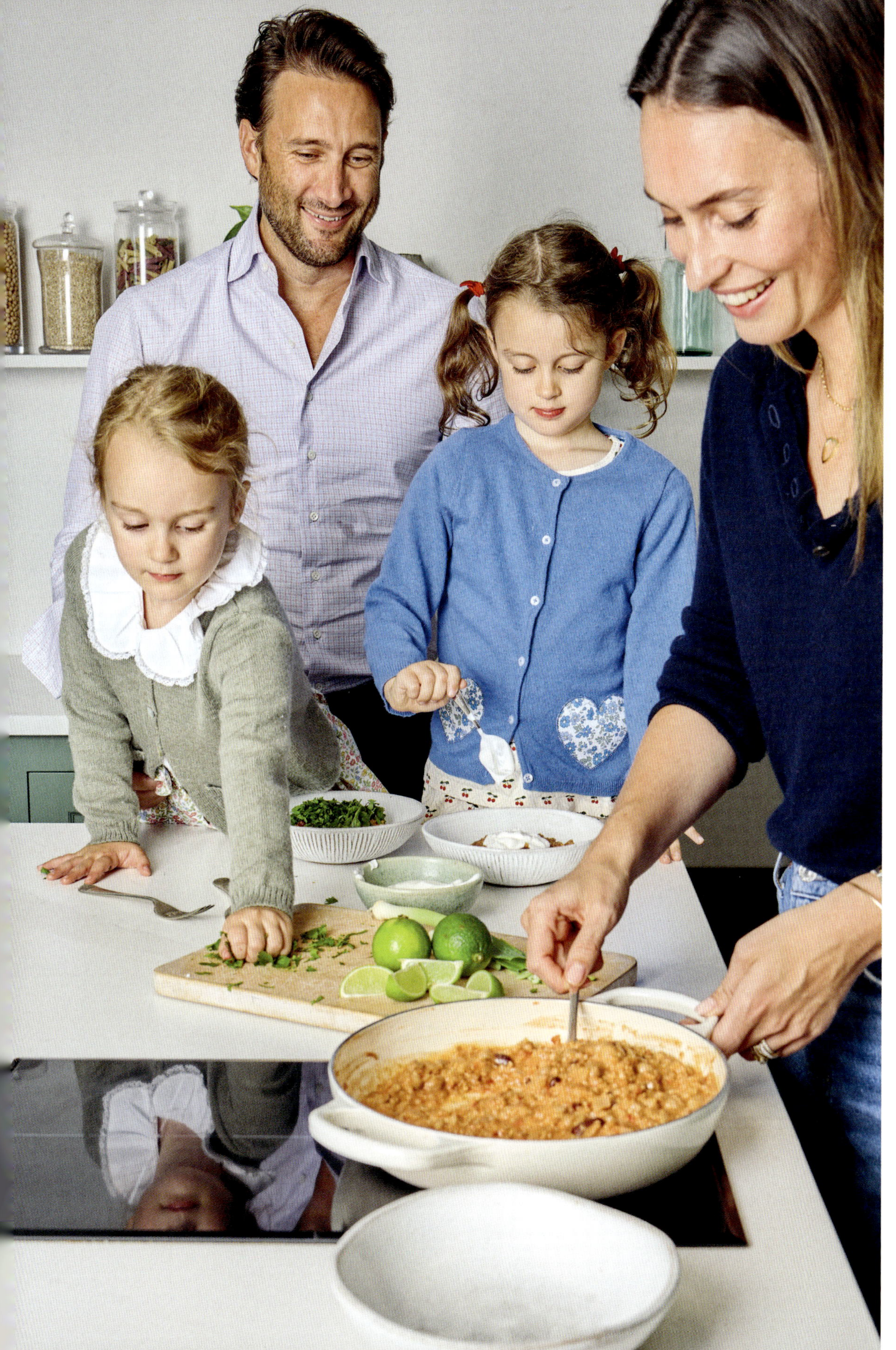

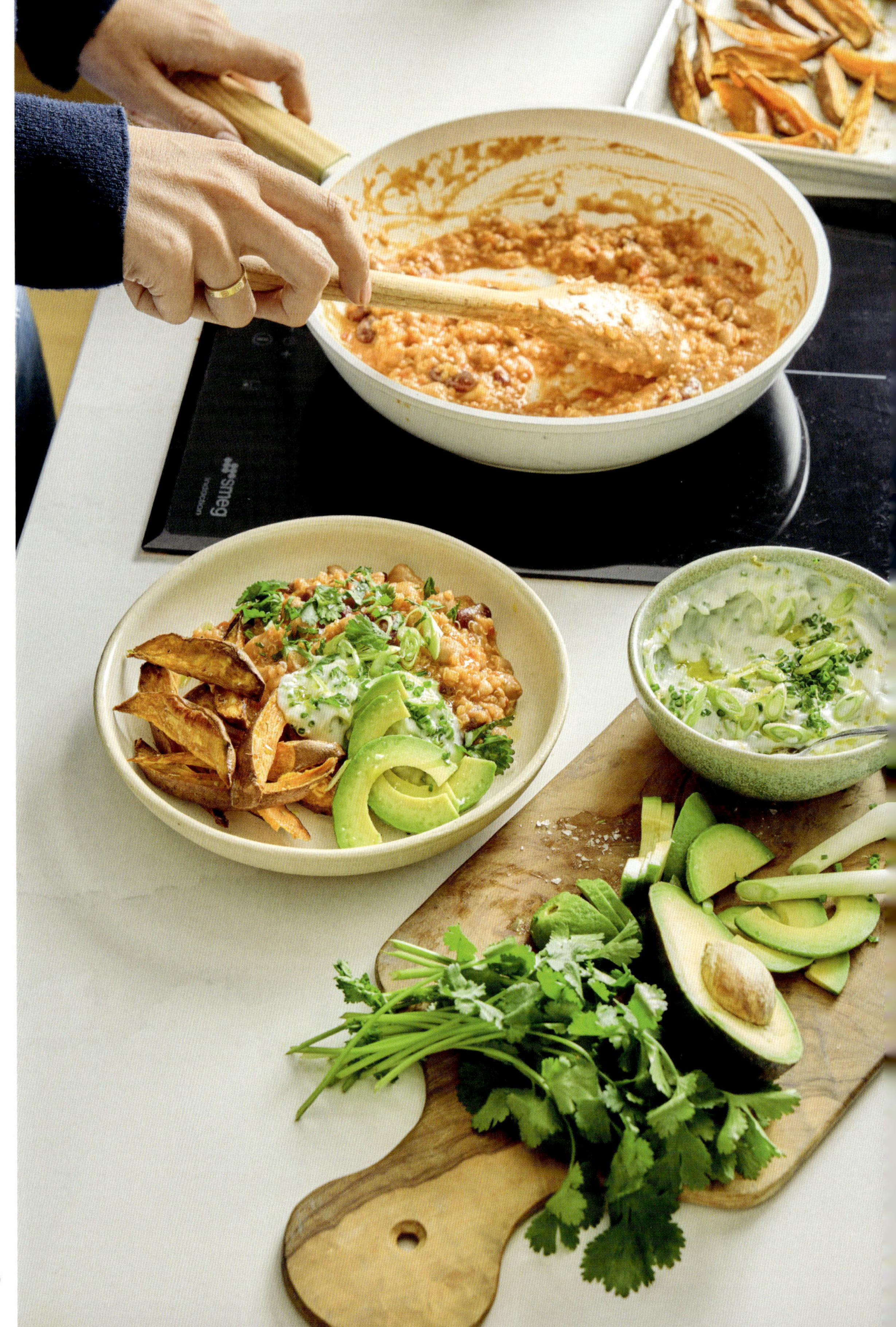

Loaded Chili Bowls with Sweet Potato Wedges

18 PLANTS

Serves 2

1 large sweet potato, peeled and
    cut into ¾ in wedges
pinch of cayenne pepper
    (optional)
olive oil
3½ oz plain yogurt
grated zest and juice of 1 lemon
1 small garlic clove, crushed
about 2–3 tablespoons chives,
    finely chopped, plus extra to
    garnish
½ bunch of green onions (about
    3 or 4), thinly sliced
1 avocado, thinly sliced
2 servings of Five-Bean and
    Quinoa Chili (see page 148)
handful of cilantro (about ½ cup),
    roughly chopped
sea salt and black pepper

This is the perfect way to transform your leftover Five-Bean Chili into something fresh and vibrant – it feels like a completely different dish with hardly any effort. The sweet potato wedges are golden and crisp around the edges, the chive yogurt is creamy and zingy, and the whole thing is piled high with herbs, avocado, and a squeeze of lemon. It's colorful, filling, and full of texture – the kind of bowl that makes leftovers feel anything but boring.

1. Preheat the oven to 350°F fan. On a large baking tray, toss together the sweet potato, cayenne pepper (if using), 1 tablespoon of olive oil, and a pinch of salt. Roast for 30–35 minutes, until tender and golden.

2. In a small bowl, mix together the yogurt, lemon zest, half of the lemon juice, garlic, chives, green onion, and season to taste. In a separate bowl, pour the remaining lemon juice over the avocado. Set both aside.

3. Gently warm up the leftover chili in a small saucepan set over a medium heat or in the microwave.

4. To serve, load two bowls with the chili, sweet potato wedges, creamy chive yogurt, and avocado. Scatter over the remaining chives and the cilantro.

Make it your own: This is delicious served with crispy tortilla chips. Swap sweet potato wedges for a baked potato. Stir a different type of bean through the chili for extra plant-points. Roast mushrooms alongside the sweet potato for extra plant-points. Swap yogurt for kefir.

Smoky Chipotle White Bean Chili

13 PLANTS

Serves 4

olive oil
4 garlic cloves, crushed
1 teaspoon cumin seeds
1 teaspoon coriander seeds,
    crushed
1 teaspoon dried oregano
2 bay leaves
1 tablespoon chipotle chili paste
1 teaspoon dried red chili flakes
2 onions, thinly sliced
2 green bell peppers, thinly sliced
1 × 20 oz jar of white beans, plus
    the stock from the jar
1 × 20 oz jar of lima beans, plus
    the stock from the jar
juice of 2 limes
sea salt

For the chipotle yogurt
4 tablespoons plain yogurt
1 teaspoon chipotle chili paste

To serve
1 avocado, thinly sliced
small handful of cilantro (about
    ⅓ cup), finely chopped

Make it your own: Serve with
some crusty bread or toasted
sourdough. Add some fresh chili
and/or green onion on top, or stir
through a handful or two
of spinach.

This is the kind of easy, flavorful dinner I turn to on cold evenings when I want something cosy and comforting but don't want to spend ages cooking. It's full of punchy flavors thanks to the garlic, coriander seeds, cumin, and chipotle, and it all comes together in one pan with very little prep. I like using jars of beans here for their thicker, creamier stock, but canned beans work too.

1. Warm 2 tablespoons of olive oil in a shallow casserole or frying pan set over a medium heat. Add the garlic, cumin, and cilantro seeds, oregano, bay leaves, chipotle paste, and chili flakes. Cook for 1–2 minutes, until fragrant.

2. Add the onion, peppers, and a pinch of salt. Cook for 15–20 minutes, stirring frequently, until softened and deeply golden.

3. Stir in both the beans, along with the stock from their jars and 14 fl oz of water, then bring to a simmer and cook for 15–20 minutes, stirring frequently, until slightly reduced.

4. Meanwhile, in a small bowl, combine the yogurt and chipotle paste, then set aside.

5. Remove the pan from the heat, stir in the lime juice and season to taste. Serve with the chipotle yogurt, avocado, and cilantro.

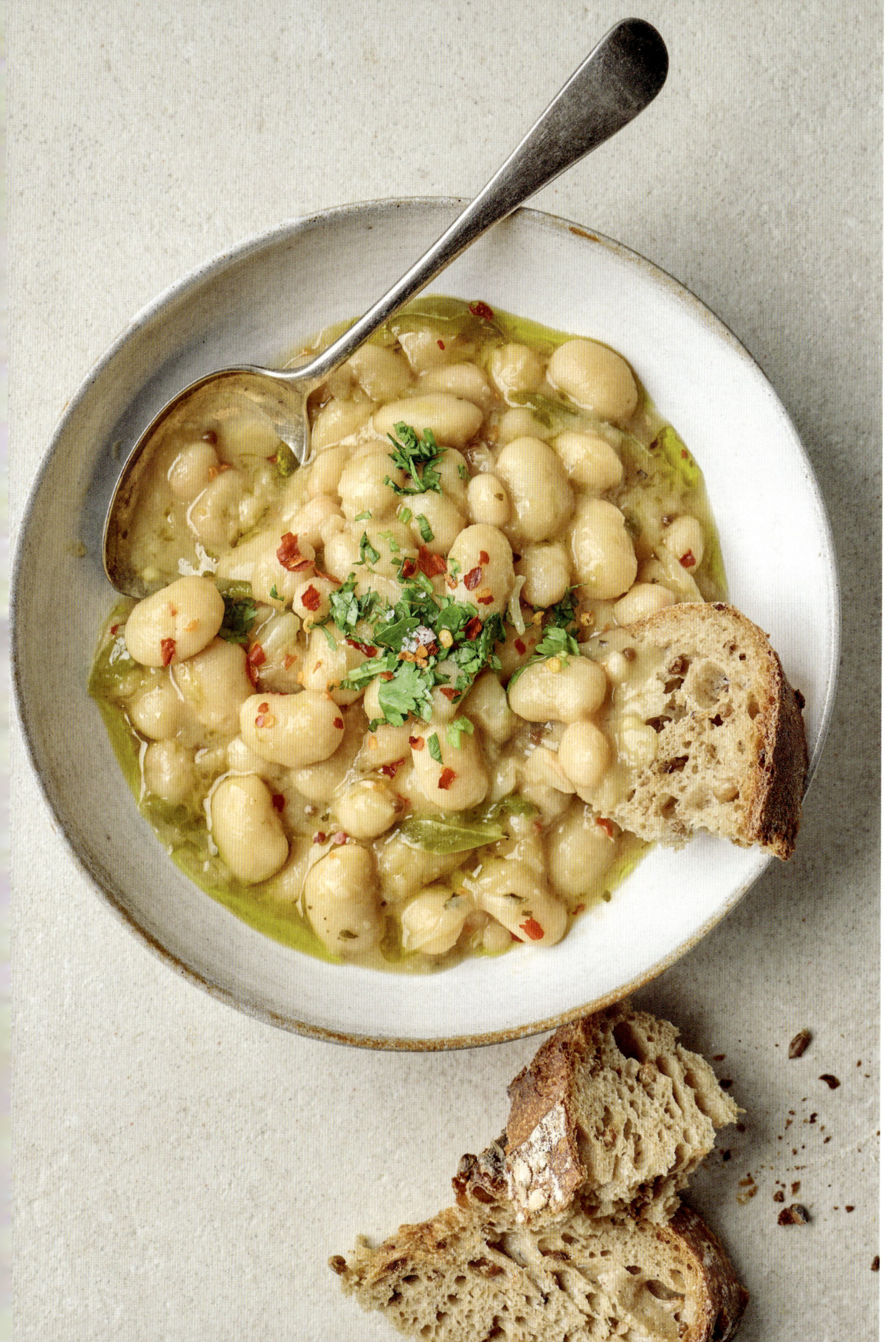

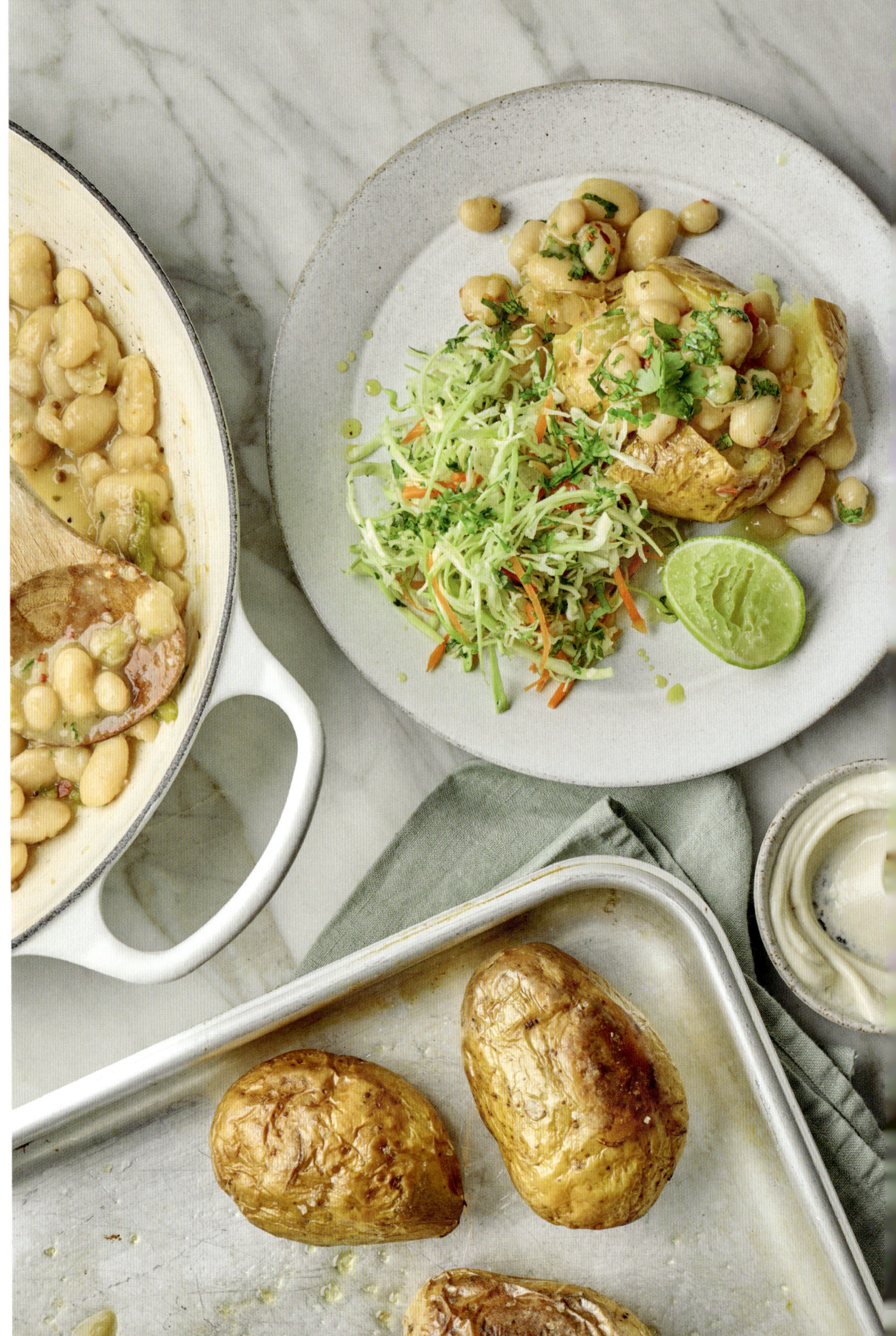

Bean Chili with Baked Potatoes and Tahini Slaw

17 PLANTS

Serves 2

2 baking potatoes
olive oil
2 servings of Smoky Chipotle
   White Bean Chili (see page
   152)
sea salt and black pepper

For the slaw

1 large carrot, julienned or
   coarsely grated
½ small white cabbage,
   shredded
1 tablespoon tahini
1 tablespoon plain yogurt
1 teaspoon Dijon mustard
1 tablespoon extra virgin olive oil
½ garlic clove, crushed
handful of cilantro (about ½ cup),
   roughly chopped, plus extra to
   serve

Topping baked potatoes is a comforting, delicious way to use your leftover Smoky Chipotle Chili. I love how the creamy slaw balances the smoky chili.

1. Preheat the oven to 350°F fan. Wash the potatoes, then prick them all over with a fork.

2. For speedy microwave baked potatoes, place on a microwave-safe plate and cook on full power for 4 minutes. Carefully turn the potatoes over – they will be hot! Cook for another 4 minutes, then push a knife into the center to check if they're tender – it should slide in easily and the potato should feel soft in the middle. If the potatoes are not quite cooked, flip them over and continue to cook in 1–2-minute bursts. To finish in the oven, rub a little olive oil into the skins and sprinkle with salt. Cook for 10–15 minutes until the skins are crisp and golden.

3. For oven-cooked potatoes, rub a little olive oil and a pinch of salt into the skins. Place directly on the middle shelf of the oven (or use a baking sheet) and cook for about 1 hour, until crisp on the outside and tender in the middle.

4. To make the slaw, toss the carrot, cabbage, and a pinch of salt in a bowl. In a separate bowl, whisk together the tahini, yogurt, mustard, olive oil, garlic, a pinch of salt, and 1 tablespoon of water to loosen – it should be the consistency of single cream. Stir through the vegetables and cilantro.

5. When the potatoes have about 10–15 minutes left, reheat the chili in a saucepan set over a medium heat. Serve the baked potatoes topped with the chili, the extra cilantro, and a generous serving of slaw alongside.

Lima Bean and Carrot Soup with Ginger and Turmeric

7 PLANTS

Serves 4

olive oil, plus extra to serve
2 garlic cloves, roughly chopped
small chunk of fresh ginger
    root (about 1 in), peeled and
    roughly chopped
1 red onion, roughly chopped
4 carrots (about 2 cups), roughly
    chopped into ¾ in chunks
1 tablespoon tomato purée
1 × 14 oz can of plum tomatoes
2 teaspoons ground turmeric
1 × 14 oz can of lima beans,
    drained and rinsed
17 fl oz hot vegetable stock
sea salt and black pepper

This is a no-fuss, one-pan wonder packed with warming spices, sweet carrots, creamy lima beans, and a good hit of ginger and turmeric to help you feel your best. Blend it until smooth or keep it chunky, depending on your mood, and finish with a drizzle of olive oil or a handful of crunchy toppings.

1. Warm a drizzle of olive oil in a large saucepan set over a medium–low heat. Add the garlic and ginger and cook for 2–3 minutes until fragrant.

2. Add the remaining ingredients and 1 teaspoon of salt. Bring to the boil, then turn down the heat and simmer for 20 minutes, until the carrots have softened.

3. Blitz with a stick blender until smooth. Season to taste and serve with an extra drizzle of oil and a crack of black pepper.

Make it your own: Serve with a sprinkling of mixed seeds, croutons (see page 102), or crunchy chickpeas. You could also add a dollop of yogurt on top, or some chili in the soup to make it extra creamy or spicy.

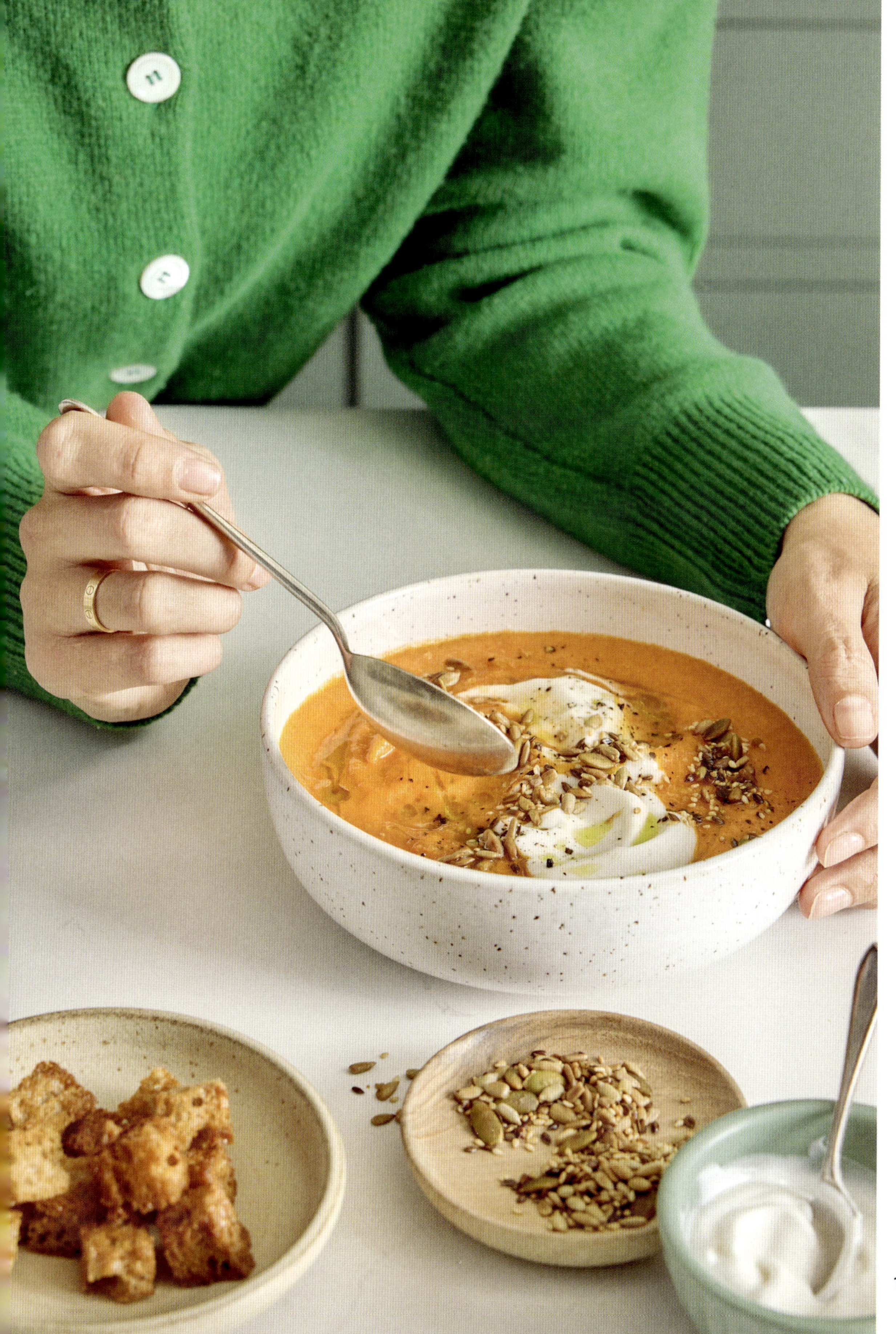

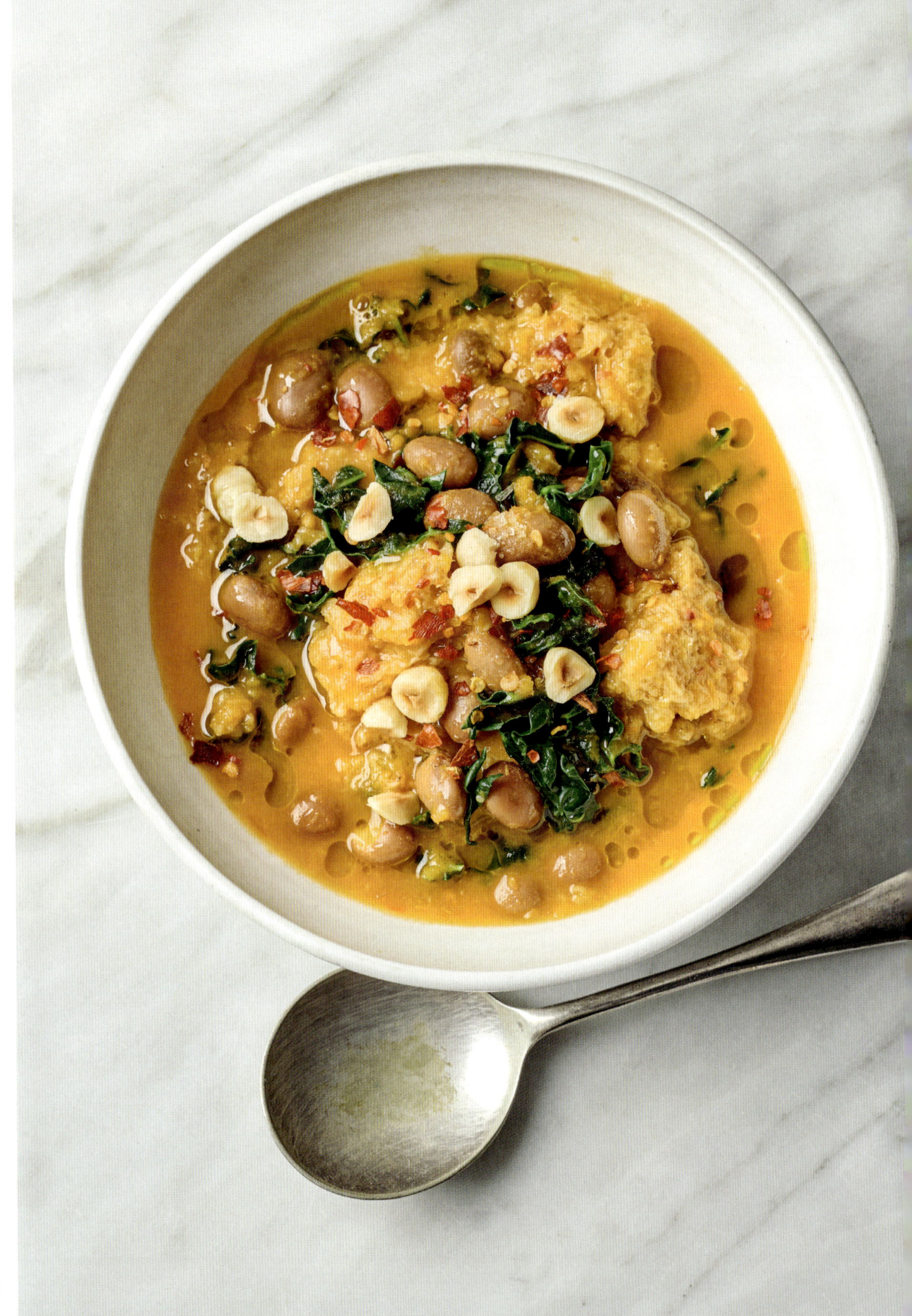

Hearty Lima Bean Soup with Cavolo Nero and Hazelnuts

10 PLANTS

Serves 2

2 servings of Lima Bean and
  Carrot Soup with Ginger and
  Turmeric (see page 156)
1 × 14 oz can of borlotti beans (or
  use cannellini beans), drained
  and rinsed
2 handfuls of cavolo nero (about
  1½ cups), sliced
2 thick slices of stale bread, cut
  into 1 in chunks
handful of hazelnuts (about
  ⅓ cup), roughly chopped
dried red chili flakes
extra virgin olive oil, to finish

Borlotti beans, cavolo nero, and crusty bread simmer in your leftover soup to create a nourishing bowl of goodness that's ready in minutes.

1. Pour the leftover soup into a saucepan set over a medium–high heat, add 14 fl oz of water and bring to a simmer.

2. Stir in the beans, cavolo nero, and bread. Simmer for 5 minutes, until the cavolo nero is cooked and the bread is soft and has soaked up the flavors.

3. To serve, divide the soup between bowls. Scatter over the hazelnuts, add a pinch of chili flakes, and a generous drizzle of extra virgin olive oil.

Make it your own: Scatter over basil. Swap the hazelnuts for walnuts or pine nuts.

Cauliflower and Coconut Curry with Lemony Rice

10 PLANTS

**Serves 4
(the rice only serves 2)**

1 small cauliflower (about
8 cups), cut into bite-sized
florets
1 red onion, cut into ¾ in slices
1⅓ cups green beans, trimmed
small chunk of fresh ginger root
(about 1 in), peeled and cut
into thin matchsticks
3 garlic cloves, thinly sliced
1 teaspoon cumin seeds
1 teaspoon mustard seeds
1 teaspoon fennel seeds
1 teaspoon ground turmeric
pinch of dried chili flakes
olive oil
generous cup of cherry
tomatoes, halved
1 × 14 fl oz can of coconut milk
juice of ½ lemon (you use the
rind in the rice)
sea salt and black pepper

For the lemony rice
½ cup basmati rice, rinsed
½ lemon, the rind peeled off in
large strips using a vegetable
peeler
7 fl oz boiling water

Make it your own: Top the
bowls with toasted coconut
flakes, add cilantro for flavor and
freshness, or stir chickpeas and
tofu through the curry with the
coconut milk for protein.

Cauliflower has always been one of my favorite veggies, and it really comes into its own in this curry, alongside the delicious lemony rice. Swap the green beans for any other quick-cook greens you have in your fridge.

1. The rice only makes two portions, so if you're not batch cooking this and are serving it for four, you'll need to double the rice quantity.

2. Preheat the oven to 420°F fan. On a very large baking tray (it needs to be large enough to hold the veg in a single layer), toss together the cauliflower, onion, green beans, ginger, garlic, cumin seeds, mustard seeds, fennel seeds, turmeric, chili flakes, 1 teaspoon of salt, and 2 tablespoons of olive oil.

3. Roast for 20–25 minutes, adding the cherry tomatoes for the final 15 minutes, until the veg are tender and charred.

4. To make the rice, put the rice, lemon rind, a pinch of salt and the boiling water into a shallow roasting tin or oven-proof dish. Cover tightly with foil and place in the oven. Cook for 15 minutes until all the water has been absorbed. Set aside to steam for 5 minutes, or until the curry is ready, and fluff through with a fork before serving.

5. To finish the curry, remove the tray of vegetables from the oven and stir in the coconut milk. Return to the oven and roast for another 5–10 minutes, until bubbling and golden. Season to taste and stir in the lemon juice.

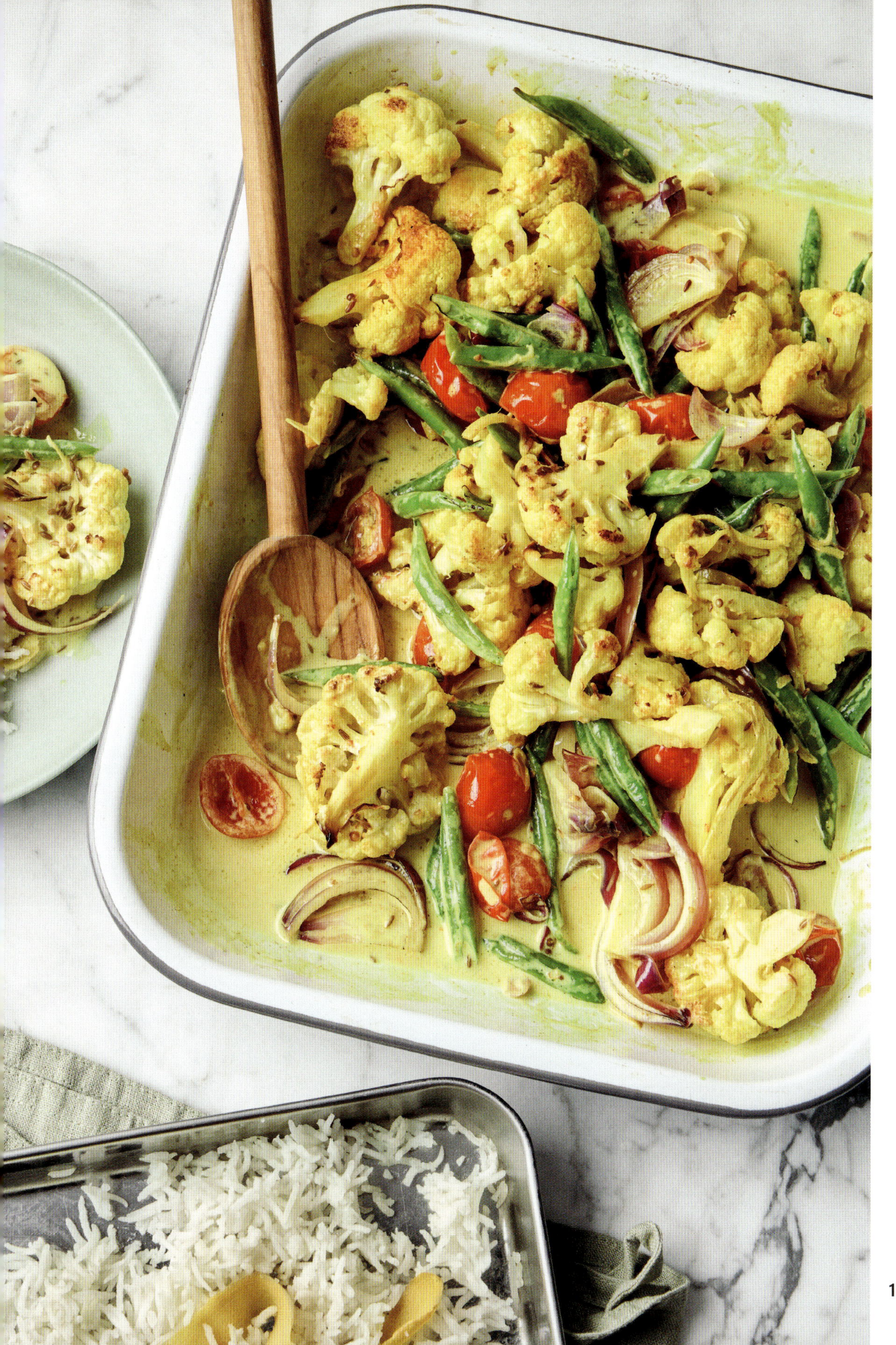

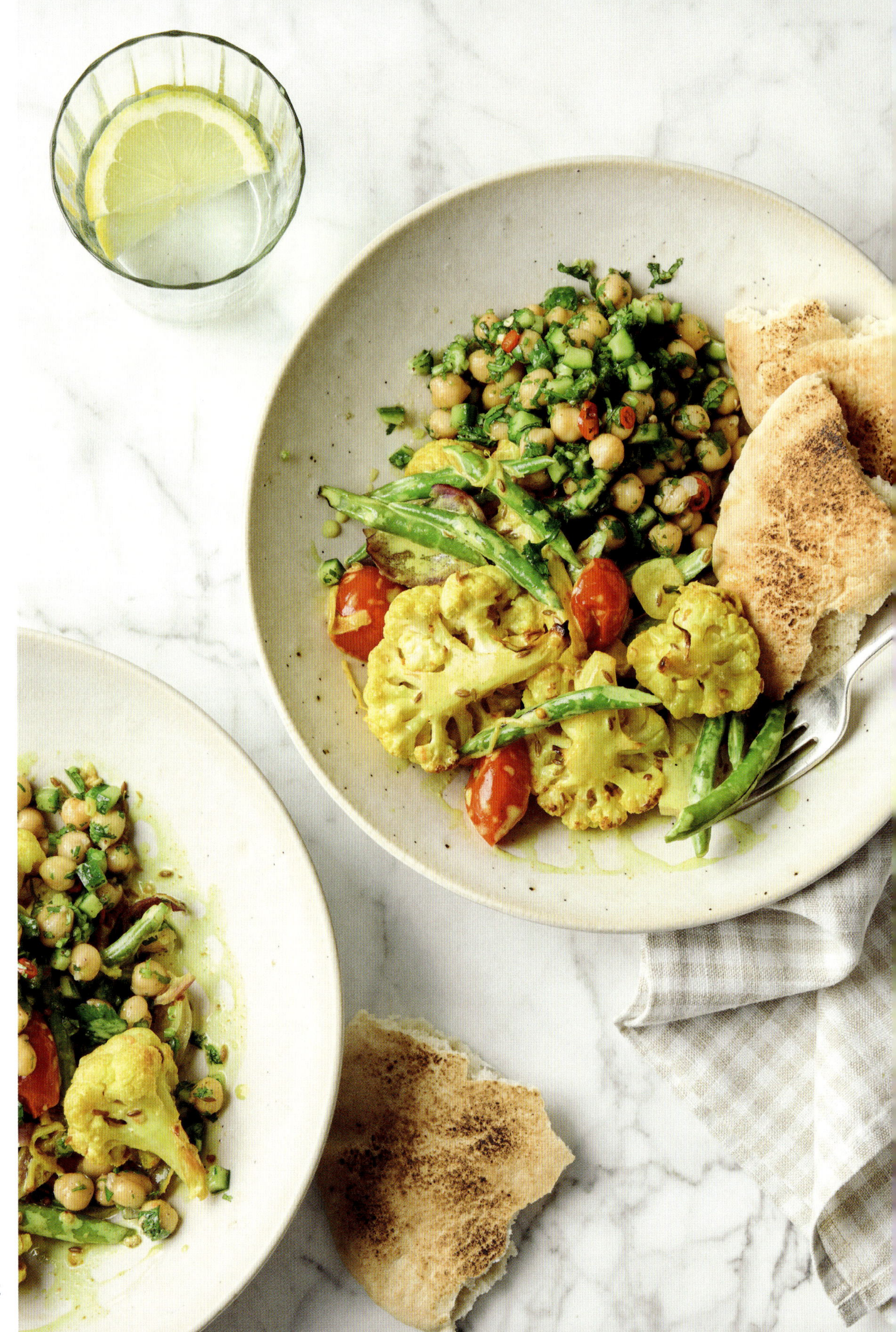

Cauliflower Curry with Chickpea Salad and Toasted Pitta

14 PLANTS

Serves 2

2 servings of Cauliflower and
  Coconut Curry (see page 160)
½ cucumber, deseeded and
  diced
1 × 14 oz can of chickpeas
  (or use 1 × 20 oz jar), drained
  and rinsed
handful of cilantro (about 1 cup),
  roughly chopped
1 bird's eye chili, finely chopped
pinch of sumac (optional)
olive oil
sea salt
2 pitta breads, toasted, to serve

For a quick second serving, try your creamy cauliflower curry with a delicious chickpea, chili, and cucumber salad with cilantro, lots of olive oil, and toasted pitta breads. It all comes together in a matter of minutes, helping you get a nourishing, no-fuss dinner on the table at the end of a busy day.

1. Gently reheat the curry in a small saucepan until bubbling.

2. To make the salad, simply combine the cucumber, chickpeas, cilantro, chili, sumac (if using), 1 tablespoon of olive oil, and a pinch of salt in a bowl.

3. To serve, divide the curry between bowls and serve with the chickpea salad and toasted pitta.

This chapter is packed with nourishing recipes that you can throw together in minutes, whether it's to make a quick breakfast before work or something delicious to take on-the-go or have as a mid-afternoon snack. They're easy recipes that will keep you feeling fueled without any fuss.

SIMPLE SNACKS AND BREAKFASTS

Blueberry Overnight Oats

———

Fruity Breakfast Muffins

———

Maple and Almond
Oaty Bites

———

Quick Crunchy Pickled Veggies

Plant-Point Granola

———

10-Minute Banana
Pancakes

———

Plant-Point
Trail Mix

Coffee Overnight Oats

———

Date, Banana, and Peanut Butter
Freezer Bites

———

Sun-Dried Tomato and White
Bean Dip

———

Miso Hummus

Blueberry Overnight Oats

6 PLANTS

Serves 2

1¼ cups rolled oats

14 fl oz oat or almond milk, plus extra to serve

¾ cup frozen blueberries

1 large banana, sliced

1 tablespoon peanut butter (use smooth or crunchy)

1 tablespoon chia seeds

2 tablespoons shelled hemp seeds

2 tablespoons plain yogurt

These overnight oats are creamy, full of goodness, and so easy: just stir everything together in the evening, and you'll have a nourishing, delicious breakfast waiting for you the next morning. My kids love them too, so I usually double the quantity to help make chaotic mornings feel a little calmer.

1. In a large bowl or jar, mix all the ingredients together, making sure that the peanut butter is fully dispersed. Stir well, then cover and refrigerate overnight.

2. In the morning, stir the oats, then add a splash of milk, if needed. Enjoy topped with extra peanut butter or a sprinkle of hemp seeds if you like.

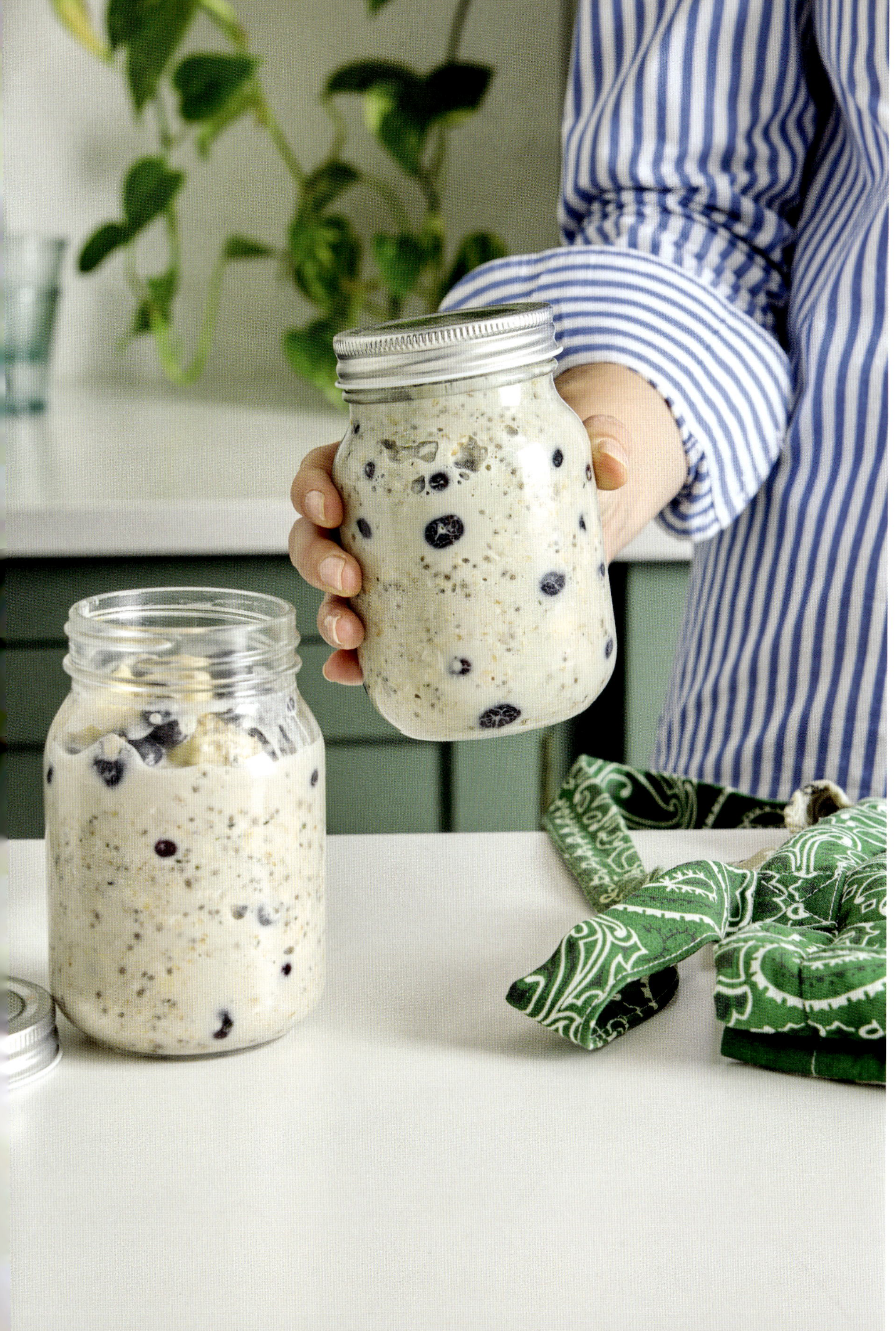

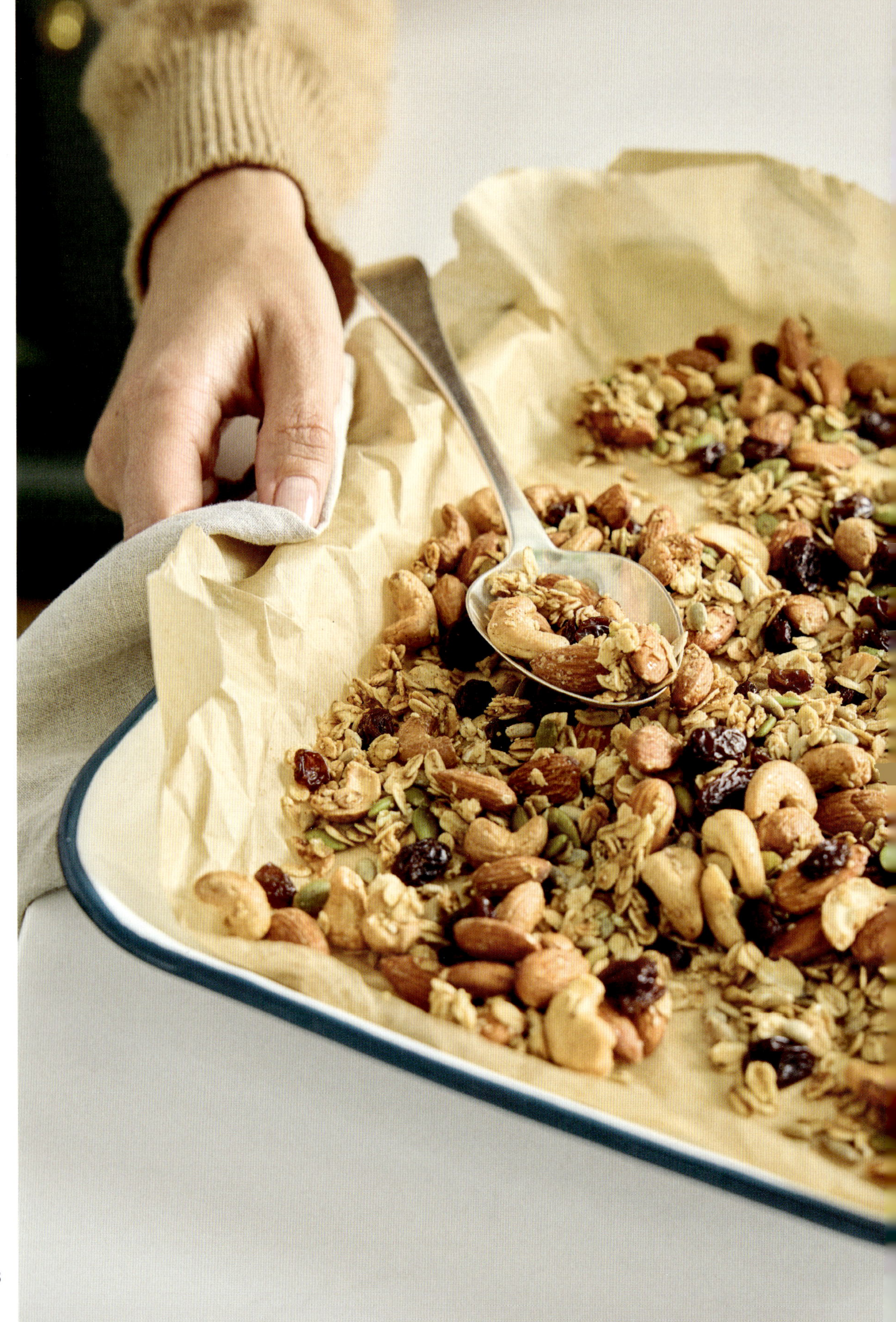

Plant–Point Granola

7 PLANTS

Fills a 50 fl oz jar (about 10-12 servings)

3¼ cups rolled oats
generous ½ cup sunflower seeds
generous ½ cup pumpkin seeds
1½ cups almonds
1½ cups cashews
½ tablespoon ground cinnamon
2 tablespoons olive oil
3½ fl oz maple syrup
pinch of sea salt (optional)
½ cup raisins

Golden, crunchy, and naturally sweetened with maple syrup, this delicious homemade granola is the easiest way to get lots of plants into your morning. I love it with creamy yogurt, fresh fruit, or just straight from the jar (trust me, it won't last long!).

1. Preheat the oven to 325°F fan. Line a large baking tray with baking parchment paper.

2. Put the oats, sunflower seeds, pumpkin seeds, almonds, cashews, cinnamon, olive oil, maple syrup, and sea salt (if using) into a large mixing bowl. Stir well until everything is coated, then tip the mix on to the baking tray.

3. Bake for 20–25 minutes, stirring halfway through, until the nuts and oats are golden.

4. Remove from the oven and let it cool before stirring in the raisins. The oats will get crunchier and crunchier as it cools.

5. Once the granola has cooled to room temperature, pour it into an airtight container; it will keep for weeks (but you'll finish it long before it stops being delicious!).

Make it your own: Add any leftover nuts and seeds, such as walnuts, pecans, and hazelnuts. You could also swap oats for rye flakes, spelt flakes etc.

Coffee Overnight Oats

Serves 2

1¼ cups rolled oats

10 fl oz oat or almond milk

1–2 shots of espresso (or 4 teaspoons instant coffee dissolved in a little hot water)

1 tablespoon almond butter

2 tablespoons plain yogurt

2 dates, roughly chopped

2 tablespoons shelled hemp seeds

1 teaspoon maple syrup (optional)

If you love coffee, you'll adore these overnight oats. They're a brilliant way to get your morning coffee fix while packing in fiber, healthy fats, and plant protein too. I usually make a batch of these just for me, while the kids stick to the blueberry version (see page 166), which keeps everyone happy and makes busy mornings a little easier.

1. In a large bowl or jar, mix all of the ingredients together, making sure that the almond butter is fully dispersed. Stir well, then cover and refrigerate overnight.

2. In the morning, stir then add a splash of milk, if needed, and enjoy the oats topped with extra almond butter or a sprinkle of hemp seeds if you like.

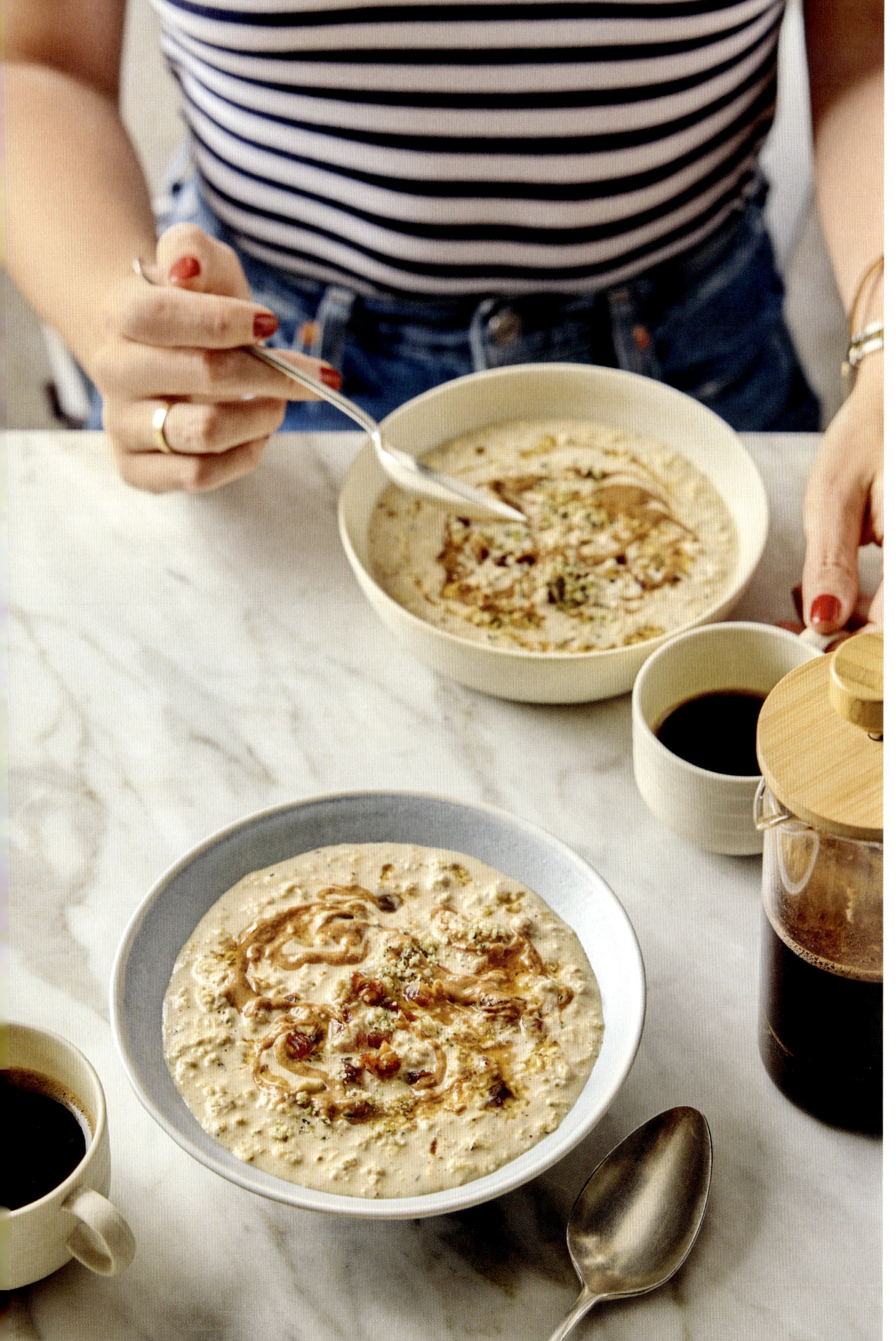

Fruity Breakfast Muffins

Makes 12

2 red apples or pears
1½ cups plain flour
1½ tsp baking powder
pinch of salt
½ cup rolled oats
½ teaspoon baking soda
½ teaspoon ground cinnamon
3 ripe bananas
3 tablespoons coconut milk
3 tablespoons coconut oil,
  melted
3 tablespoons maple syrup

These muffins are full of simple, nourishing ingredients. They're perfect for breakfast, as a snack, or whenever you fancy something a little bit cosy. I love them warm from the oven with a drizzle of nut butter on top, and they never last long in our house, so I usually make a double batch.

1. Preheat the oven to 325°F fan. Line a 12-hole muffin tray with paper cases.

2. Core one apple and cut it into small cubes. Set aside.

3. Sift the flour into a large bowl with the baking powder and a pinch of salt, then mix in the oats, baking soda and cinnamon.

4. In a separate bowl, mash the bananas until smooth, then stir in the coconut milk, coconut oil, and maple syrup. Combine the wet and dry ingredients, then fold in the apple cubes. Mix well and pour the batter into the muffin cases.

5. Cut the remaining apple into thin slices and place three slices on top of each muffin. Bake for 20–25 minutes, until golden and a knife inserted into the center comes out clean. Cool in the tray for 10 minutes, then transfer to a wire rack to cool completely or enjoy warm.

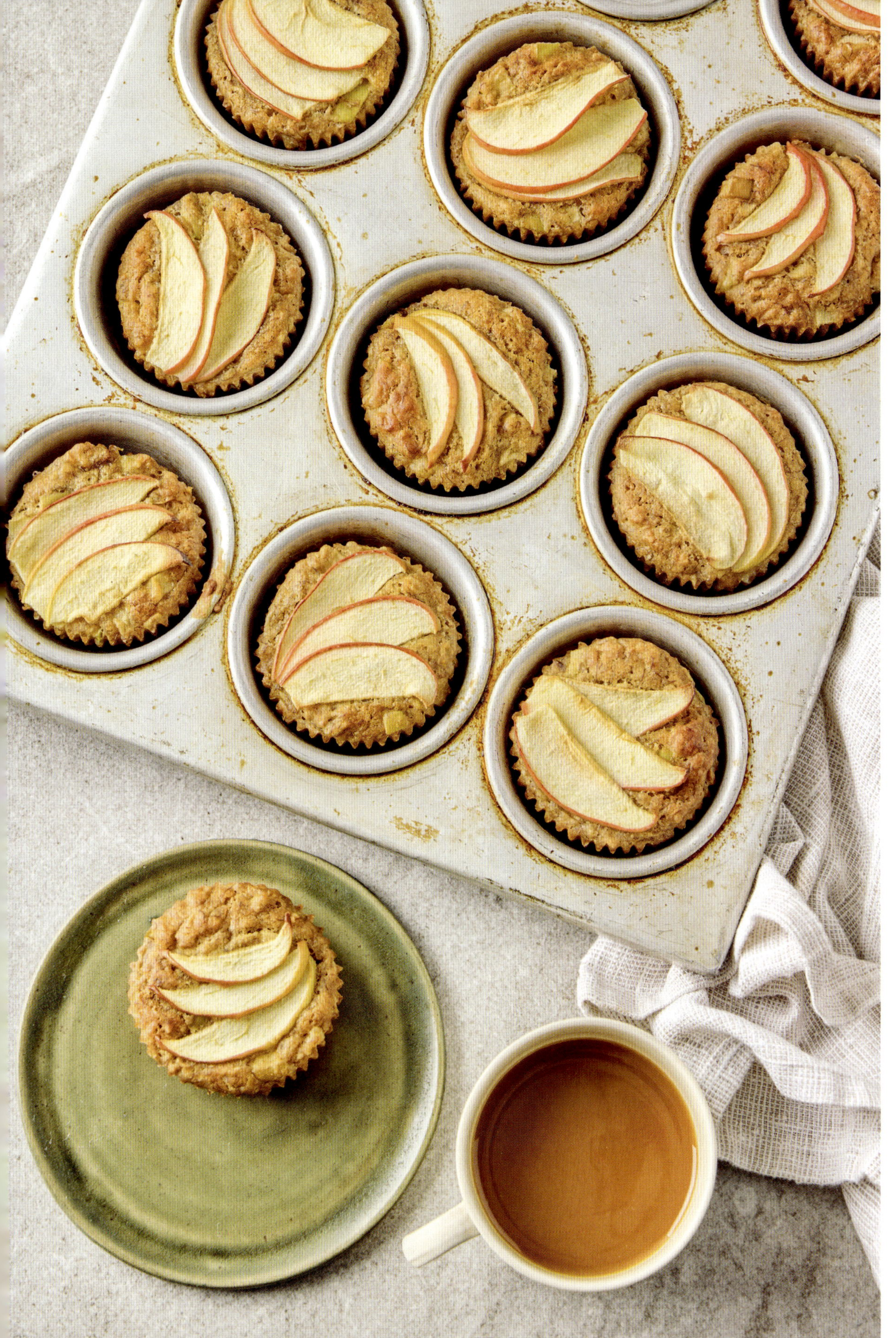

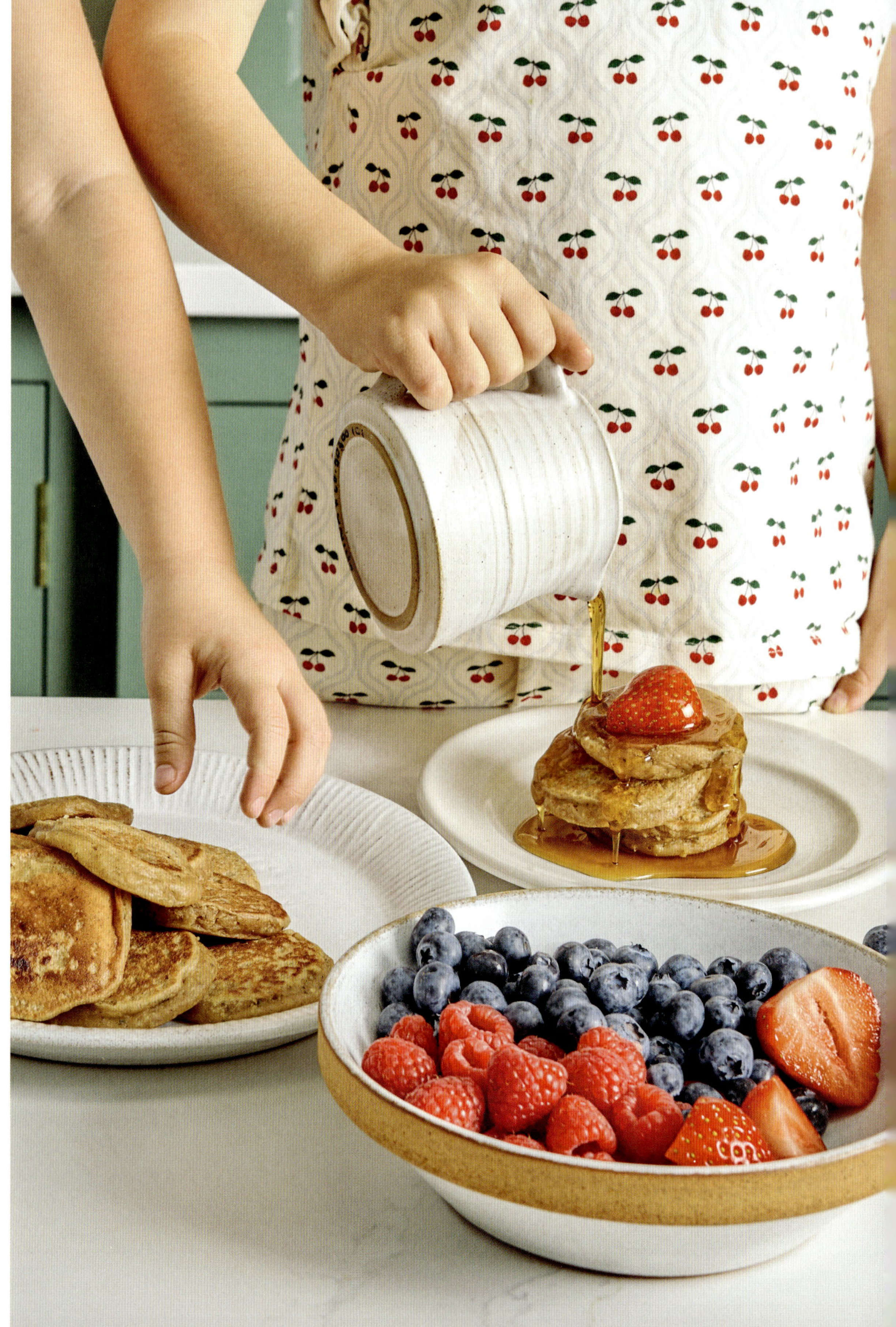

10-Minute Banana Pancakes

Serves 4 (makes about 16 mini pancakes)

1 small ripe banana
1 tablespoon smooth peanut
   butter
¼ cup rolled oats
¼ cup plain flour
¼ tsp baking powder
pinch of salt
1 tablespoon shelled hemp seeds
2½ fl oz almond or oat milk
1 tablespoon olive oil
1 tablespoon maple syrup
   (optional)
coconut oil, for frying
sea salt

To serve (optional)
maple syrup
nut butter
berries or other fresh fruit
plain yogurt

These little pancakes are naturally sweet, soft in the middle, and full of goodness. They make the perfect breakfast or snack, with just the right balance of sweetness and satisfaction. The batter is a little sticky, so make sure to grease your pan well and you'll get golden, fluffy pancakes every time.

1. Place the banana, peanut butter, oats, flour, baking powder, hemp seeds, milk, olive oil, and maple syrup, plus a tiny pinch of salt, in a small food processor or mini chopper and blitz for 2–3 minutes until you have a smooth batter.

2. Heat a little coconut oil in a non-stick frying pan set over a medium heat. Once warm, add a tablespoon of batter for each pancake, gently spreading it into circles with your spoon – you want them to be about 2 in wide. Cook for 2–2 ½ minutes on each side, flipping once you see little holes appearing all over the batter.

3. Serve immediately, either plain or with a drizzle of maple syrup, some nut butter, fresh fruit, yogurt, or anything else that takes your fancy!

Note: You do need a good non-stick pan for these, as the batter can be a bit sticky.

Date, Banana, and Peanut Butter Freezer Bites

4 PLANTS

Makes 12–16 (depending on size)

18 Medjool dates (about 2¼ cups), pitted and halved
4 heaped tablespoons smooth, spreadable peanut butter (or swap for another nut butter)
2 ripe bananas, thinly sliced
5 oz dark chocolate (70 percent cocoa solids or more)
pinch of flaky sea salt (optional)

I am obsessed with these. They started as a viral trend on social media and I wasn't sure if they'd live up to the hype, but they most definitely do and I've been making them on repeat for over a year! They're the easiest, most delicious way to get more fiber into your day, naturally sweet, and so satisfying: chewy dates, creamy nut butter, and soft banana slices, all coated in a rich layer of dark chocolate with a sprinkle of sea salt. They taste like dessert but are packed with goodness – perfect straight from the freezer when you need a little sweet fix.

1. Line a small, freezer-friendly baking tray with baking parchment paper.

2. Press the dates on to the paper to form one even layer – I do mine in about five rows with the dates just touching each other.

3. Spread or drizzle the nut butter gently over the dates using a spoon, then layer the banana slices on top.

4. Gently melt the dark chocolate in the microwave set to a low power, or in a heatproof bowl set above a pan of simmering water (don't let the bowl touch the water). Pour it over the banana and spread evenly.

5. Freeze for at least 1 hour, then sprinkle over a pinch of flaky sea salt (if using), slice, and enjoy!

To store: Keep the slices in the freezer.

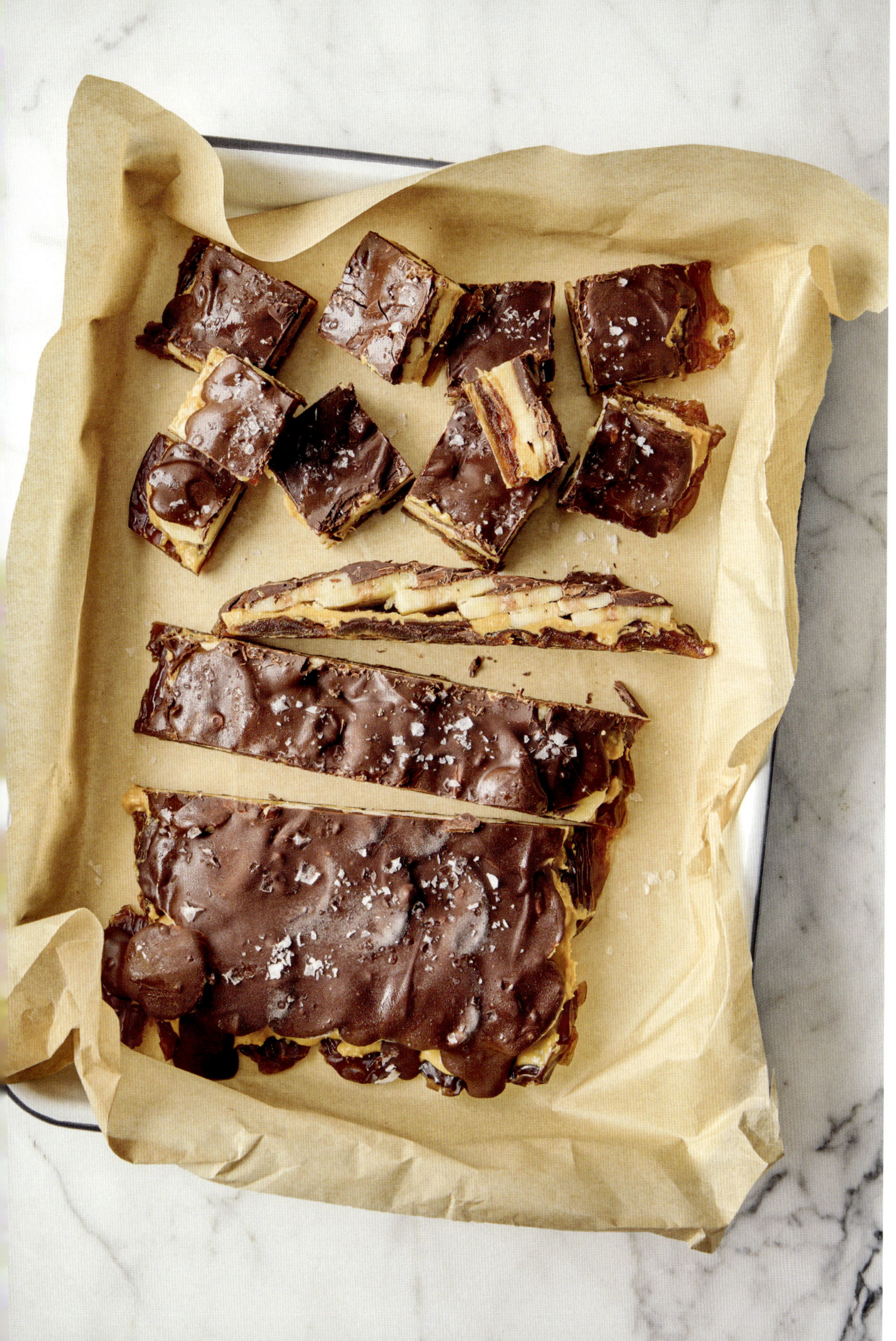

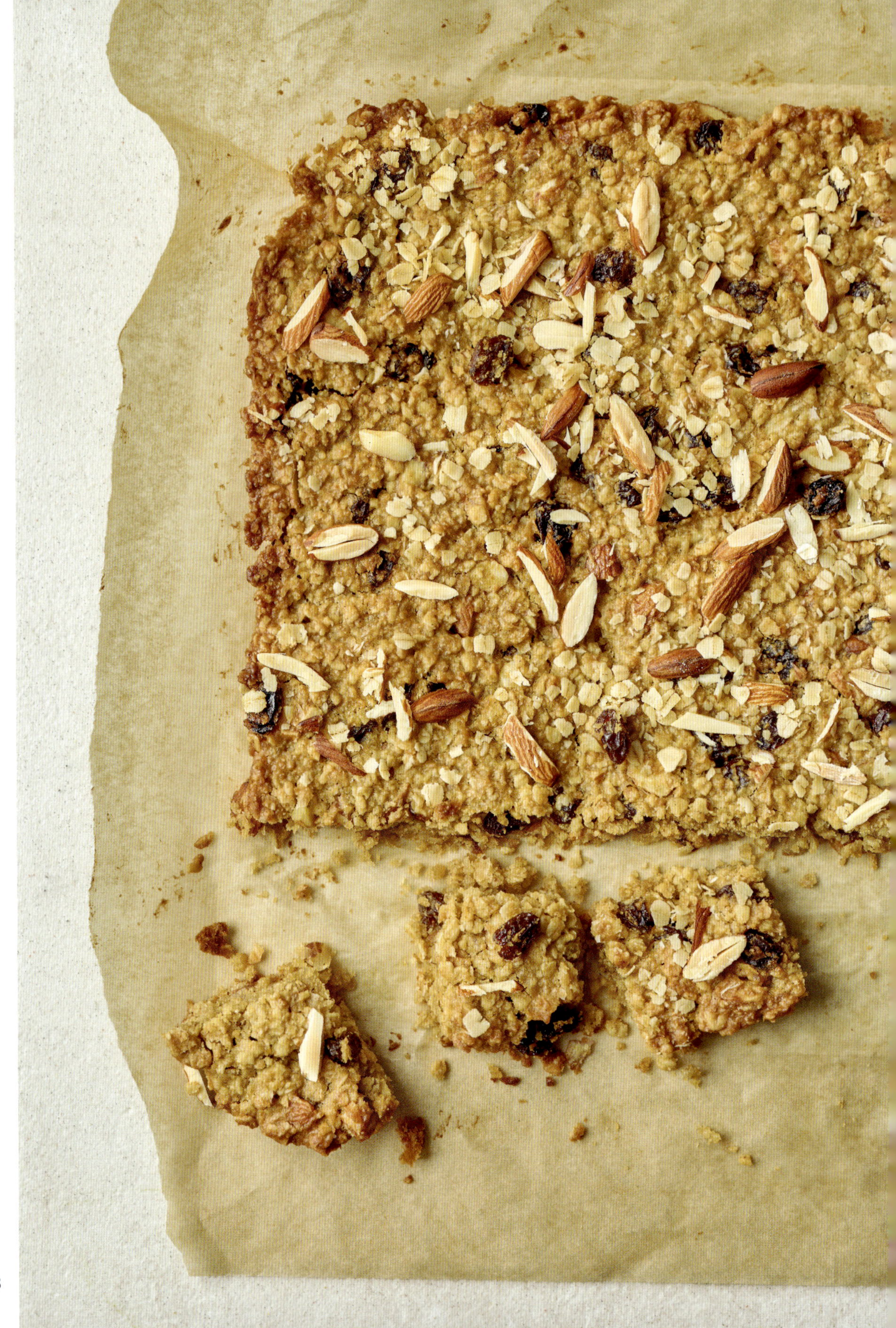

Maple and Almond
Oaty Bites

6 PLANTS

Makes 16 bites

6 tablespoons olive oil, plus extra
  for greasing the tin
1 × 14 oz can of chickpeas,
  drained and rinsed
3½ fl oz maple syrup
½ teaspoon ground cinnamon
2 tablespoons smooth peanut
  butter
1¼ cups rolled oats, plus an extra
  handful to finish
1 cup almonds, roughly chopped
½ cup raisins
sea salt

These are such a great snack to have for busy weeks. They feel like a treat, but they're packed with goodness. I know adding the chickpeas sounds strange, but it helps create the soft, chewy texture, and you can't taste them alongside the oats, maple syrup, and nut butter.

1. Preheat the oven to 350°F fan. Use a little olive oil to grease a 8 × 8 in brownie tin and line it with baking parchment paper.

2. Put the chickpeas, olive oil, maple syrup, cinnamon, peanut butter, oats, and a pinch of salt into a food processor and blitz until smooth.

3. Tip the mixture into a bowl and stir through the almonds and raisins. Transfer to the brownie tin, pressing it into the corners and flattening with the back of a spoon, so it's firm and even. Scatter over the extra handful of oats.

4. Bake for 25 minutes, until golden, then leave to cool completely in the tin before lifting out and slicing into 16 squares (if you don't let them cool completely they may crack).

Make it your own: Swap almonds for hazelnuts and/or peanut butter for almond butter. You can also add chunks of dark chocolate.

Plant-Point Trail Mix

Fills a 1.5L jar

1½ cups almonds
1½ cups pecans or cashews
¾ cup pumpkin seeds
¾ cup sunflower seeds
1½ cups coconut flakes
½ teaspoon ground ginger
 (optional)
2 tablespoons olive oil
2 tablespoons maple syrup
pinch of sea salt
1¼ cups raisins or halved dried
 apricots (or use a mix of both!)

This is my go-to for an easy snack or something to scatter over breakfast bowls. It's crunchy, with the perfect amount of sweetness. Plus, it's such a great way to up your plant points. You can add or substitute any nuts and seeds you already have in your cupboard.

1. Preheat the oven to 325°F fan. Line a large baking tray with baking parchment paper.

2. Add the almonds, pecans, pumpkin seeds, sunflower seeds, coconut flakes, ground ginger (if using), olive oil, maple syrup, and sea salt to a large bowl. Mix together until evenly combined, then pour on to the baking tray and spread out.

3. Bake for 15–20 minutes, stirring halfway through, until everything has a deep golden color.

4. Remove from the oven and let the trail mix cool completely, then stir in the raisins. Store in an airtight container; it will keep for up to a week.

Make it your own: You could also add dried cherries, cranberries, mulberries, dried mango, or cacao nibs.

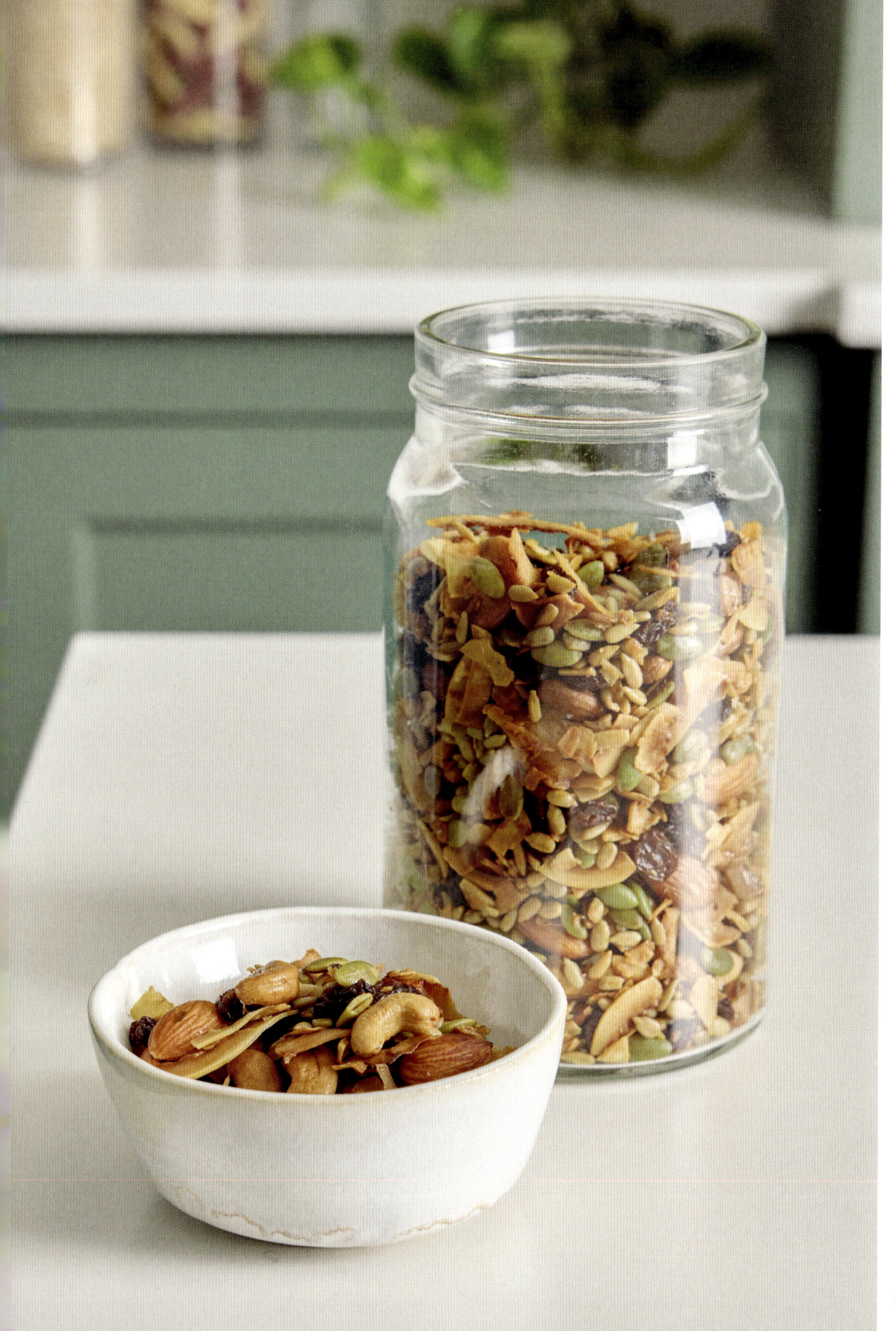

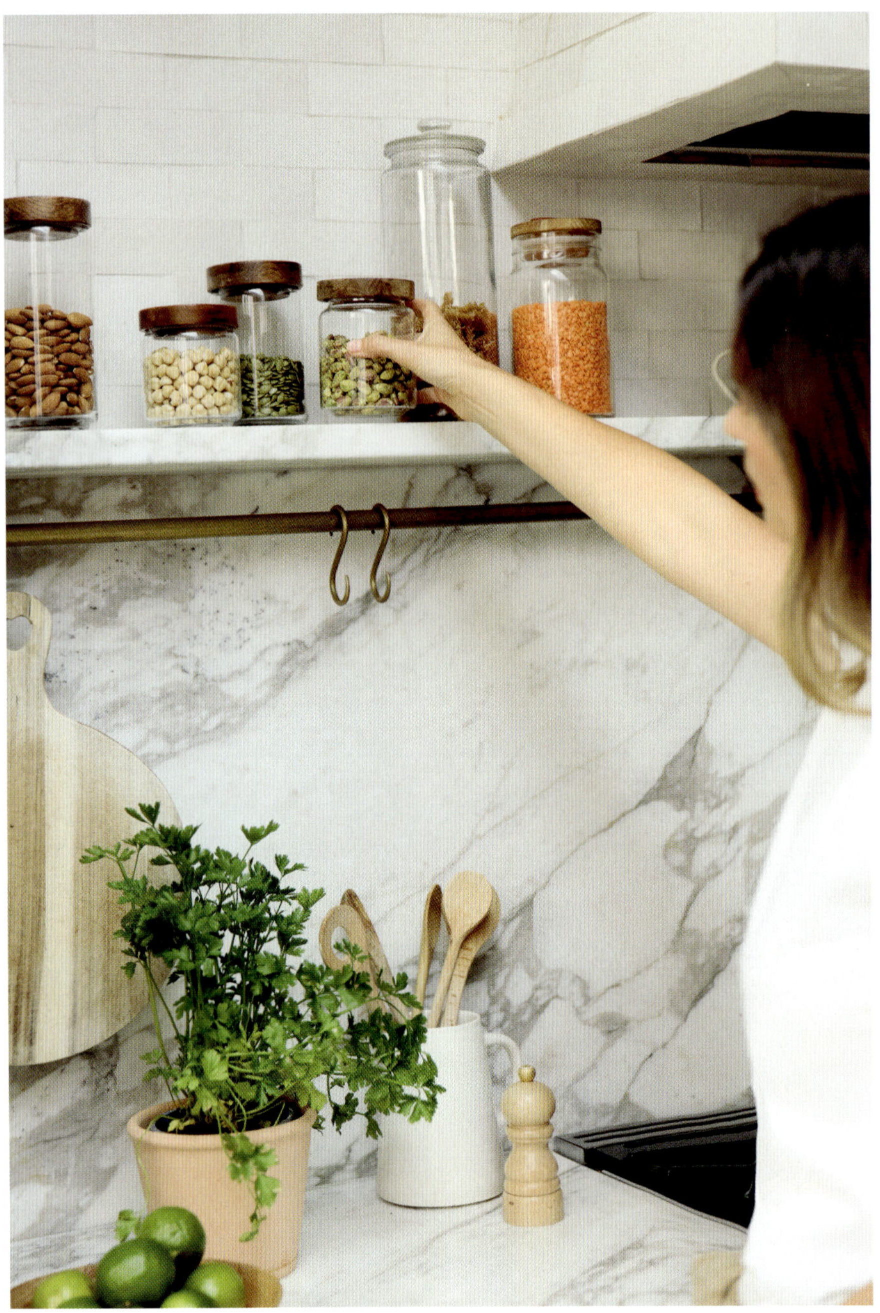

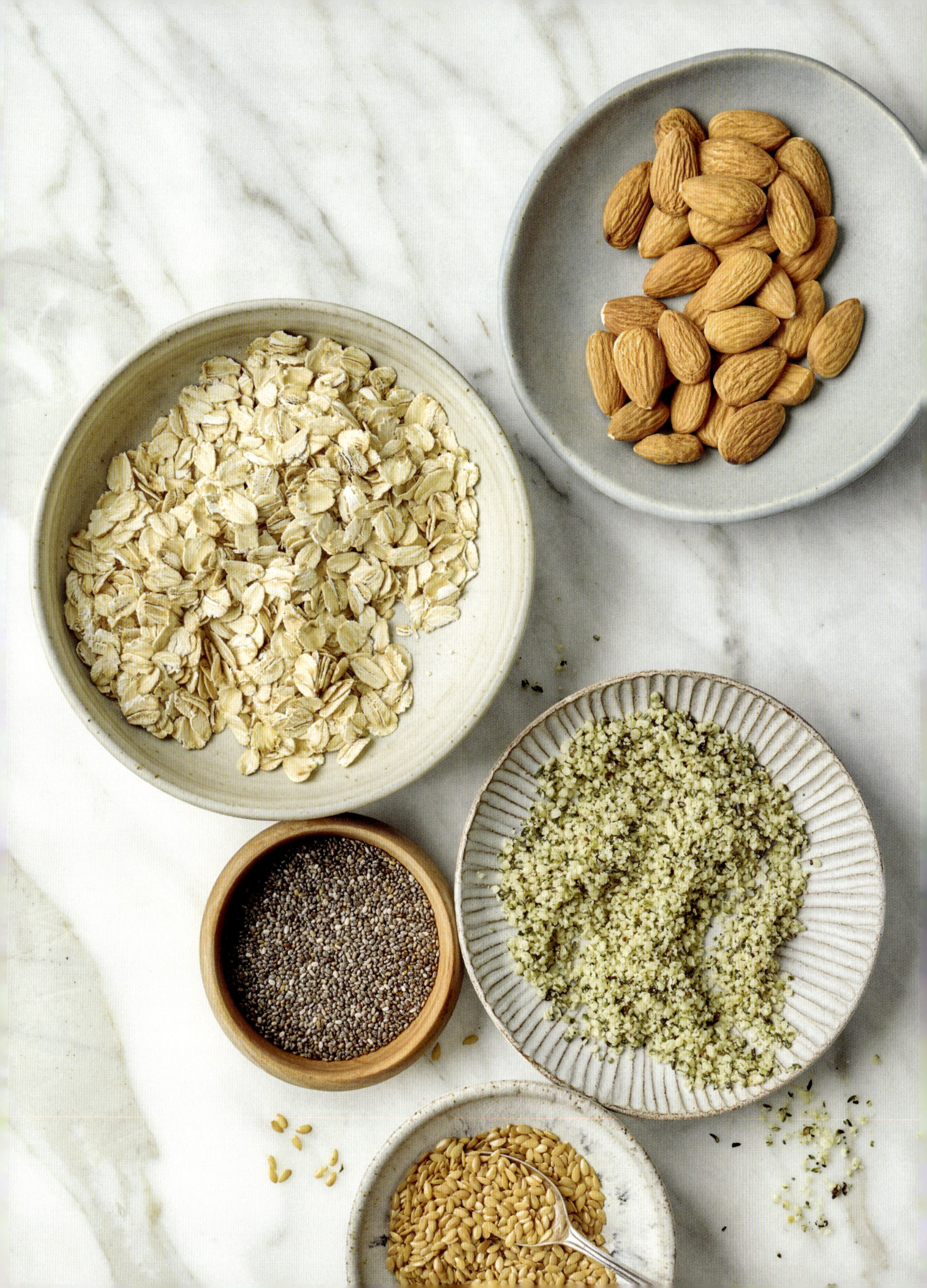

Sun-Dried Tomato and White Bean Dip

Serves 4

1 × small jar of sun-dried
   tomatoes (about 10 oz) drained
1 × 14 oz can of white beans
   (cannellini, haricot or lima
   beans all work well), drained
   and rinsed
2 tablespoons tahini
1 tablespoon almond butter,
   (optional)
juice of 1 lemon
1 small garlic clove
extra virgin olive oil, for drizzling
sea salt and black pepper

This dip is a brilliant way to eat up any leftover raw veg – serve it with sticks of celery, cucumber, cauliflower, whatever you have to hand. It's even better topped with a big handful of fresh herbs like basil, dill, or chives – just use whatever you have going spare. I always drizzle over a little extra virgin olive oil and a sprinkle of flaky salt before serving.

1. In a food processor, combine all the ingredients along with 2 tablespoons of water. Blitz until smooth and season generously, to taste.

2. To serve, drizzle generously with extra virgin olive oil and add a pinch of flaky sea salt and a crack of black pepper.

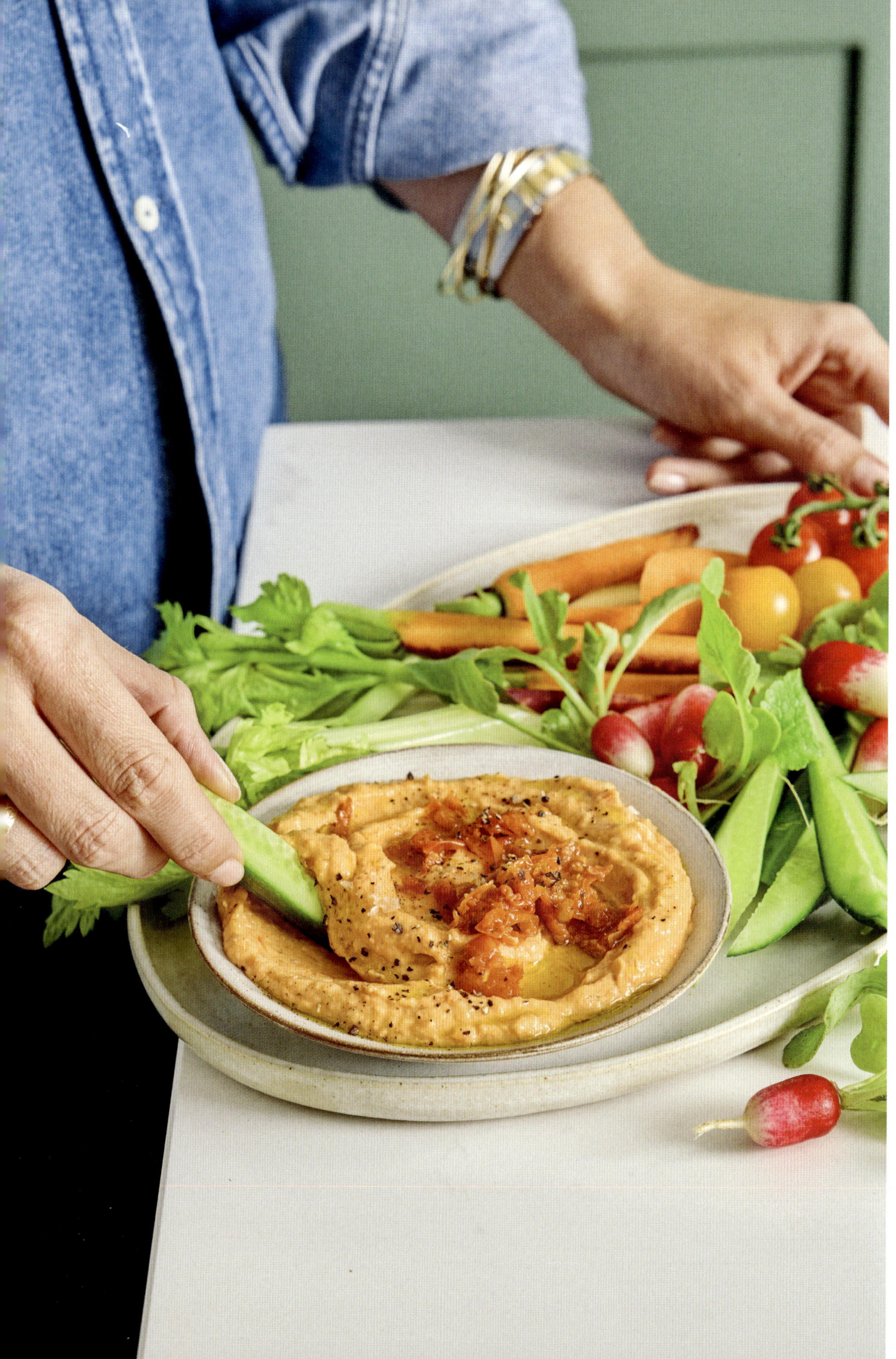

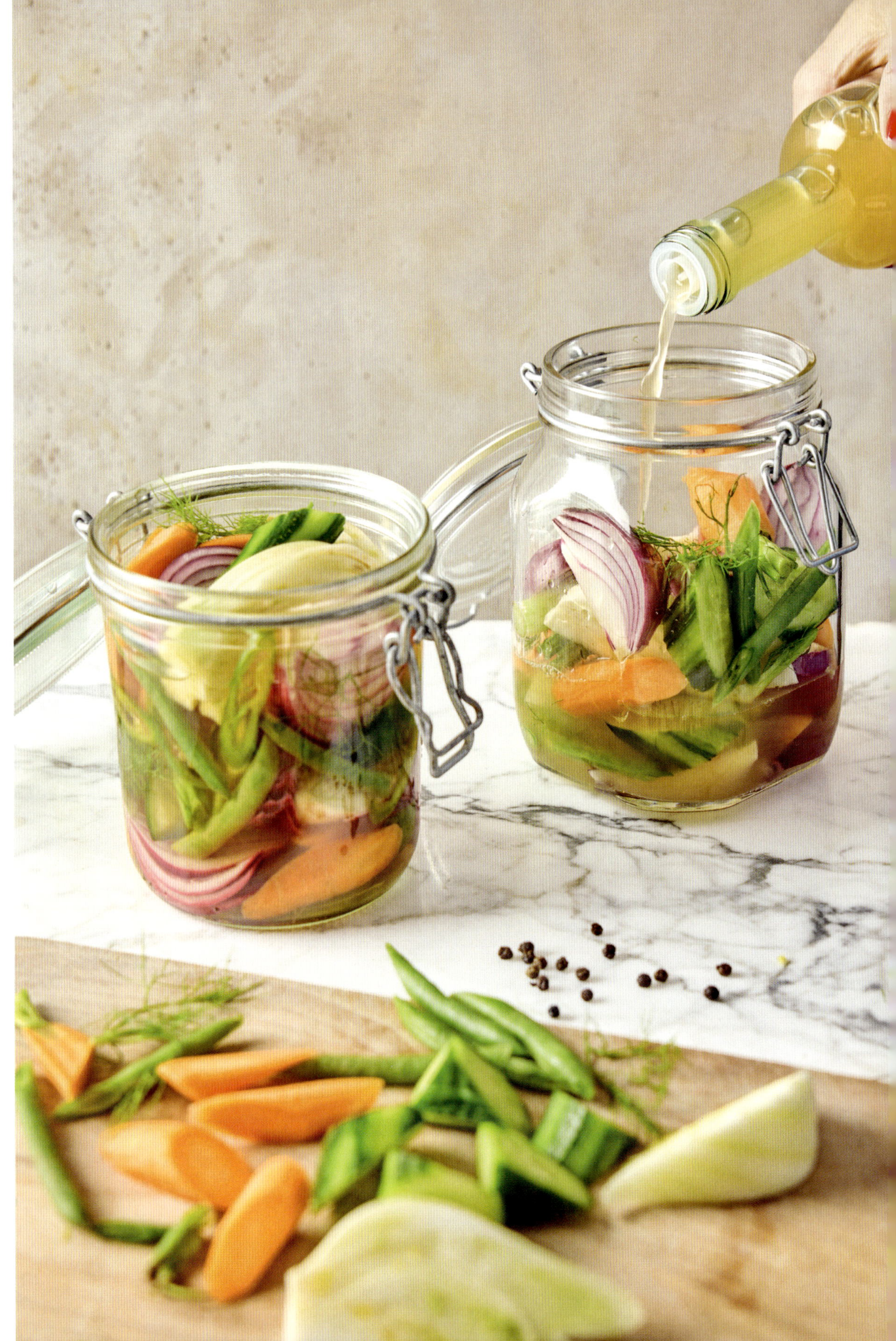

Quick Crunchy Pickled Veggies

4 PLANTS

Fills about 2 x 17 fl oz jars

2.2 lb mixed vegetables
    (cauliflower, carrots, cucumber,
    fennel, red onion, green beans)
3 jalapeños, thinly sliced
9 fl oz white wine vinegar
2 fl oz apple cider vinegar
9 fl oz water
2 bay leaves
10 black peppercorns
1 tablespoon sea salt
1 tablespoon maple syrup

These crunchy, tangy and lightly spicy pickled veg make a delicious snack straight from the jar. They're also a brilliant addition to salads, sandwiches, or avocado toast.

1. Start by chopping all the vegetables into small, bite-sized pieces, making sure that everything is a similar size so that they pickle evenly.

2. Pour the white wine vinegar, apple cider vinegar, and water into a saucepan, then add the bay leaves, peppercorns, salt and maple syrup. Bring to a gentle boil, then remove from the heat and set aside briefly to cool.

3. Pack the vegetables into one large or two medium glass jars, then carefully pour over the pickling liquid, making sure everything is fully submerged; then seal the jar and give it a gentle shake to distribute everything evenly. Leave to cool to room temperature.

4. Once cooled, transfer the jars to the fridge. The pickles will be crisp, tangy, and ready to eat the next day. They keep well for 3 to 4 weeks, so you can enjoy them any time.

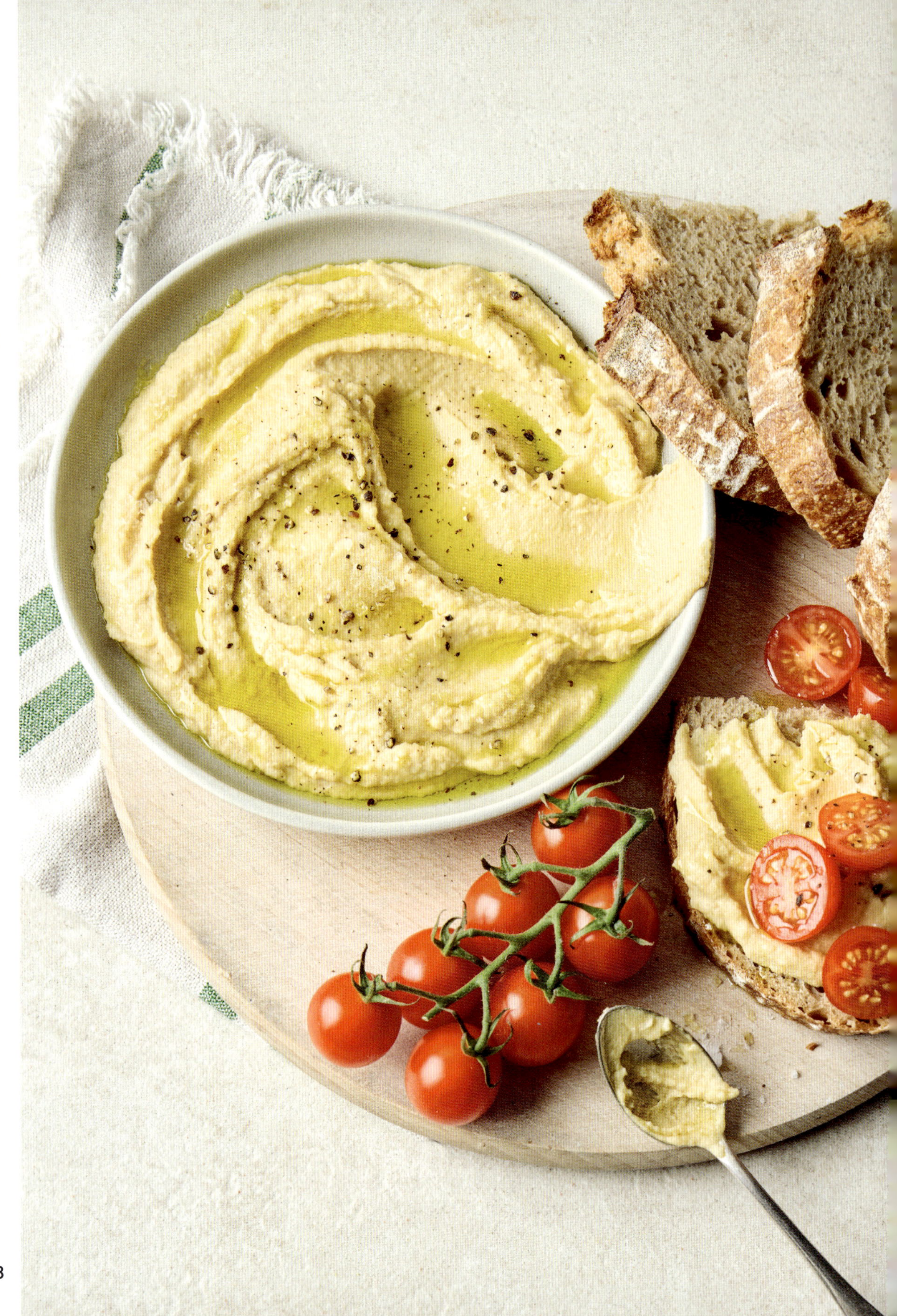

Miso Hummus

4 PLANTS

Serves 4

1 × 14 oz can of chickpeas,
    drained and rinsed
1 tablespoon peanut butter
1 tablespoon white miso paste
juice of 1 lime
1 teaspoon maple syrup
extra virgin olive oil
sea salt and black pepper
pinch of dried red chili flakes, to
    serve (optional)

This hummus is rich, thick, and packed with a deep, savory flavor from the miso. For an easy, 5-minute lunch, simply pile on to sourdough with cherry tomatoes and a drizzle of extra virgin olive oil.

1. Put the chickpeas, peanut butter, miso, lime juice, maple syrup, 3 tablespons of extra virgin olive oil, and 4–5 tablespoons of cold water into a high-speed blender and blitz for a few minutes, until completely smooth.

2. Taste before adding any salt – the miso is already salty, as is the peanut butter, so I generally find you don't want any salt.

3. To serve, drizzle with a little extra virgin olive oil and sprinkle over a pinch of chili flakes (if using) or some black pepper. Store in an airtight container in the fridge for up to 5 days.

Tip: For extra creamy hummus, remove the chickpea skins before blending. To do this simply, place the chickpeas in a large bowl and cover with plenty of cold water. Gently massage until the skins come off, then carefully pour the water through a colander. Refill and repeat the process to remove as many skins as possible.

With eight weeks of easy-to-follow meal plans, this chapter will
prevent the eternal worry around the question of what's for dinner.
Each weekly plan contains six suppers and two lunches, plus a
shopping list. The plans are flexible enough to give you space to head
out for dinner or grab lunch elsewhere, but have the structure to help you
get organized and make mealtimes stress-free. Even better, each plan
ensures you eat your 30-plants-a-week without even thinking.

MEAL PLANS

LUNCH

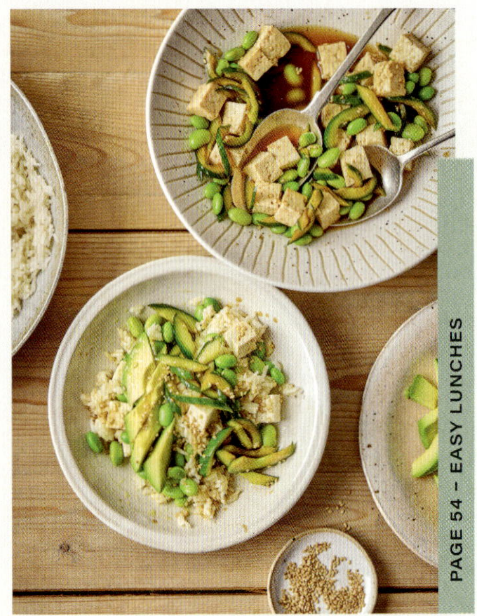

PAGE 54 – EASY LUNCHES

Cucumber and Tofu Bowls 5

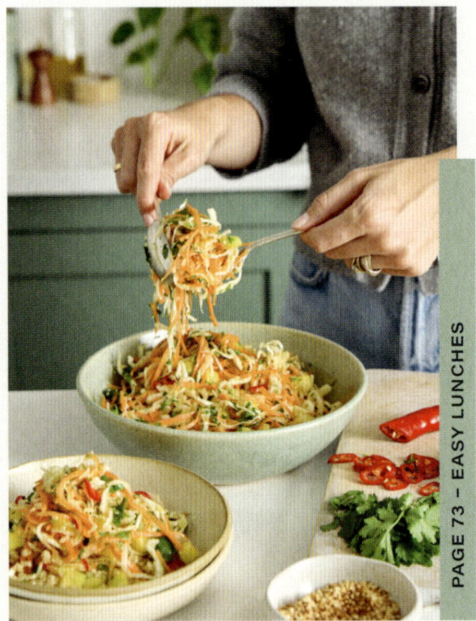

= PLANT COUNT

PAGE 73 – EASY LUNCHES

Cabbage and Mango Salad 8

DINNER

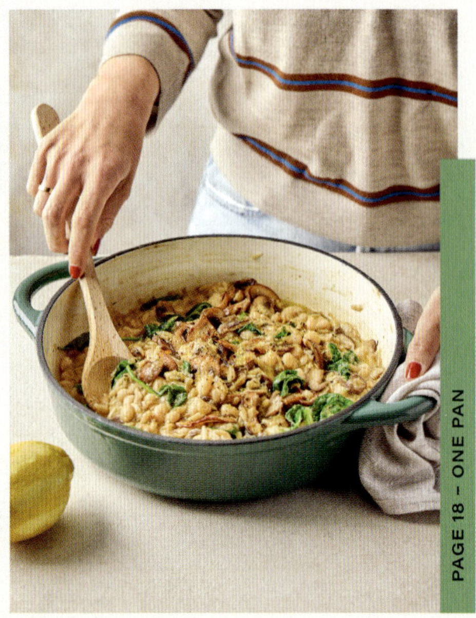

PAGE 18 – ONE PAN

Mushroom Orzo Risotto 7

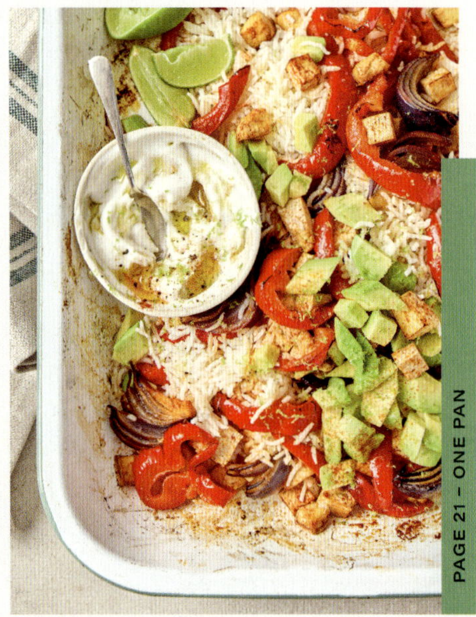

PAGE 21 – ONE PAN

Fajita–Style Tofu Traybake 8

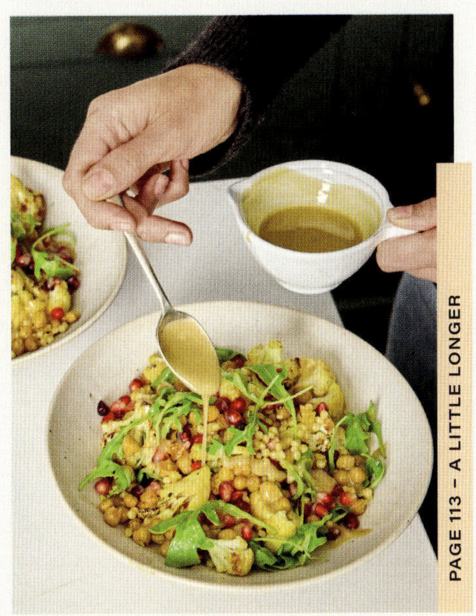

Giant Couscous Salad   10

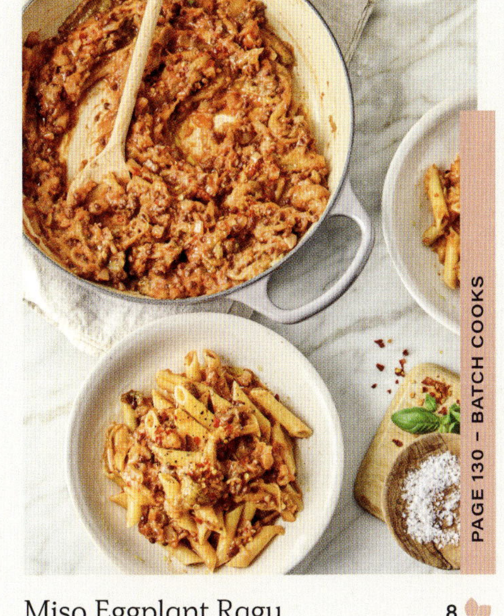

Miso Eggplant Ragu   8

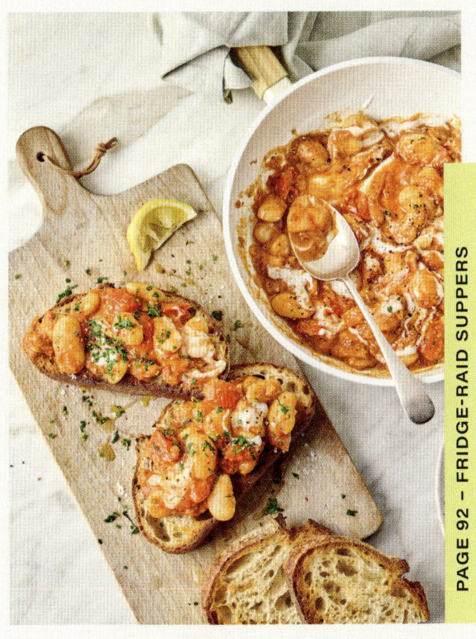

Fancy Lima Beans   5

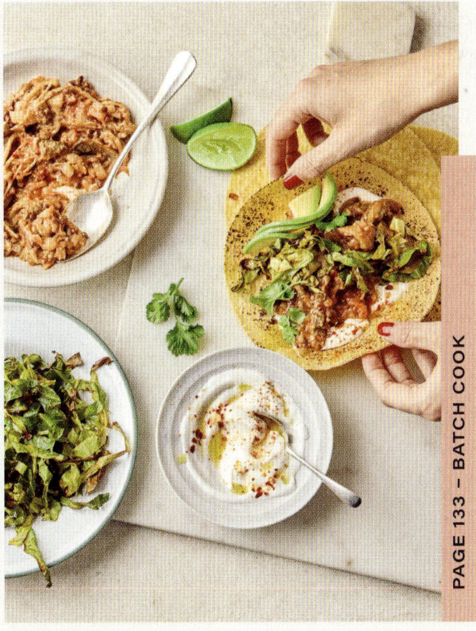

Eggplant Tortillas   14

WEEK O2

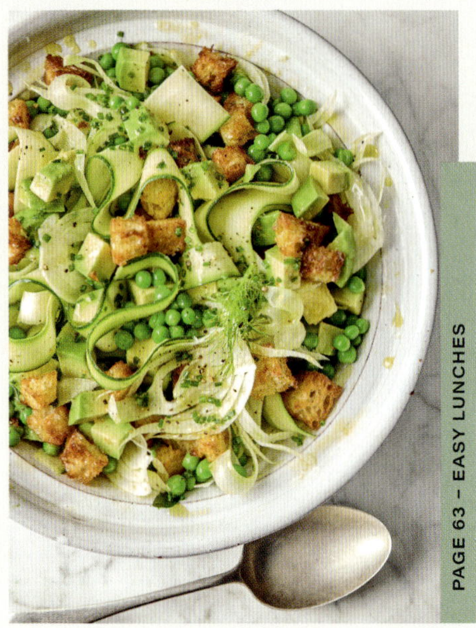

Plant-Packed Salad 7

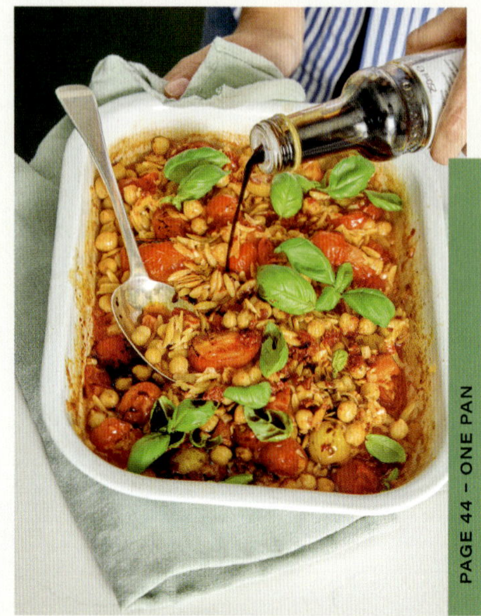

Chickpea and Harissa Orzo 8

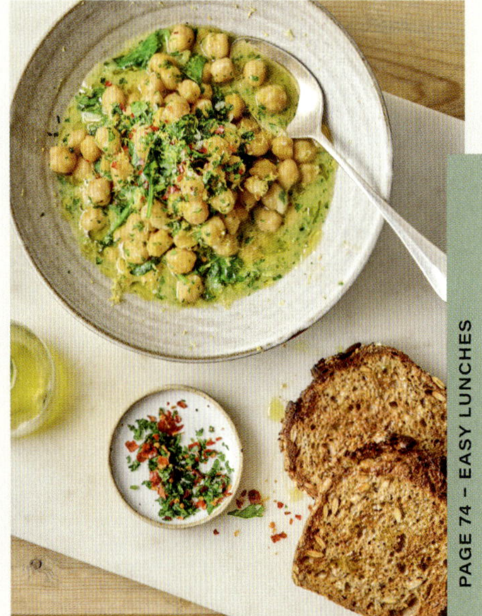

= PLANT COUNT

Garlic and Parsley Chickpeas 6

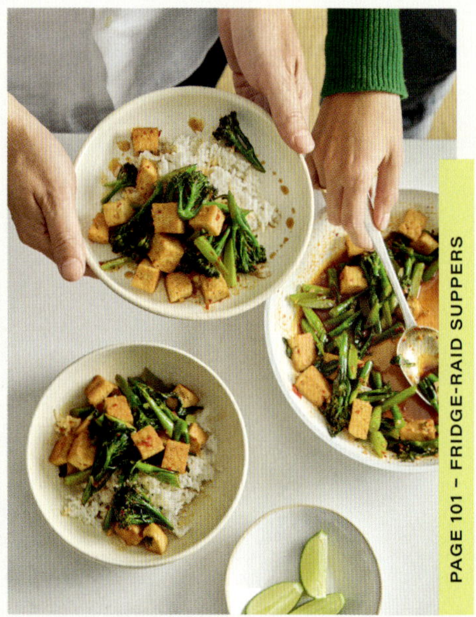

Stir-Fried Harissa Tofu 6

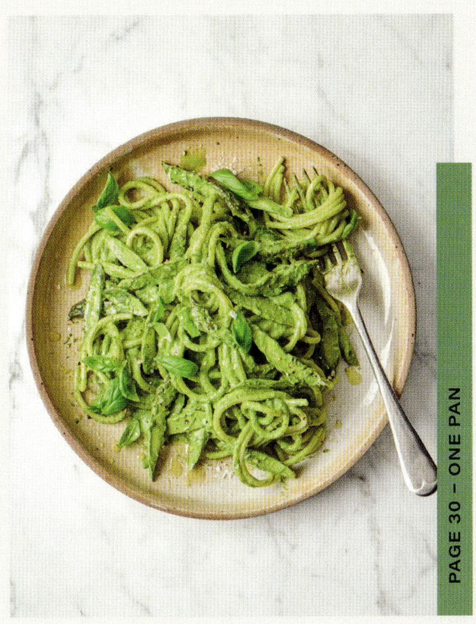

Walnut and Basil Spaghetti 7

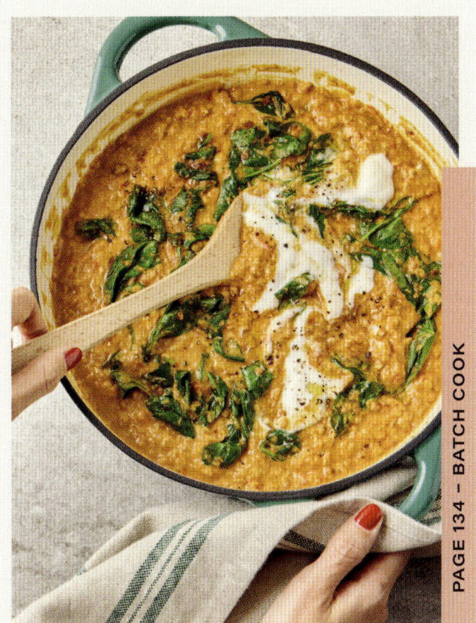

Creamy Coconut Lentils 10

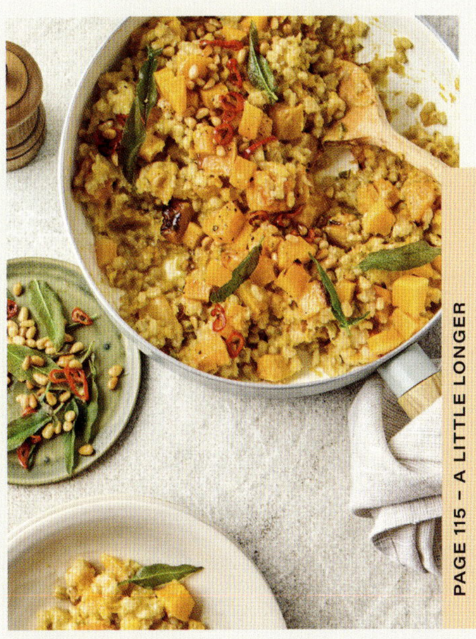

Squash and Pearl Barley Risotto 7

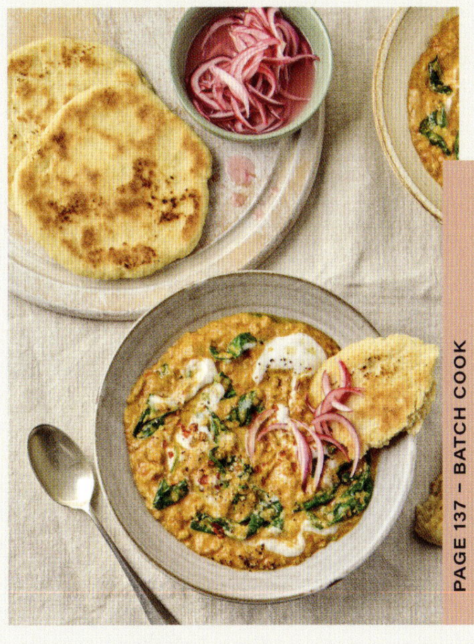

Coconut Lentils with Flatbreads 10

LUNCH

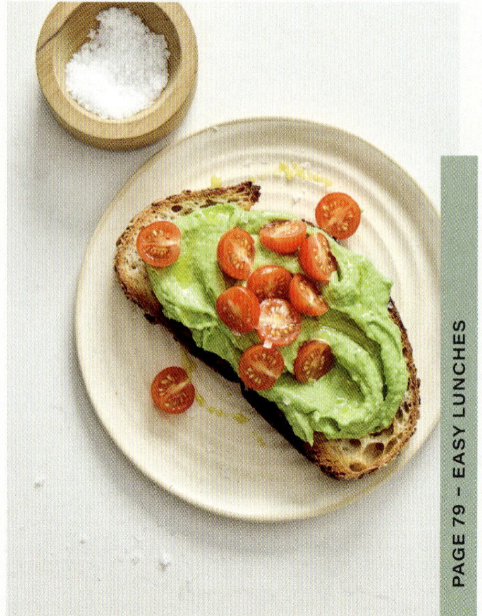

PAGE 79 – EASY LUNCHES

Avocado and Jalapeño Hummus 7 🌿

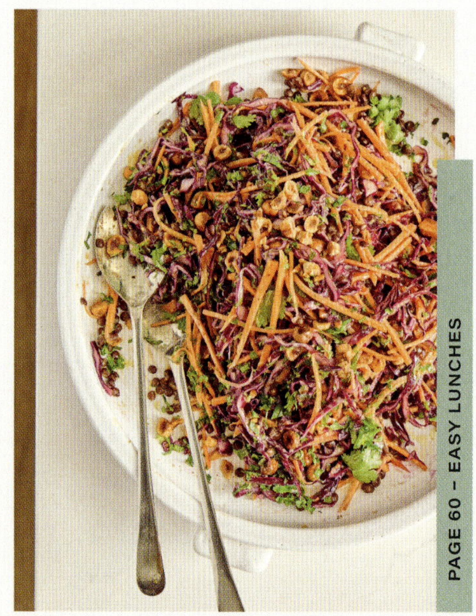

= PLANT COUNT

PAGE 60 – EASY LUNCHES

Hazelnut and Lentil Salad 6 🌿

DINNER

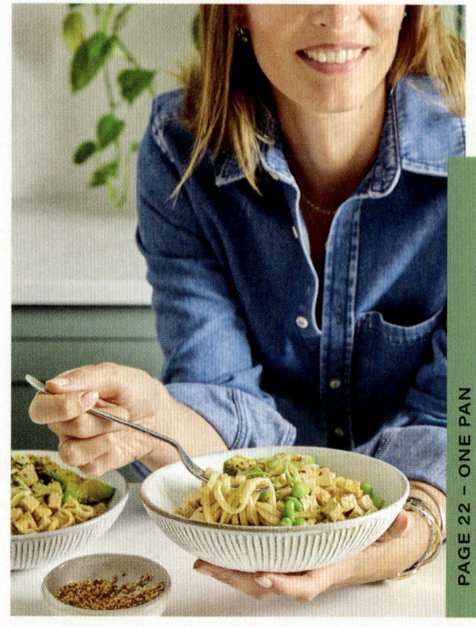

PAGE 22 – ONE PAN

Ginger and Tahini Noodles 9 🌿

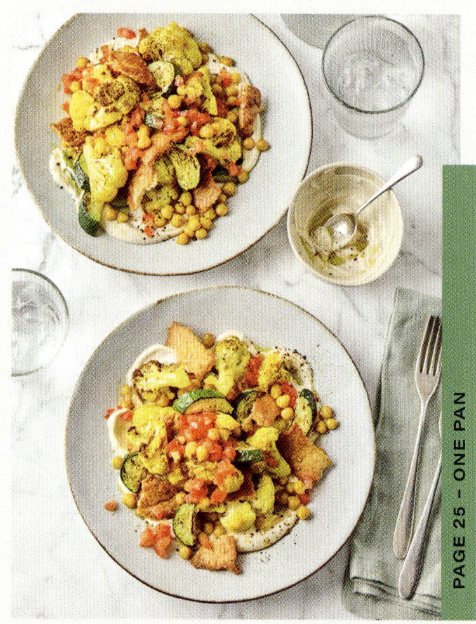

PAGE 25 – ONE PAN

Pitta and Cauliflower Salad 8 🌿

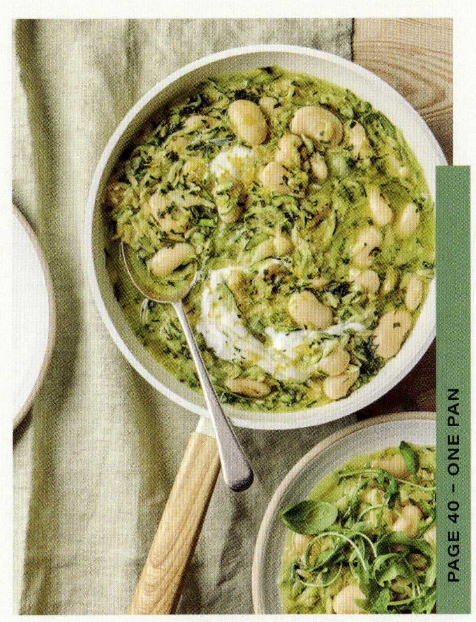

Lima Bean and Zucchini Orzo

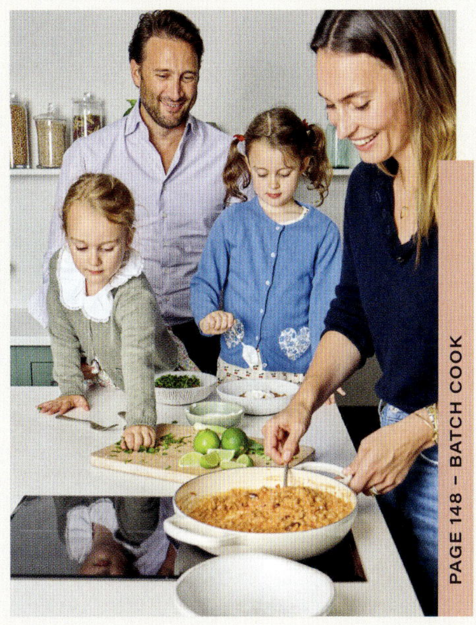

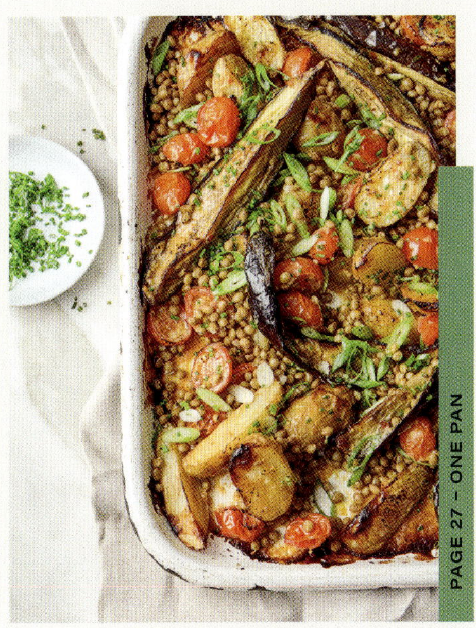

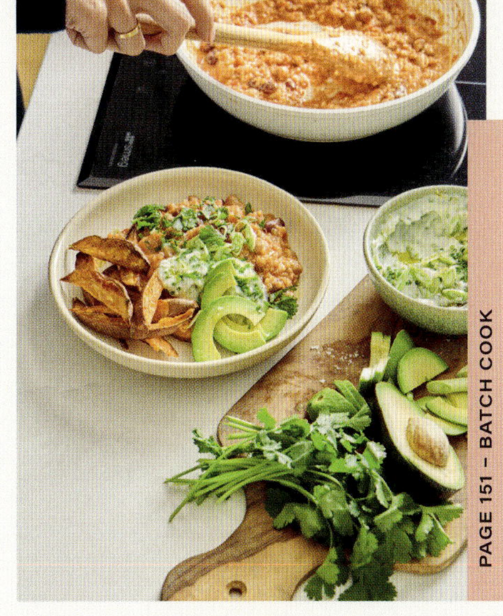

WEEK 04

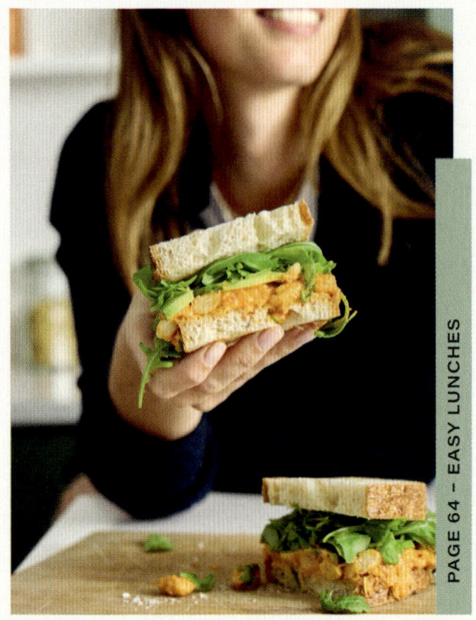

Spicy Lima Bean Sandwich 6

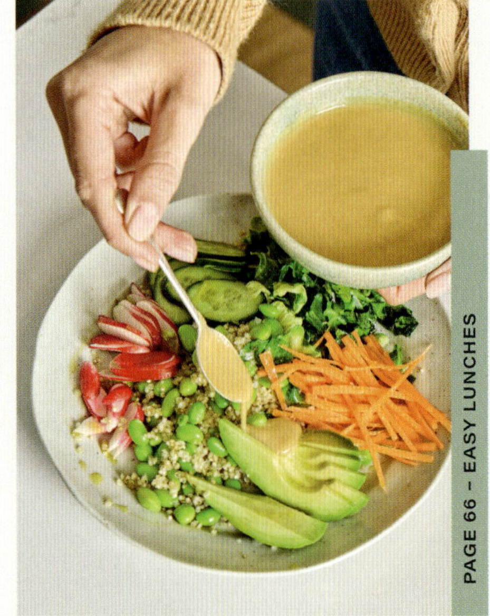

= PLANT COUNT

Miso Quinoa Salad 8

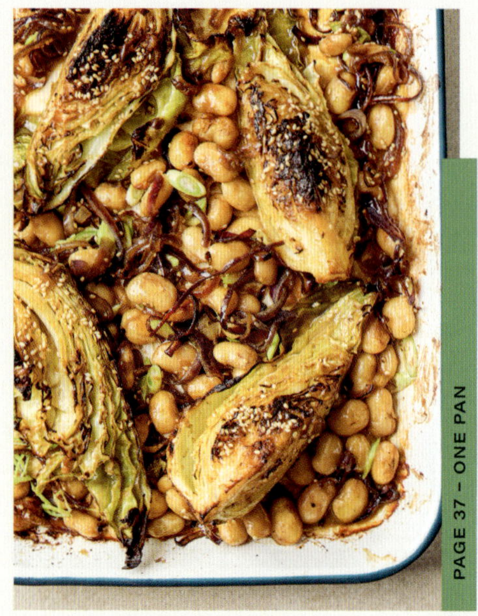

Miso-Roasted Cabbage 7

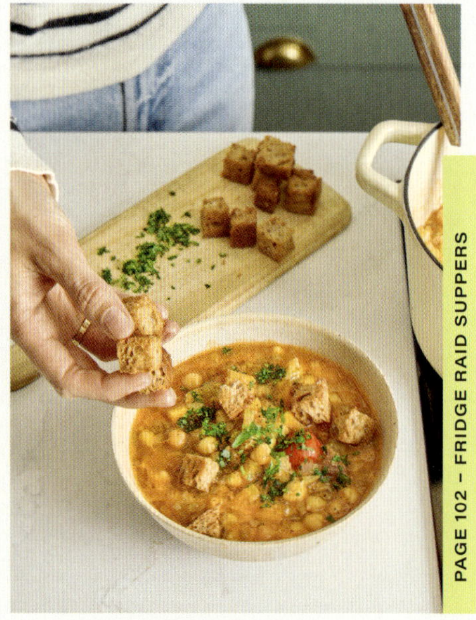

Chunky Chickpea Soup 9

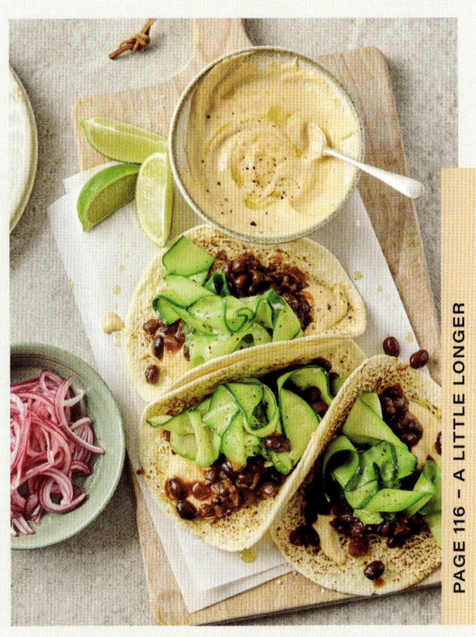
PAGE 116 – A LITTLE LONGER

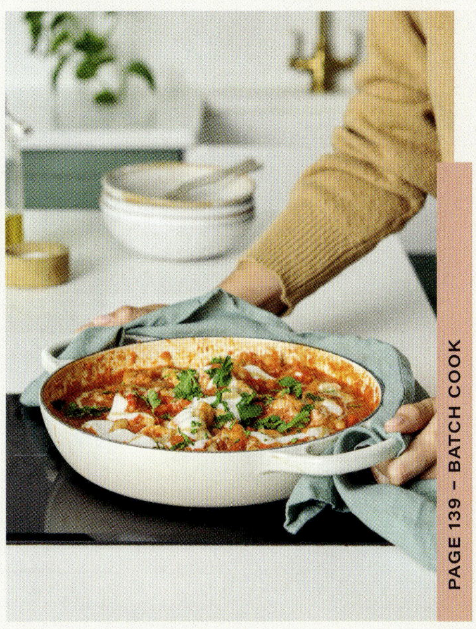
PAGE 139 – BATCH COOK

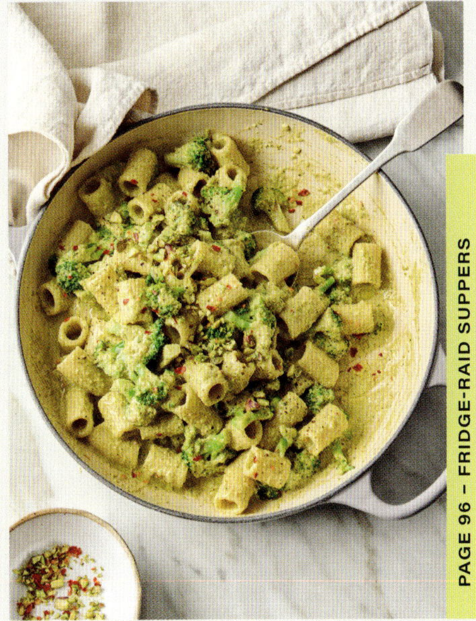
PAGE 96 – FRIDGE-RAID SUPPERS

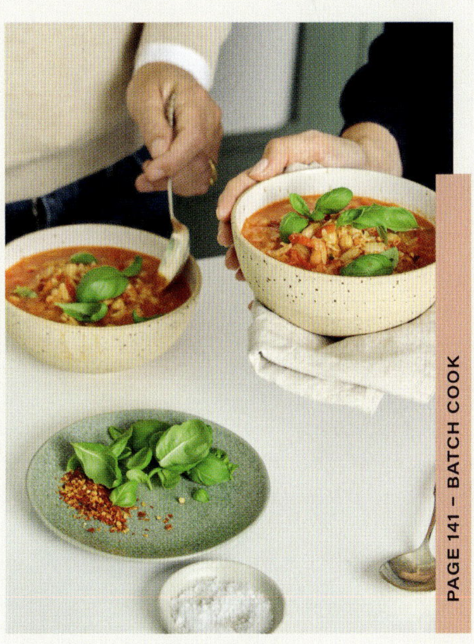
PAGE 141 – BATCH COOK

WEEK 05

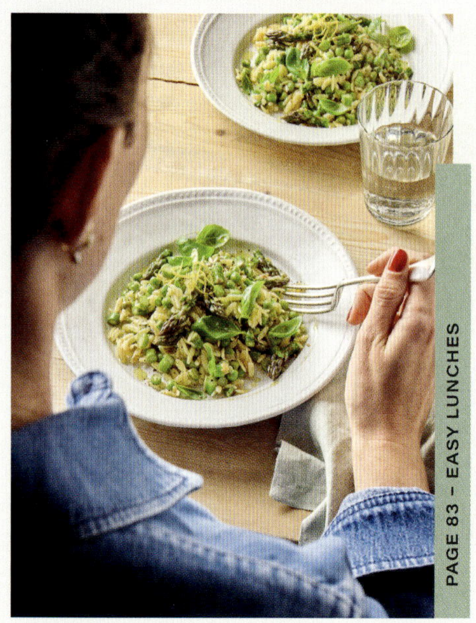

Lemony Pea Orzo   6

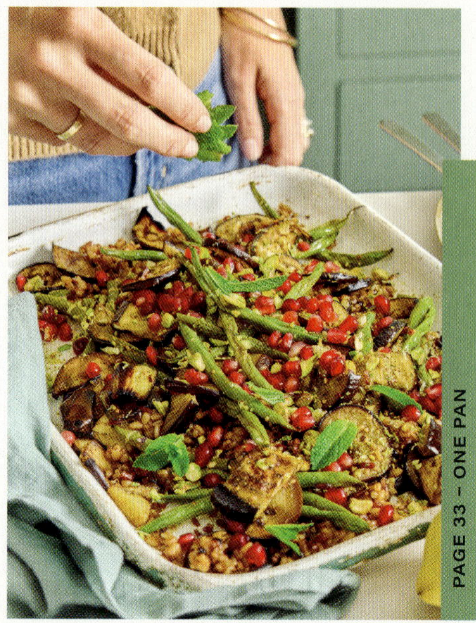

Warm Eggplant Salad   9

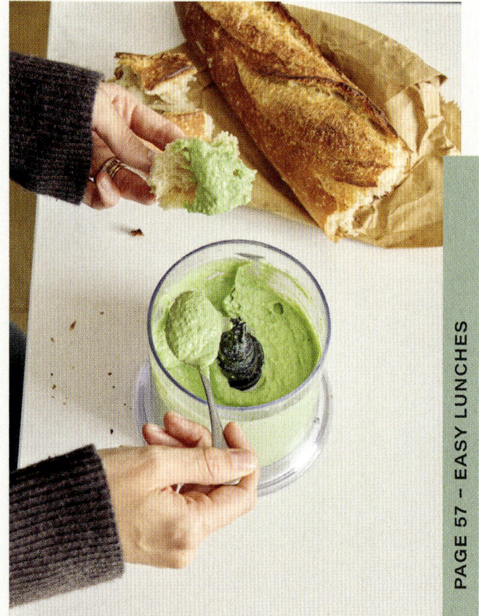

Whipped Greens   7

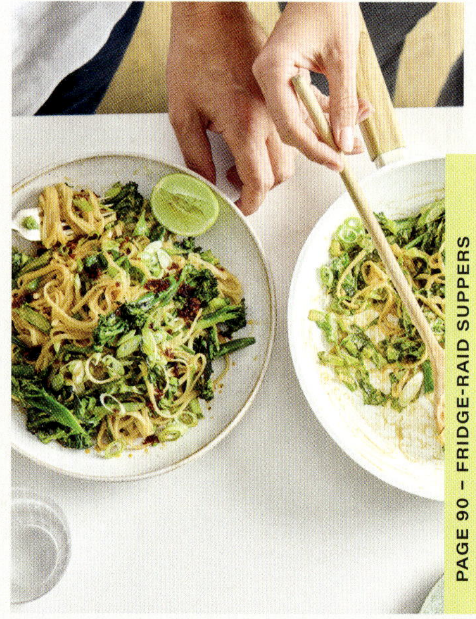

My Go-To Noodles   7

= PLANT COUNT

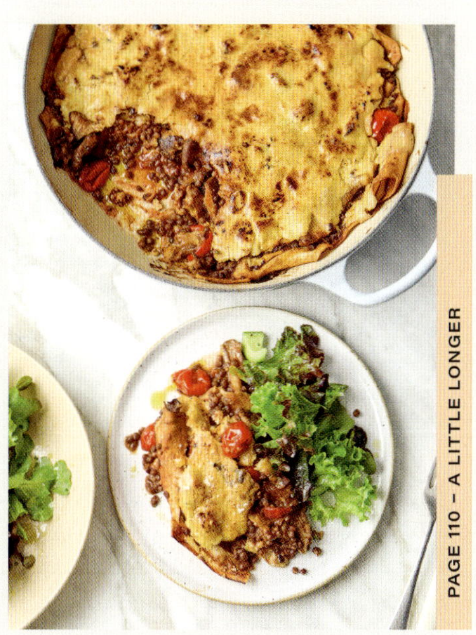

Lazy Mushroom Lasagne   8

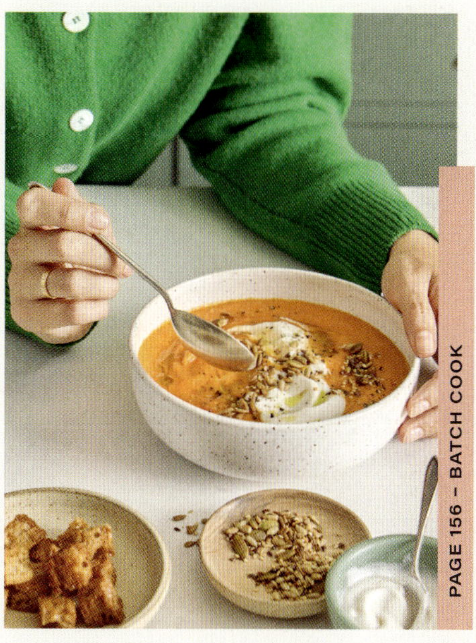

Lima Bean and Carrot Soup   7

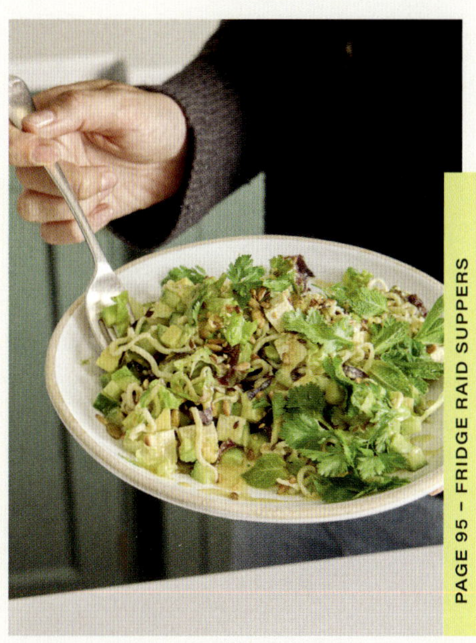

Herby Avocado Noodle
Salad   10

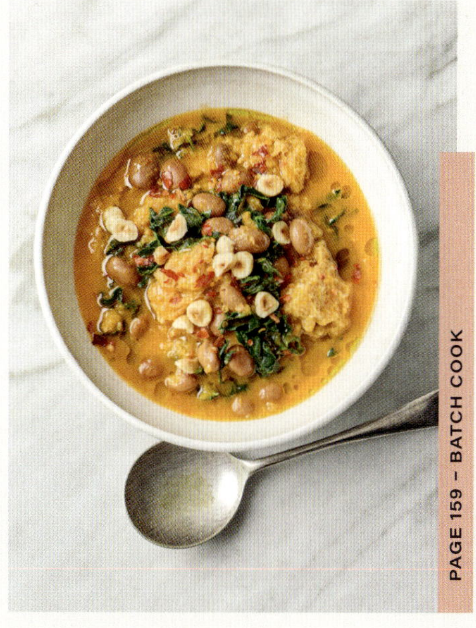

Lima Bean Soup with
Cavolo Nero   10

WEEK 06

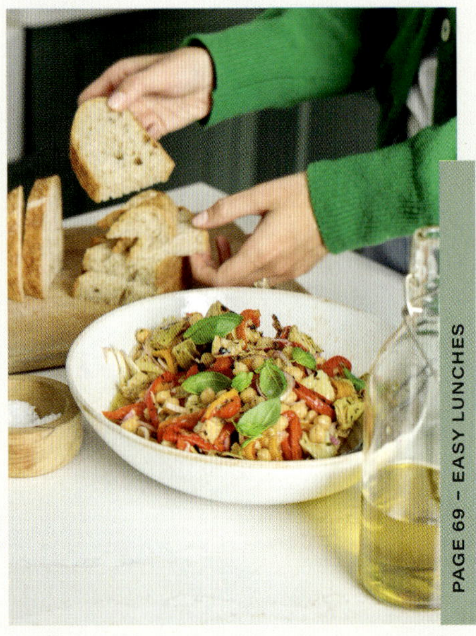

Artichoke and Red Pepper Salad 6

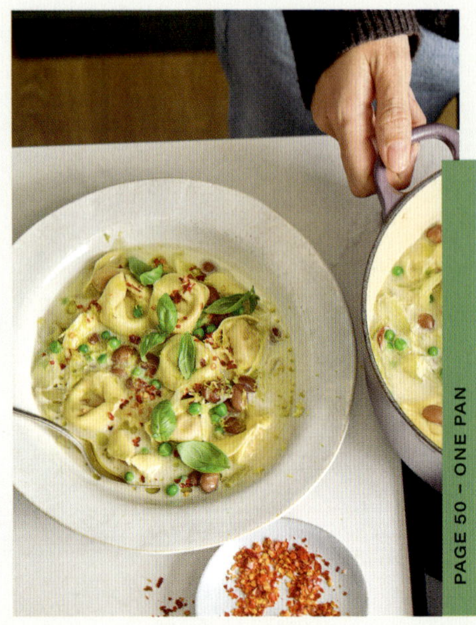

Tortelloni and Bean Broth 7

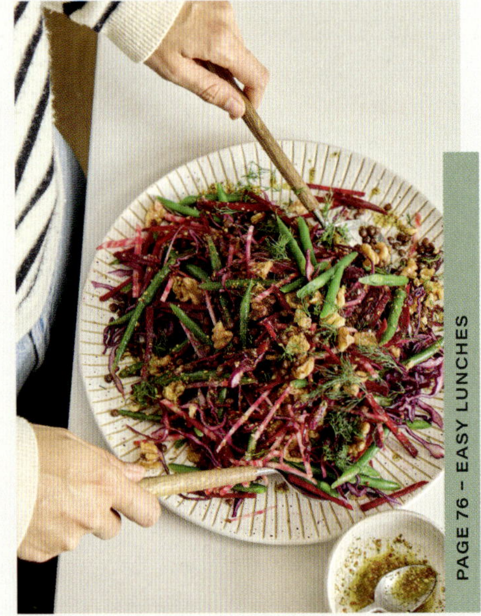

Beet and Green Bean Salad 7

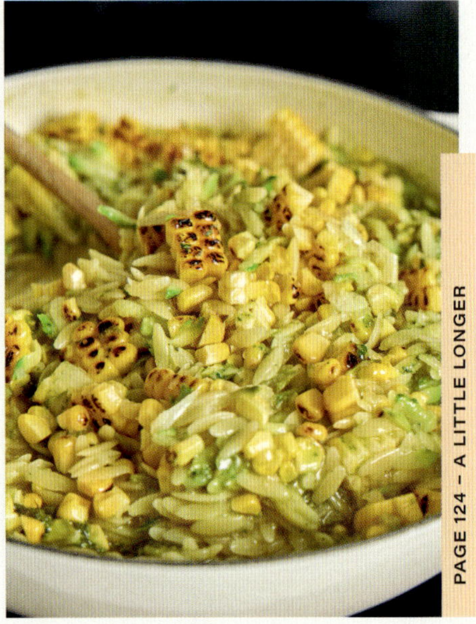

Corn and Zucchini Orzo 8

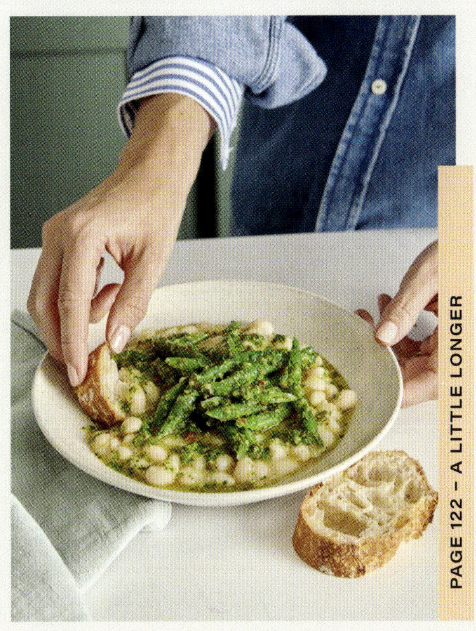

Chimichurri Green Beans 7

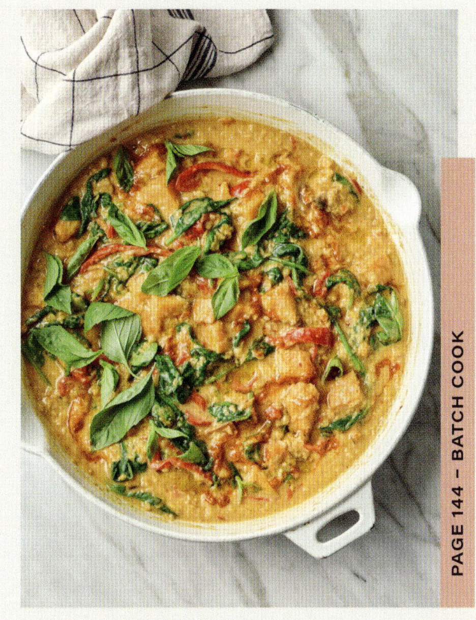

Sweet Potato Thai Curry 10

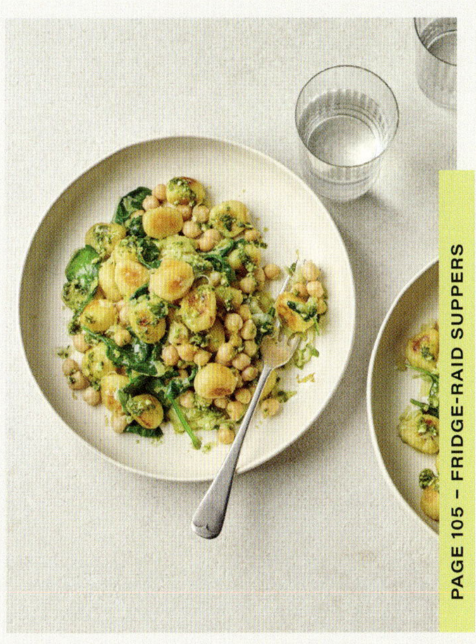

Leek and Chickpea Gnocchi 5

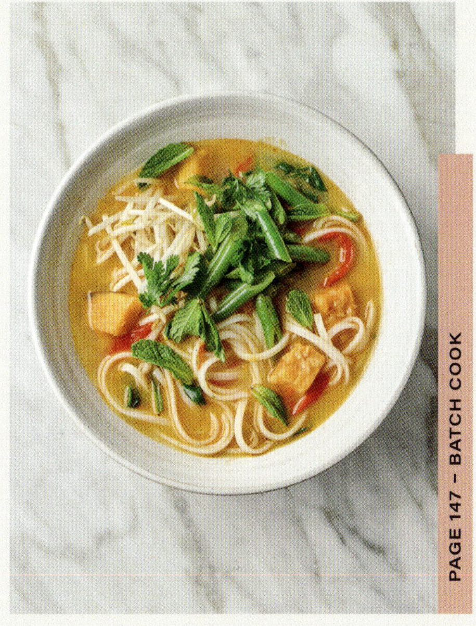

Speedy Thai Noodles 14

WEEK 07

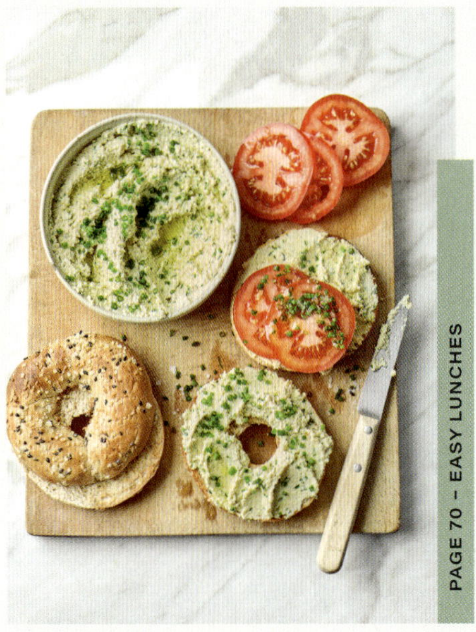

Garlic and Chive Cream Cheese 4

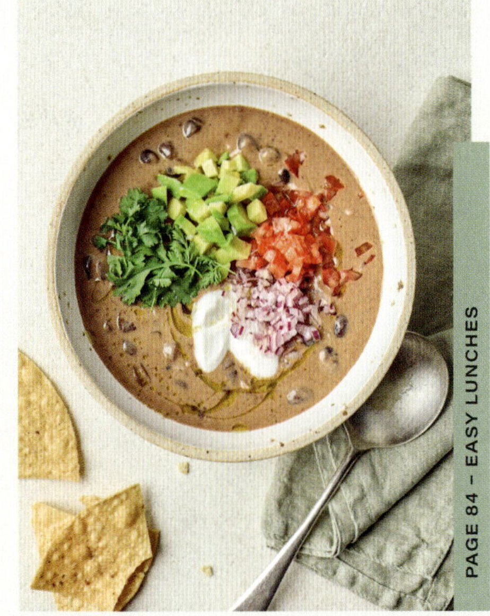

Chunky Black Bean Soup 9

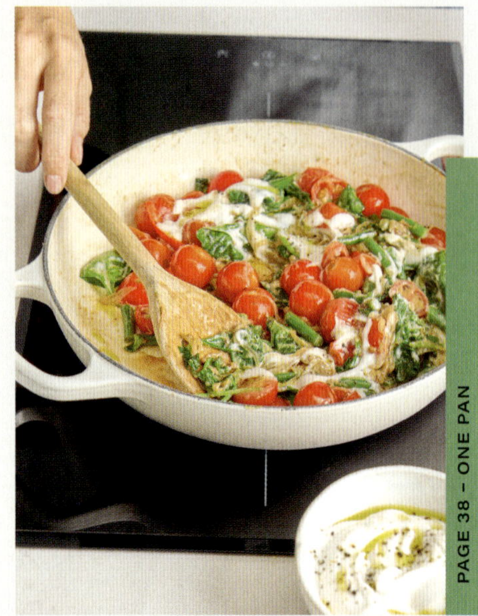

Tomato and Spinach Curry 9

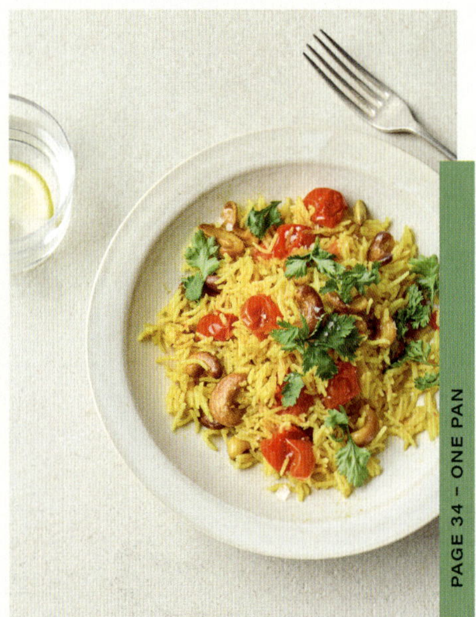

Cashew Pilau Rice 8

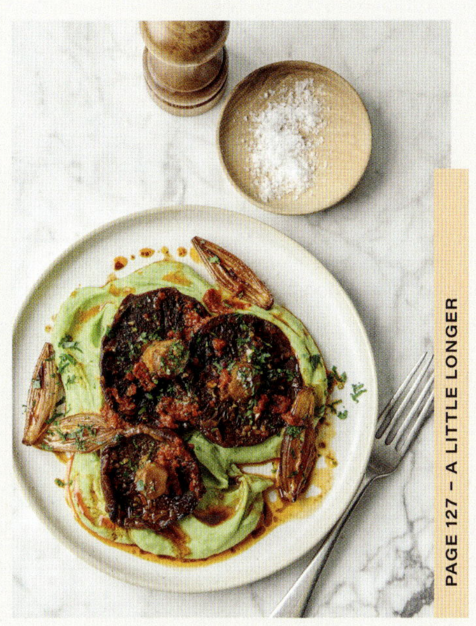

Mushrooms with Lima Bean Mash 8

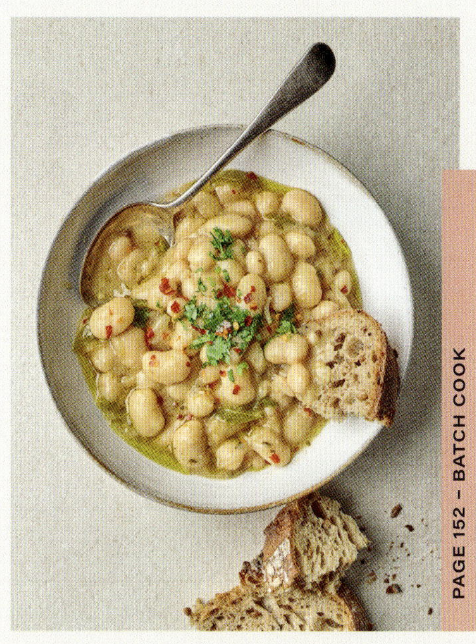

Smoky White Bean Chili 13

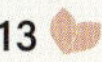

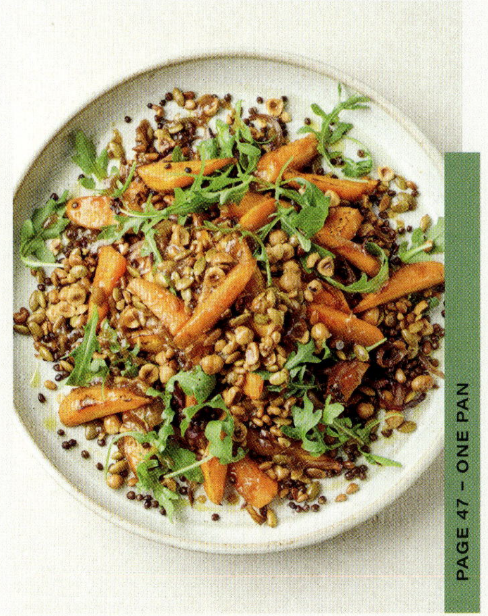

Roasted Carrot Salad 10

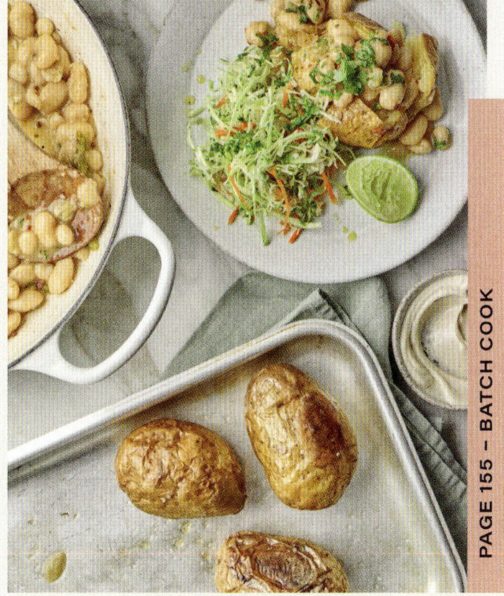

Chili with Baked Potatoes 17

WEEK 08

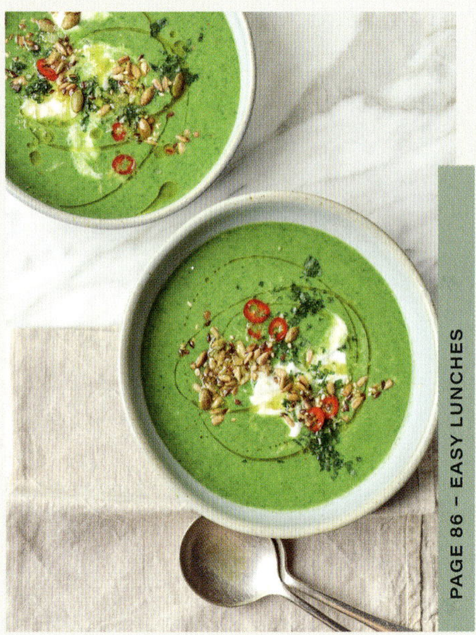

Pea and Spinach Soup   6

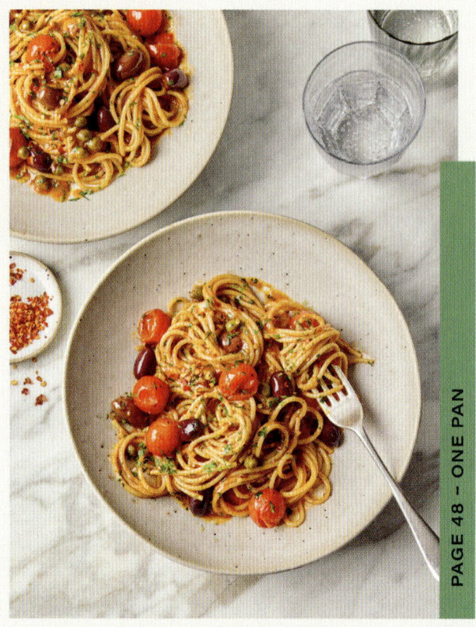

Olive and Tomato Spaghetti   6

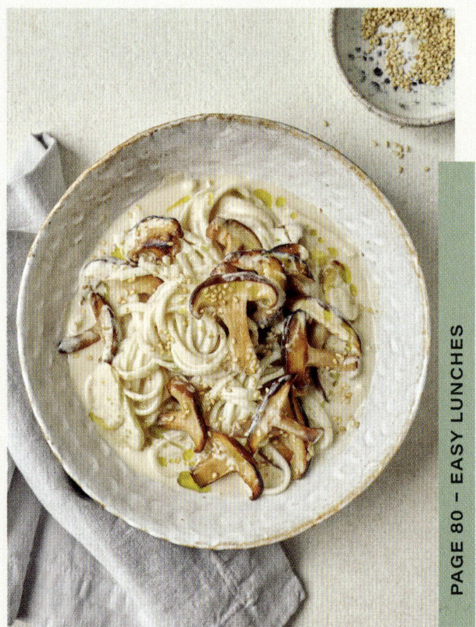

Miso and Mushroom Noodles   7

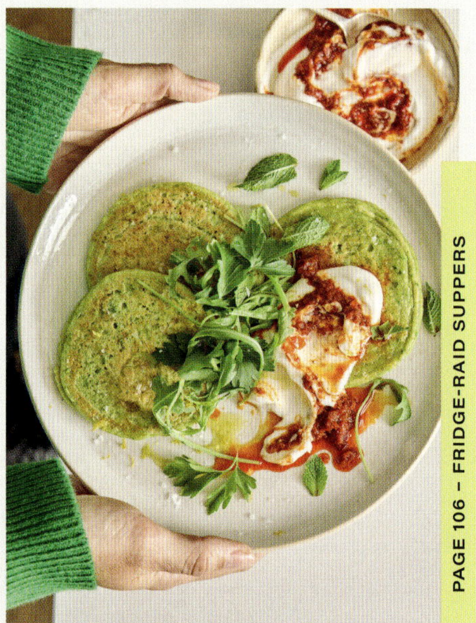

Pea and Chickpea Pancakes   6

= PLANT COUNT

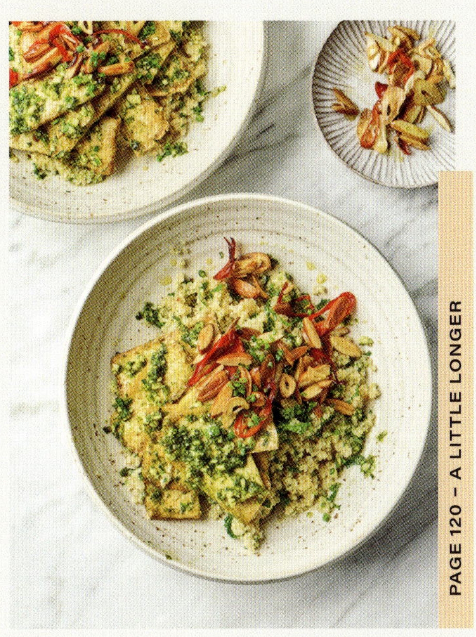

Pesto Tofu   9

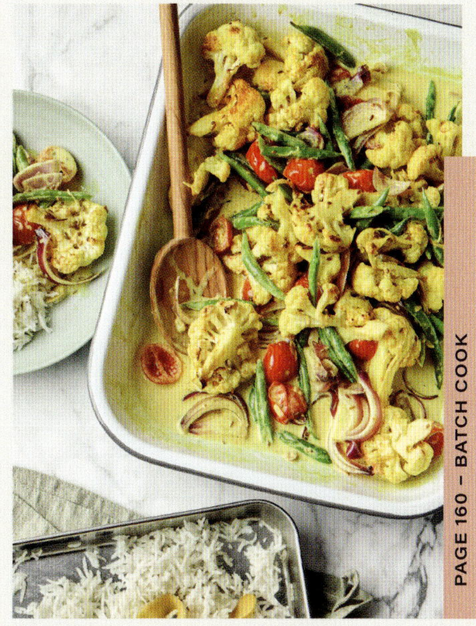

Cauliflower and Coconut Curry   10

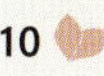

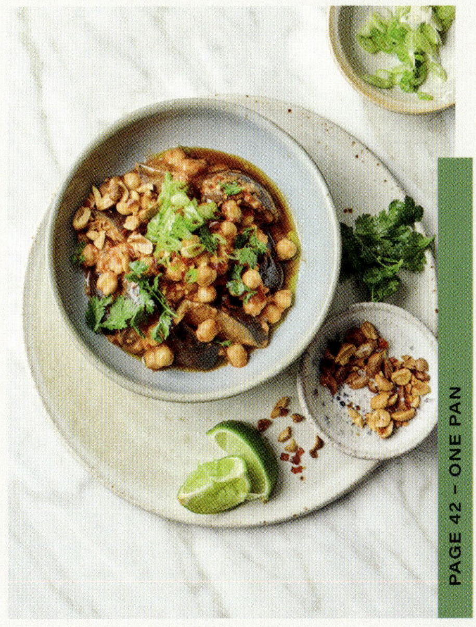

Satay-Style Eggplant Stew   8

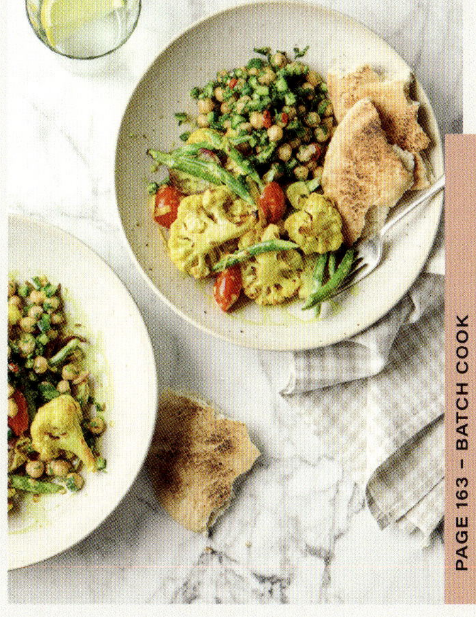

Curry with Chickpea Salad   14

WEEK 01

37 ❧

FRESH INGREDIENTS

- ☐ 2 × blocks of firm tofu (about 20 oz)
- ☐ Plain yogurt (about 7 oz)

Vegetables

- ☐ 3 onions
- ☐ 1 red onion
- ☐ 1 basket of mixed mushrooms (e.g. chestnut and shiitake, 9 oz)
- ☐ 2 red bell peppers
- ☐ 1 small cucumber
- ☐ 1 cauliflower
- ☐ 1 white cabbage
- ☐ 2 carrots
- ☐ cherry tomatoes (5 oz)
- ☐ 4 eggplant
- ☐ Mixed salad leaves (2 oz)
- ☐ Baby spinach (2 oz)
- ☐ 3–4 ripe avocados

Fruit

- ☐ 3 lemons
- ☐ 2–3 limes
- ☐ 1 ripe mango
- ☐ Pomegranate seeds (5 oz)

Herbs and aromatics

- ☐ 2 garlic bulbs (you'll need about 12 cloves)
- ☐ 1 red chili
- ☐ Cilantro (about 2 oz)

FROZEN INGREDIENTS

- ☐ Edamame (3½ oz)

CUPBOARD STAPLES

- ☐ Oat or almond milk (at least 3½ fl oz)

Grains, pulses, and other cans

- ☐ Jasmine rice (3½ oz)
- ☐ Basmati rice (3½ oz or 1 × 9 oz cooked pouch)
- ☐ Giant couscous (3½ oz)
- ☐ Quinoa (3 oz)
- ☐ Orzo (3½ oz)
- ☐ Pasta or other grain for serving with pulled eggplant
- ☐ Chickpeas (1 x 14 oz can)
- ☐ White beans (1 x 14 oz can)
- ☐ Butter beans (1 x 14 oz can)
- ☐ Beluga or green lentils (1 x 14 oz can)

Oils, vinegars, and condiments

- ☐ Olive oil
- ☐ Rice vinegar or apple cider vinegar (at least 4 tablespoons)
- ☐ Soy sauce or tamari (3½ fl oz)
- ☐ White miso paste (4 teaspoons)
- ☐ Tomato passata (1 x 24 oz jar)
- ☐ Tomato purée (1 tablespoon)
- ☐ Tahini (2 tablespoons)
- ☐ Almond butter (1 tablespoon)
- ☐ Maple syrup (at least 7 tablespoons)

Dried herbs and spices

- ☐ Dried thyme (1 teaspoon)
- ☐ Smoked paprika (3 teaspoons)
- ☐ Ground cumin or cumin seeds (3 teaspoons)
- ☐ Ground turmeric (1 teaspoon)
- ☐ Chili flakes (to taste)
- ☐ Vegetable stock cubes (at least 2 cubes or 17 oz)
- ☐ Sea salt (flaky, if possible)
- ☐ Black pepper

Nuts and seeds

- ☐ Sesame seeds (5 tablespoons)

Breads and wraps

- ☐ Crusty bread (2 slices)
- ☐ Whole-wheat tortillas (4 small or 2 large)

Scan here to download a copy of this week's meal plan and shopping list: 

FRESH INGREDIENTS

- ☐ 1 × block of firm tofu (about 10 oz)
- ☐ Plain yogurt (about 11 oz)

Vegetables

- ☐ 1 small fennel bulb
- ☐ 1 zucchini
- ☐ 2 shallots
- ☐ 2 red onions
- ☐ 1 onion or extra shallot (for the risotto)
- ☐ 2 garlic bulbs (you'll need around 24 cloves)
- ☐ cherry tomatoes (9 oz)
- ☐ 1 small butternut squash or pumpkin (about 28 oz)
- ☐ Asparagus (about 4½ oz)
- ☐ Tenderstem broccoli (7 oz)
- ☐ Spinach (about 11 oz)
- ☐ Baby spinach (3½ oz)

Fruit

- ☐ 1 avocado
- ☐ 3–4 limes
- ☐ 1–2 lemons

Herbs and aromatics

- ☐ Small chunk of fresh ginger root (about 1 oz)
- ☐ Basil (about 2 oz), plus extra to serve
- ☐ Flat-leaf parsley (about 1 oz)
- ☐ Sage (about 1 oz)
- ☐ 4 red chilis
- ☐ Chives (1 oz)

FROZEN INGREDIENTS

- ☐ Frozen peas (7 oz)

CUPBOARD STAPLES

- ☐ Almond milk (3½ fl oz)

Grains, pulses, and other cans

- ☐ Orzo (6 oz)
- ☐ Spaghetti or pasta of choice (6 oz for 2 servings)
- ☐ Pearl barley (4½ oz)
- ☐ Red split lentils (7 oz)
- ☐ Rice (11 oz uncooked or 6 portions)
- ☐ Chickpeas (1 × 14 oz can + 1 × 20 oz jar)
- ☐ Chopped tomatoes (1 × 14 oz can)
- ☐ Coconut milk (1 × 14 fl oz can)
- ☐ 6 oz plain flour
- ☐ insert 3 tsp baking powder

Oils, vinegars, and condiments

- ☐ Olive oil
- ☐ Extra virgin olive oil
- ☐ Tamari or soy sauce (3 tablespoons)
- ☐ Apple cider vinegar (2 tablespoons)
- ☐ Rice vinegar (1 tablespoon)
- ☐ Balsamic vinegar (1–2 tablespoons)
- ☐ Harissa paste (about 3 tablespoons)
- ☐ White miso paste (1 tablespoon)
- ☐ Maple syrup (1 tablespoon, plus optional drizzle for pickled onions)

Dried herbs and spices

- ☐ Medium curry powder (2 teaspoons)
- ☐ Dried red chili flakes (½ teaspoon)
- ☐ Vegetable stock cubes (at least 1 cube or 24 oz)
- ☐ Nutritional yeast (2 tablespoons)
- ☐ Sea salt (fine and flaky, if possible)
- ☐ Black pepper

Nuts and seeds

- ☐ Walnuts (about 2 oz)
- ☐ Pine nuts (about 1 oz)

Breads and wraps

- ☐ Crusty bread (4 slices)

Scan here to download a copy of this week's meal plan and shopping list:

SHOPPING LIST

FRESH INGREDIENTS

- [ ] 1 x block of firm tofu (about 10 oz)
- [ ] Plain yogurt (about 14 oz)

Vegetables

- [ ] 3 zucchini
- [ ] 1 small cauliflower (about 28 oz)
- [ ] 1 red onion
- [ ] 1 small red cabbage
- [ ] 2 carrots
- [ ] 1 large eggplant
- [ ] Baby potatoes (10½ oz)
- [ ] 1 large bunch of green onions
- [ ] 1 tomato
- [ ] 1 large sweet potato
- [ ] 1 garlic bulb
- [ ] Large chunk of fresh ginger root (about 2 oz)
- [ ] Cherry tomatoes (10½ oz)
- [ ] Arugula (about 2 oz)
- [ ] Spinach (2 oz)

Fruit

- [ ] 7 limes
- [ ] 3 lemons
- [ ] 3 avocados

Herbs and aromatics

- [ ] Cilantro (about 2 oz)
- [ ] Basil (about 1 oz, plus extra to garnish)
- [ ] Chives (about 1 oz)
- [ ] 1–2 red chilis (to taste)
- [ ] 2 jalapeños (about 1 oz)

FROZEN INGREDIENTS

- [ ] Edamame (3½ oz)

CUPBOARD STAPLES

Grains, pulses, and other cans

- [ ] Quinoa (2½ oz)
- [ ] Orzo (2 servings, about 6 oz)
- [ ] Noodles (2 servings, about 6 oz) — rice, soba, or whole-wheat
- [ ] White beans or chickpeas (1 × 14 oz can)
- [ ] Chickpeas (2 × 14 oz cans)
- [ ] Cooked puy lentils (1 × 9 oz pouch)
- [ ] Brown lentils (1 × 14 oz can)
- [ ] Lima beans (1 × 18 oz jar)
- [ ] Mixed beans (2 × 14 oz cans)
- [ ] Chopped tomatoes (1 × 14 oz can)
- [ ] Coconut milk (1 × 14 fl oz can)

Oils, vinegars, and condiments

- [ ] Olive oil
- [ ] Extra virgin olive oil
- [ ] Sesame oil (if wished, for stir-frying)
- [ ] Tahini (9 tablespoons)
- [ ] White miso paste (2 tablespoons)
- [ ] Tamari or soy sauce (1 tablespoon, plus extra to serve)
- [ ] Maple syrup (about 4 tablespoons)
- [ ] Smooth peanut butter (2 oz)

Dried herbs and spices

- [ ] Ground turmeric (1 teaspoon)
- [ ] Ground cumin (1 teaspoon)
- [ ] Dried red chili flakes (1 teaspoon)
- [ ] Cayenne pepper (pinch, optional)
- [ ] Vegetable stock cubes (at least 1 cube or 9 oz)
- [ ] Sea salt
- [ ] Black pepper

Nuts and seeds

- [ ] Hazelnuts or peanuts (2 oz)
- [ ] Sesame seeds (handful, plus extra to garnish)

Breads and wraps

- [ ] Crusty sourdough (to serve with hummus)
- [ ] Whole-wheat pitta breads (2)

WEEK 04

38 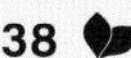

FRESH INGREDIENTS

- [ ] Plain yogurt (about 7 oz)

Vegetables

- [ ] 1 small hispi cabbage (about 16 oz)
- [ ] 5 carrots
- [ ] 1 zucchini
- [ ] 1 small head of broccoli (about 9 oz)
- [ ] 3 celery sticks
- [ ] 1 onion
- [ ] 2 red onions
- [ ] 2–3 green onions
- [ ] 2 shallots
- [ ] 2 Romano peppers
- [ ] 2 red chili
- [ ] 2 servings of salad veg for the quinoa bowls (choose any of the following: tomatoes, radishes, cucumber, zucchini, pre-roasted beets, carrots)
- [ ] Arugula or salad leaves (about 3½ oz)

Fruit

- [ ] 2 lemons
- [ ] 2 limes
- [ ] 1–2 avocados

Herbs and aromatics

- [ ] 2 garlic bulbs (at least 14 cloves)
- [ ] Small chunk of fresh ginger root (about 1 oz)
- [ ] Basil (about 2 oz)
- [ ] Flat-leaf parsley (about 1 oz)
- [ ] Cilantro (about 2 oz)

FROZEN INGREDIENTS

- [ ] Edamame (3½ oz)

CUPBOARD STAPLES

Grains, pulses, and other cans

- [ ] Quinoa (4 oz)
- [ ] Red lentils (2 oz)
- [ ] Orzo (6 oz)
- [ ] Pasta (about 6 oz for 4 servings; short pasta, like fusilli or rigatoni, works well)
- [ ] Brown rice, pasta or baked potatoes (optional, to serve with stew)
- [ ] Chickpeas (2 × 14 oz cans)
- [ ] Lima beans (2 × 14 oz cans)
- [ ] Black beans (1 × 14 oz can)
- [ ] Haricot or cannellini beans (1 × 14 oz can)
- [ ] Cherry tomatoes (1 × 14 oz can)
- [ ] Chopped tomatoes (1 × 14 oz can)

Oils, vinegars, and condiments

- [ ] Olive oil
- [ ] Extra virgin olive oil (4 tablespoons)
- [ ] White miso paste (about 5 tablespoons)
- [ ] Tahini (about 4 tablespoons)
- [ ] Tamari or soy sauce (2 tablespoons)
- [ ] Maple syrup (about 4 teaspoons)
- [ ] Apple cider vinegar (1 tablespoon)
- [ ] Harissa paste (1½ tablespoons)

Dried herbs and spices

- [ ] Smoked paprika (2 teaspoons)
- [ ] Dried red chili flakes (optional, to serve)
- [ ] Vegetable stock (at least 2 cubes or 24 oz)
- [ ] Sea salt
- [ ] Black pepper

Nuts and seeds

- [ ] Shelled pistachios (2 oz + extra to serve)
- [ ] Cashews (3½ oz)
- [ ] Sesame seeds (sprinkle to finish)

Breads and Wraps

- [ ] 1 loaf bread (6 slices)
- [ ] Tortillas (4)

WEEK 05   43 

= PLANT COUNT

FRESH INGREDIENTS

- ☐ 1 × block of firm tofu (10 oz)
- ☐ Plain yogurt (about 3 ½ oz)

Vegetables

- ☐ 2 shallots
- ☐ 1 red onion
- ☐ 4 carrots
- ☐ Asparagus (7 oz)
- ☐ Green beans (7 oz)
- ☐ Quick-cook veg (e.g. shredded cabbage, Tenderstem broccoli, cavolo nero, 11 oz)
- ☐ Cavolo nero (about 3½ oz)
- ☐ Mixed mushrooms (e.g. oyster, shiitake, or portobello, 16 oz)
- ☐ 1 small cucumber
- ☐ 1 baby gem lettuce
- ☐ 2 celery sticks
- ☐ 2 small eggplant (about 11 oz total)

Fruit

- ☐ 4 lemons
- ☐ 1 avocado
- ☐ Pomegranate seeds (about 3 oz)

Herbs and aromatics

- ☐ 2 garlic bulbs
- ☐ Large chunk of fresh ginger root (about 2 oz)
- ☐ Basil (about 2 oz)
- ☐ Mint (about ½ oz)
- ☐ Mixed herbs (about 2 oz, mint and cilantro are good)
- ☐ Bay leaf
- ☐ Bunch of green onions (optional)

FROZEN INGREDIENTS

- ☐ Peas (7 oz)
- ☐ Edamame (3½ oz)

CUPBOARD STAPLES

- ☐ 1 × block of silken tofu (about 11 oz)
- ☐ Capers (2 tablespoons, optional)

Grains, pulses, and other cans

- ☐ Orzo (4½ oz)
- ☐ Lasagne sheets (8 sheets, about 6 oz)
- ☐ Rice noodles (2 servings, about 6 oz)
- ☐ Spelt, soba, or rice noodles (2 servings, about 6 oz)
- ☐ Mixed grains (1 x 9 oz cooked pouch)
- ☐ Lima beans (1 × 14 oz cans)
- ☐ Beluga lentils (1 × 14 oz can)
- ☐ Plum tomatoes (1 × 14 oz can)
- ☐ Cherry tomatoes or chopped tomatoes (1 × 14 oz can)
- ☐ Borlotti or cannellini beans (1 × 14 oz can)

Oils, vinegars, and condiments

- ☐ Olive oil
- ☐ Extra virgin olive oil
- ☐ Sesame oil or olive oil (for noodles)
- ☐ Tamari or soy sauce (2 tablespoons)
- ☐ Tomato purée (2 tablespoons)
- ☐ White miso paste (3 tablespoons)
- ☐ Apple cider vinegar (1 tablespoon)
- ☐ Tahini (2 tablespoons)
- ☐ Almond or peanut butter (2 tablespoons)
- ☐ Maple syrup (about 4 tablespoons)
- ☐ Crispy chilli oil (optional)

Dried herbs and spices

- ☐ Dried oregano (1 teaspoon)
- ☐ Ground turmeric (2 teaspoons)
- ☐ Za'atar (1 tablespoon, plus extra to serve, optional)
- ☐ Dried red chili flakes (2 pinches, plus extra to serve, optional)
- ☐ Vegetables stock cubes (at least 1 cube or 17 oz)
- ☐ Nutritional yeast (4 tablespoons)
- ☐ Bay leaf
- ☐ Sea salt
- ☐ Black pepper

Nuts and seeds

- ☐ Cashews (3½ oz)
- ☐ Pistachios (2 oz)
- ☐ Hazelnuts (1 oz)
- ☐ Mixed seeds (2 oz, plus extra to serve)

Breads and wraps

- ☐ Small loaf of bread
- ☐ about 3½ oz stale bread

WEEK 06 47 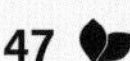

FRESH INGREDIENTS

- [ ] 1 × 9 oz package of tortelloni
- [ ] 2 servings of gnocchi (about 18 oz)
- [ ] Plain yogurt (2 tablespoons)

Vegetables

- [ ] 2 small or 1 large beets (about 9 oz)
- [ ] 1 red cabbage
- [ ] 2 corn on the cob
- [ ] 1 zucchini
- [ ] 2 celery sticks
- [ ] 2 Romano peppers
- [ ] 2 sweet potatoes (about 11 oz)
- [ ] 3 leeks
- [ ] 2 shallots
- [ ] 1 onion
- [ ] 1 red onion
- [ ] Green beans (14 oz)
- [ ] Beansprouts (3½ oz)
- [ ] Spinach (8 oz)

Fruit

- [ ] 5 lemons
- [ ] 1 lime

Herbs and aromatics

- [ ] 2 bird's eye chilis
- [ ] 2 red chilis
- [ ] 2 garlic bulbs
- [ ] Small chunk of fresh ginger root (about 1 oz)
- [ ] Flat-leaf parsley (about 1 oz)
- [ ] Basil (about 2½ oz)
- [ ] Dill (about ½ oz)
- [ ] Cilantro (about 1 oz)
- [ ] Thai basil (about 1 oz)
- [ ] Chives (about ½ oz)
- [ ] Mint (about ½ oz)

FROZEN INGREDIENTS

- [ ] Peas (6 oz)

CUPBOARD STAPLES

- [ ] Marinated artichokes (1 x 9 oz jar)
- [ ] Flame-roasted red peppers (1 x 9 oz jar)

Grains, pulses, and other cans

- [ ] Orzo (6 oz)
- [ ] 2 servings of spelt noodles (or rice noodles)
- [ ] Dried red lentils (3½ oz)
- [ ] Chickpeas (2 × 14 oz cans)
- [ ] Borlotti beans (1 × 14 oz can)
- [ ] Puy or beluga lentils (1 × 9 oz pouch or 1 × 14 oz can)
- [ ] White beans (1 × 20 oz jar)
- [ ] Coconut milk (2 × 14 fl oz cans)

Oils, vinegars, and condiments

- [ ] Olive oil
- [ ] Extra virgin olive oil
- [ ] Apple cider vinegar (5 tablespoons)
- [ ] Wholegrain mustard (1 teaspoon)
- [ ] Vegetable stock cube (at least 3 cubes or 52 oz)
- [ ] Tamari or soy sauce (optional)
- [ ] Red Thai curry paste (3 tablespoons)
- [ ] Pesto (3 tablespoons)

Dried herbs and spices

- [ ] Dried red chili flakes (optional)
- [ ] Cayenne pepper (optional)
- [ ] Sea salt
- [ ] Black pepper

Nuts and seeds

- [ ] Walnuts (2½ oz)
- [ ] Almonds (2 oz)
- [ ] Hazelnuts (1 oz)
- [ ] Dukkah (2 tablespoons, optional)

Breads and wraps

- [ ] Crusty sourdough, flatbread, or toasted pitta bread (for serving)

WEEK 07

39 🌿

Scan here to download a copy of this week's meal plan and shopping list:

FRESH INGREDIENTS

- ☐ 1 × block of firm tofu (about 10 oz)
- ☐ Plain yogurt (about 6 oz)

Vegetables

- ☐ 4 carrots
- ☐ 2 green bell peppers
- ☐ 3 red onions (including 1 large one)
- ☐ 3 banana shallots (about 7 oz)
- ☐ 3 shallots
- ☐ 2 onions
- ☐ 2 baking potatoes
- ☐ 1 large tomato
- ☐ Cherry tomatoes (18 oz)
- ☐ 6 large portobello mushrooms
- ☐ 1 small white cabbage
- ☐ Green beans (3½ oz)
- ☐ Arugula (about 1 oz)

Fruit

- ☐ 3 limes
- ☐ 2 avocados

Herbs and aromatics

- ☐ 2 red chilis
- ☐ 1 bird's eye chili (or you can use dried red chili flakes)
- ☐ 2 garlic bulbs
- ☐ Small chunk of fresh ginger root (about 1 oz)
- ☐ Cilantro (about 4½ oz)
- ☐ Basil (about 1 oz)
- ☐ Chives (about 1 oz)

CUPBOARD STAPLES

Grains, pulses, and other cans

- ☐ 2 servings of basmati rice (about 2 oz for two people)
- ☐ Black beans (1 × 14 oz can)
- ☐ Beluga or brown lentils (1 × 14 oz can)
- ☐ White beans (1 × 14 oz can and 1 × 20 oz jar)
- ☐ Lima beans (2 × 14 oz cans and 1 × 20 oz jar)

- ☐ Coconut milk (1 × 14 fl oz can)

Oils, vinegars, and condiments

- ☐ Olive oil
- ☐ Extra virgin olive oil
- ☐ Sesame oil (optional, for noodles)
- ☐ Balsamic vinegar (4 tablespoons)
- ☐ Apple cider vinegar (2 tablespoons)
- ☐ Tahini (1 tablespoon)
- ☐ Maple syrup (3 tablespoons)
- ☐ Harissa paste (2 tablespoons)
- ☐ Chipotle chili paste (4 teaspoons)
- ☐ Dijon mustard (1 teaspoon)
- ☐ White miso paste (2 teaspoons)

Dried herbs and spices

- ☐ Vegetable stock cube (½)
- ☐ Cardamom pods (2 pods)
- ☐ Bay leaves (3)
- ☐ Ground turmeric (½ teaspoon)
- ☐ Cumin seeds (3 teaspoons)
- ☐ Coriander seeds (about 4 teaspoons)
- ☐ Dried oregano (1 teaspoon)
- ☐ Dried red chili flakes (1 teaspoon plus extra for serving)
- ☐ Sea salt
- ☐ Black pepper

Nuts and seeds

- ☐ Cashews (about 2 oz)
- ☐ Hazelnuts (about 2 oz)
- ☐ Pine nuts (about 2 oz)
- ☐ Pumpkin seeds (about 2 oz)

Breads and wraps

- ☐ Tortilla chips (optional)

🌿 = PLANT COUNT

WEEK 08 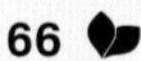 66

Scan here to download a copy of this week's meal plan and shopping list: 

FRESH INGREDIENTS

- ☐ 1 × block of firm tofu (about 10 oz)
- ☐ Plain yogurt (7 oz)

Vegetables

- ☐ 2 red onions
- ☐ 1 small cauliflower (about 28 oz)
- ☐ 1 eggplant
- ☐ 1 small cucumber
- ☐ Cherry tomatoes (7 oz)
- ☐ Spinach (7 oz)
- ☐ Green beans (7 oz)
- ☐ Mushrooms (any kind, 7 oz)
- ☐ 1 small bunch of green onions
- ☐ Salad leaves (for serving)

Fruit

- ☐ 4 lemons
- ☐ 1 lime

Herbs and aromatics

- ☐ 2 bulbs of garlic
- ☐ 2 red chilis
- ☐ Flat-leaf parsley (about 1 oz)
- ☐ Cilantro (about 2 oz)
- ☐ Mixed soft herbs (about 1 oz)
- ☐ Large chunk of fresh ginger root (about 2 oz)

FROZEN INGREDIENTS

- ☐ Peas (7 oz)

CUPBOARD STAPLES

- ☐ 1 × block of silken tofu (about 11 oz)
- ☐ Plant-based milk (4¼ fl oz)
- ☐ Capers (1 tablespoon)
- ☐ Kalamata olives (2 oz)
- ☐ Plain flour (80g)
- ☐ 3 tsp baking powder

Grains, pulses, and other cans

- ☐ Quinoa (3½ oz)
- ☐ Basmati rice (3½ oz)
- ☐ Chickpeas (3 × 14 oz cans)
- ☐ Lima beans (1 × 14 oz can)
- ☐ Noodles (any kind; 2 servings, about 6 oz)
- ☐ Spaghetti (2 servings, about 6 oz total)
- ☐ Cherry tomatoes (1 × 14 oz can)
- ☐ Chopped tomatoes (1 × 14 oz can)
- ☐ Coconut milk (1 × 14 fl oz can)

Oils, vinegars, and condiments

- ☐ Olive oil
- ☐ Extra virgin olive oil
- ☐ Sesame oil
- ☐ Smooth peanut butter (4 tablespoons)
- ☐ Tamari or soy sauce (4 tablespoons)
- ☐ White miso paste (2 tablespoons)
- ☐ Maple syrup (2 teaspoons)
- ☐ Harissa paste (2 tablespoons)
- ☐ Pesto (2 heaped tablespoons)

Dried herbs and spices

- ☐ Dried red chili flakes (pinch)
- ☐ Ground turmeric (1 teaspoon)
- ☐ Cumin seeds (1 teaspoon)
- ☐ Mustard seeds (1 teaspoon)
- ☐ Fennel seeds (1 teaspoon)
- ☐ Dried oregano (1 teaspoon)
- ☐ Sumac (optional)
- ☐ Sea salt
- ☐ Black pepper

Nuts and seeds

- ☐ Almonds (2¾ oz)
- ☐ Roasted peanuts (small handful)

Breads and wraps

- ☐ Pitta breads (2)

Acknowledgements

The last 14 years have been full of ups and downs, highs and lows. I've learned so much and loved (almost) every second. I know how incredibly lucky I am to have spent over a decade doing something I love so deeply. It's a real privilege to chase a dream and see it slowly take shape, even with all the inevitable backward steps along the way. It hasn't been easy, but I couldn't feel prouder that we've been able to turn Deliciously Ella, allPlants, and *The Wellness Scoop* into three meaningful, purpose-driven businesses, all focused on sharing simple ways to live a healthier life for our community.

I'm also endlessly thankful to have been on this journey with the most brilliant people. I may have started out alone, but it's now a huge team effort and nothing I do would be possible without the incredible people I get to work with. The book might have my name on the cover, but it's anything but a solo pursuit.

Huge thanks go to Jo, who completely outdid herself testing every recipe and making sure they're all spot on. To Liberty for some amazing testing too. Claudie, for designing each page so beautifully and bringing the vision to life. Imogen, the best editor and all-round support, who has so brilliantly brought the last few books together. Nicky, for such incredible attention to detail in finessing the pages to bring the book together. Clare, for the gorgeous photos; Sophia, for making the cover shoot so much fun; Tamara and Katie, for the delicious food styling (and the amazing set lunches!); and Hannah, for the beautiful props. The shoots were a joy to be a part of, a real highlight of this year.

Thank you to everyone at Hodder and Yellow Kite for your unwavering support, and to Cathryn – eight books on and still going strong.

And finally, to my family, the heart of everything: Matthew, Skye, and May. I'm forever grateful for you all.

About the Author

Ella Mills is a bestselling author, entrepreneur, and the founder of Deliciously Ella, one of the UK's fastest-growing plant-based food businesses. Following her experience of ill health in 2011, Ella started deliciouslyella.com to share her journey of cooking delicious, natural, plant-based food. As her audience grew, she launched a popular recipe app before writing what became the fastest-selling debut cookbook in the UK. Her first book, *Deliciously Ella*, was a *Sunday Times* number 1 bestseller, a *New York Times* bestseller, and has been translated into 30 languages. She has since published six more *Sunday Times* bestselling books, selling over 1.5 million copies in the UK alone.

Alongside her husband, Matthew, she has transformed Deliciously Ella into a leading plant-based brand. They have launched multiple ranges of natural, plant-based snacks and granolas, now stocked in over 10,000 stores across the UK and abroad. Together they've sold over 130 million products, with one sold every second.

Ella also co-hosts *The Wellness Scoop* podcast, which reached over 2 million downloads in its first five months. She and Matthew recently started a second plant-based business, allPlants, which has already sold 5 million products in just 18 months, further shaping the future of plant-based food.

Ella and Matthew live in the countryside with their daughters Skye and May, and their dogs Austin and Cookie.

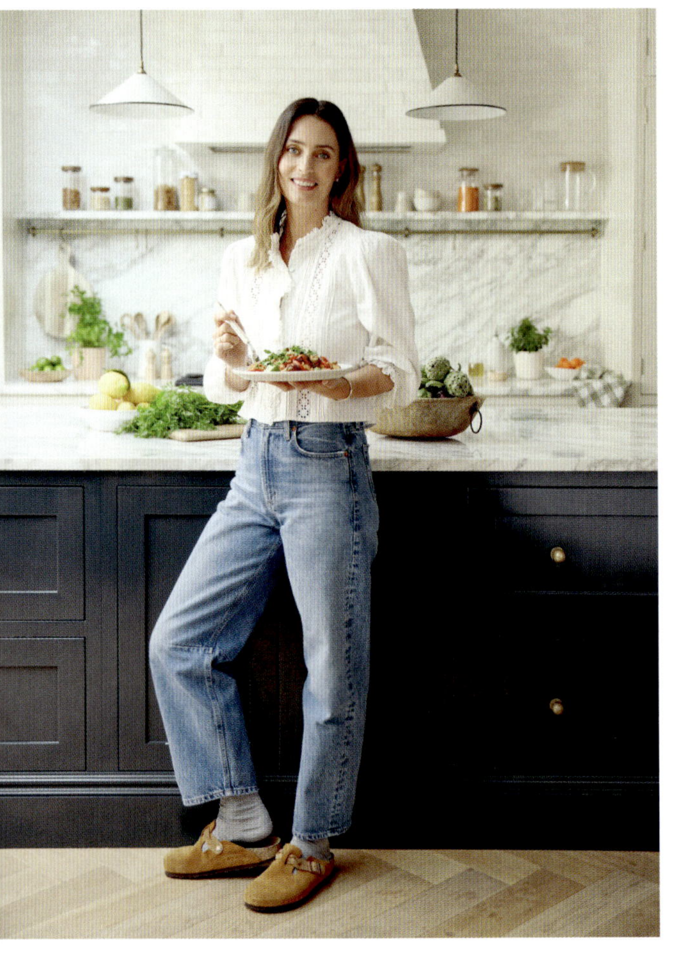

First published in Great Britain in 2025 by Yellow Kite
An imprint of Hodder & Stoughton
An Hachette UK company

1

A CIP catalogue record for this title is available from
the British Library

Hardback ISBN: 978 1 399 75395 1

Editor: Imogen Fortes
Design and art direction: Claudie Dubost
Page make-up and layout: Nicky Barneby
Food styling: Tamara Vos
Food styling assistant: Katie Smith
Prop styling: Hannah Wilkinson
Senior Production Controller: Rachel Southey

Colour origination by Alta Image, London
Printed and bound in Italy by LegoSpA

Hodder & Stoughton policy is to use papers that
are natural, renewable and recyclable products and
made from wood grown in sustainable forests. The
logging and manufacturing processes are expected
to conform to the environmental regulations of the
country of origin.

Yellow Kite
Hodder & Stoughton Ltd
Carmelite House
50 Victoria Embankment
London
EC4Y 0DZ

www.yellowkitebooks.co.uk
www.hodder.co.uk

Notes

The information and references contained herein are
for informational purposes only. They are designed
to support, not replace, any ongoing medical advice
given by a healthcare professional and should not be
construed as the giving of medical advice nor relied
upon as a basis for any decision or action. Readers
should consult their doctor before altering their diet,
particularly if they are on a set diet prescribed by
their doctor or dietician.

If you enjoyed cooking
from this book, you might
be interested in the other
Deliciously Ella titles:

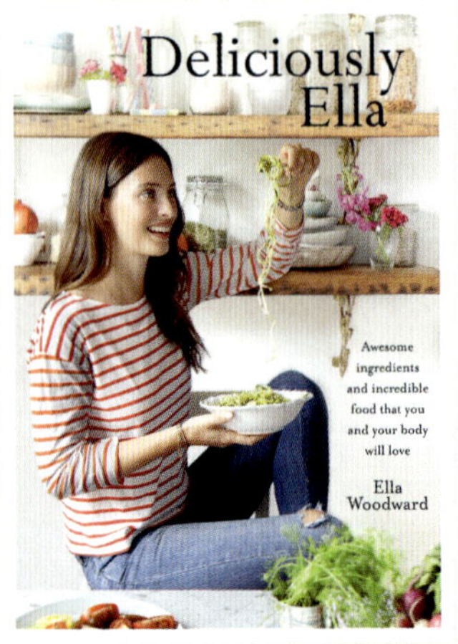

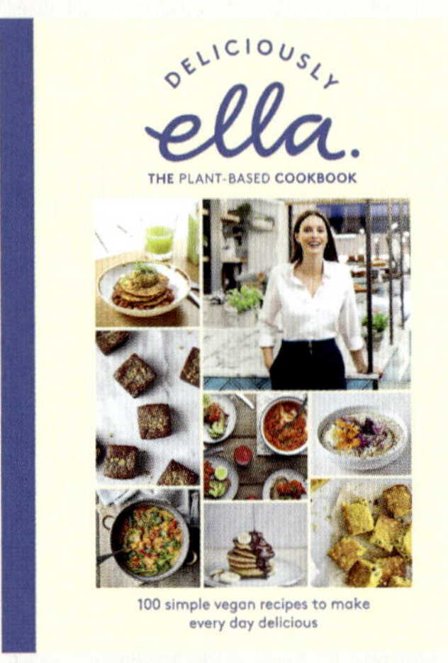

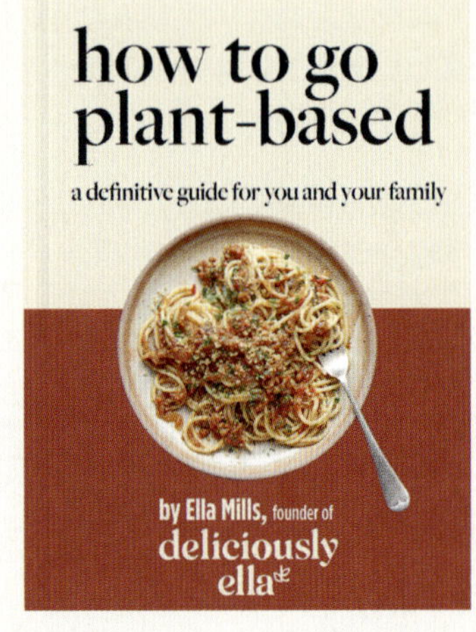

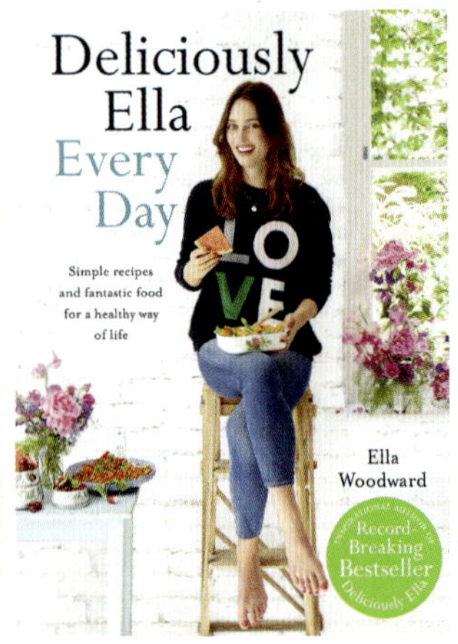

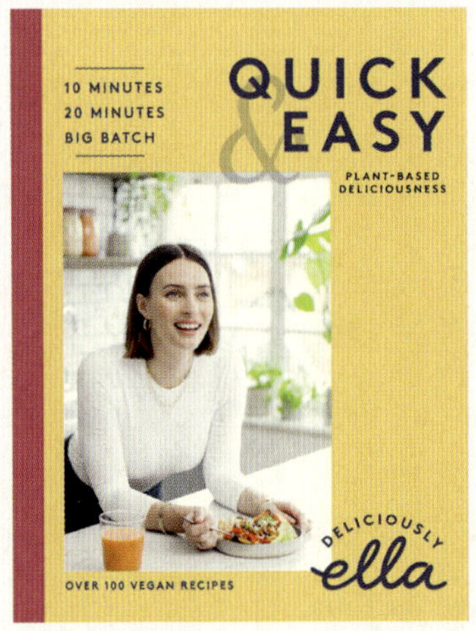

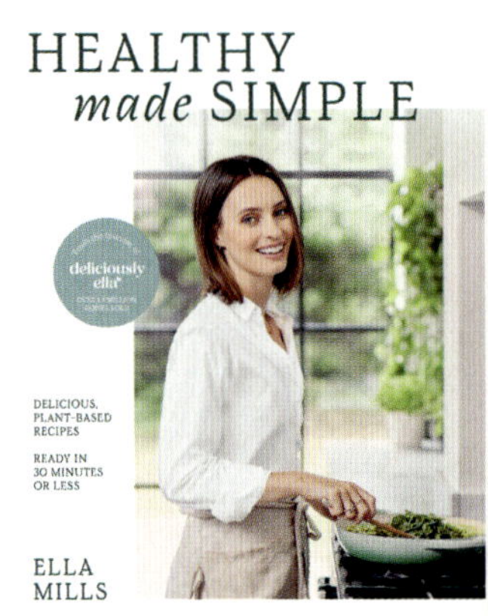